INTERNAL WORLD
AND
EXTERNAL REALITY

Object Relations Theory Applied

Commentary

Otto Kernberg's definition of object relations places it squarely within the context of Freudian thinking. His integrative approach has taken the standard analytic technique itself as a baseline from which parameters into the treatment of more regressive conditions with modified methods take their departure to create a hierarchy within a broadened perspective of psychoanalysis. He has rightly compared this to K.R. Eissler's attempt to create a similar continuum. The difference between the earlier attempt and the present one, I would say, is made possible precisely by the advances in object relations investigations. In the end, Kernberg links the regressive phenomena he describes with the developmental phases of the child, particularly as described by Margaret Mahler and her co-workers.

The blueprint that emerges is lucid, logical, and persuasive. I believe it will have a major impact in speeding the integrative work it undertakes.

Mark Kanzer, M.D.

Otto Kernberg's is one of those fertile and indefatigable minds that has become a household name within psychoanalysis, and for good reason. As this third book of his so clearly demonstrates, he has a way in his successive writings of covering a far-ranging array of topics of major theoretical and clinical concern to all of us and of integrating the separate pieces so that they build toward one coherent and unifying structure which bears his particular and always identifiable imprint. This book has the proper unity and cumulating impact that any book making a significant statement needs to have....

The solid middle of the book contains statements as lucid and comprehensive as any Kernberg has presented of his views on the nature of both normal narcissism and pathological narcissism, and of the technical implications of these views for the theory of psychoanalytic technique as well as (comparatively) for the theory of technique of psychoanalytic psychotherapy.

I cannot say that I always agree with Kernberg in all particulars. But my point here is not to take sides or to draw the lines of my own arguments. It is simply to state that Otto Kernberg is among those major authors with whose ideas every thoughtful worker within our field needs to be thoroughly familiar indeed. This present book is another demonstration of that fact.

Robert A. Wallerstein, M.D.

INTERNAL WORLD AND EXTERNAL REALITY

Object Relations Theory Applied

Otto F. Kernberg, M.D.

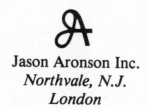

Jason Aronson Inc.
Northvale, N.J.
London

THE MASTER WORK SERIES

First softcover edition 1994

Copyright © 1985, 1983, 1980 by Otto F. Kernberg

Library of Congress Cataloging-in-Publication Data

ISBN: 1-56821-311-5
Library of Congress Catalog Card Number: 84-45723

Manufactured in the United States of America. Jason Aronson Inc. offers books and cassettes. For information and catalog write to Jason Aronson Inc., 230 Livingston Street, Northvale, New Jersey 07647.

To Paulina

CONTENTS

PREFACE

Basic to Freud's understanding of the human mind were the concepts of drives and conflict. Elaborations and extensions of his theory have since taken two distinct directions, that of ego psychology and that of object relations theory. In the past, these two approaches have been assumed to be opposed. However, my experience with patients presenting severe types of psychopathology has led me to theoretical conclusions and a clinical method that in my view renders this dichotomy invalid. I have found an object relations theory based upon and consistent with ego psychology clinically most useful. In my previous books I described the development of this theory; the present volume focuses on its application.

The book starts with a brief review of the clinical and research findings that led me to the theoretical conclusions that constitute the basis of my present stance. I then critically examine alternative object relations theories, particularly those of Melanie Klein and Fairbairn, and follow with a comprehensive summary of Jacobson's contributions and an analysis of the links between her work, Mahler's, and my own.

The remainder of the book illustrates the applications of my object relations theory to normal and pathological individuals, couples, and groups.

Part II should be of particular interest to the clinician, for it deals with psychoanalytic technique and the technique of psychoanalytic psychotherapy. The clinician will also find here an exploration of the controversial issue of the distinctions to be drawn between psychoanalysis and psychoanalytic psychotherapy.

Part III focuses on regression in groups and organizations, and on the interaction between groups and their leadership. These are subjects relevant not only to mental health professionals in administrative positions but also to the psychoanalyst, who, as a participant in professional societies and institutes, is exposed to the vicissitudes of group processes. These processes, in spite of the powerful effect they have on the functioning of all involved, often go unnoticed. The analysis of the interaction between individuals and groups will be of particular interest to social psychologists and family and group therapists.

In part IV the focus is on the couple. I view the couple as an entity and describe how it interacts with its milieu. A study of the couple inevitably leads to a consideration of love, and in this section I attempt to formulate a psychoanalytic theory of sexual love that takes into account both Freud's dual-instinct theory and my own view of the centrality of internalized object relations.

It has been my intention that the contents and format of this book will permit the reader to gain a comprehensive grasp of my theoretical and clinical approach. Some of the chapters were written specifically for this volume and have not appeared before; the other chapters, although based on articles previously published, have been significantly reworked.

ACKNOWLEDGMENTS

I wish to offer thanks to the teachers, colleagues, and friends who have given impetus to my work. Among these, I am particularly indebted to the following: Dr. Ignacio Matte-Blanco, former Chairman of the Department of Psychiatry at the University of Chile, in Santiago, Chile, first drew my attention to the importance of the British object relations schools and also taught me the value of examining theories rather than merely accepting or rejecting them. From the same Department of Psychiatry, Dr. Ramón Ganzaraín aroused my interest in group dynamics, and Dr. Carlos Whiting in the psychopathology of couples.

At Johns Hopkins Hospital, the late Dr. John Whitehorn introduced me to the culturalist personality schools and Dr. Jerome Frank to research in individual and group psychotherapy. Also in Baltimore, the late Dr. Lawrence Kubie convinced me of the importance of a systems approach in conceptualizing the structural theory in psychoanalysis.

At The Menninger Foundation, the late Dr. Herman Van der Waals stimulated my interest in the vicissitudes of normal and pathological narcissism, and Dr. Ernst Ticho and Dr. Robert Wallerstein sharpened my understanding of psychotherapeutic theory and technique and the clinical and research implications of the differences between psychoanalysis and psychotherapy. Dr. John Sutherland from Edinburgh was responsible for my undertaking a careful scrutiny of Fairbairn's clinical and theoretical contributions.

In New York, Dr. Margaret Mahler and the late Dr. Edith Jacobson generously gave of their time to criticize my work. It was Dr. Mahler who encouraged me to link my studies of borderline conditions with their theories. Various aspects of the ideas in this book have been reviewed and criticized rigorously by Dr. Harold Blum, Dr. Arnold Cooper, Dr. William Grossman, Dr. Donald Kaplan, Dr. Paulina Kernberg, and Dr. Robert Michels. I wish to thank them heartily and to absolve them from any responsibility for the results.

I am very grateful to the publishers and editors for making the following materials available to me.

Chapter 1 is a modified version of a paper that will be appearing in *The Course of Life: Psychoanalytic Contributions Toward Understanding Personality Development. Vol. III, Adulthood and the Aging Process.* DHEW Pub. No. (ADM) 79–786, edited by S. I. Greenspan and G. H. Pollock. Adelphi, Md.: The Mental Health Study Center, National Institute of Mental Health (1980). Chapter 3 is a modified and up-dated version of a paper that first appeared in the *International Journal of Psycho-Analysis,* 50:317–333 (1969). Chapter 5 is a modified version of a paper that first appeared in the *Journal of the American Psychoanalytic Association,* 27: 793–819 (1979). Chapter 6 is a revised version of a chapter that first appeared in *Rapprochement: The Critical Subphase of Separation-Individuation,* edited by R. F. Lax, J. A. Burland, and S. Bach, and published by Jason Aronson (1980). Chapter 9 is a revised version of a paper that first appeared in the *Journal of the American Psychoanalytic Association,* 27 (supplement): 207–239 (1979). Chapter 10 is a modified version of a chapter in *Curative Factors in Dynamic Psychotherapy,* edited by Samuel Slipp and to be published by McGraw-Hill Book Company. Chapter 11 is a modified version of an article that first appeared in the *Journal of Personality and Social Systems* (in press). Chapter 12 is a revised version of a paper that first appeared in the *International Journal of Group*

Psychotherapy, 28: 3–25 (1978). Chapter 13 is a revised version of a paper that first appeared in *Psychiatry,* 42: 24–39 (1979). Chapter 14 is a revised version of a paper that first appeared in the *Journal of the American Psychoanalytic Association,* 25: 81–114 (1977). Chapter 15 derives from two papers that first appeared in the *Psychoanalytic Quarterly,* 49: 27–47; 78–108 (1980).

With a sense of dedication beyond the line of duty, Mrs. Shirley Grunenthal, Ms. Virginia Van Horne, and Miss Louise Taitt transformed a jungle of typescript pages into recognizable chapters. Mrs. Grunenthal also served as my research arm and librarian and met innumerable deadlines as she typed and retyped the manuscript. Miss Anna-Mae Artim, my administrative assistant, in addition to coordinating all aspects of preparing the book, vigilantly protected my time for writing it and, in ways still mysterious to me, repeatedly brought order out of chaos. I offer my deep appreciation and gratitude for her help.

Finally, I am profoundly indebted to Mrs. Natalie Altman, my editor, who managed to significantly reduce the gap between my thinking and my writing and, in her unwavering determination to explore the internal consistency of the logic of the manuscript, helped to transform it into what I hope is a more precise and readable document. If I am now able to communicate my ideas clearly to the reader of this book, this is to no small extent a tribute to Mrs. Altman's work.

Part One

OBJECT RELATIONS THEORY EXAMINED

Chapter One

The Conceptualization
of Intrapsychic Structures:
An Overview

Back in the nineteen-fifties "borderline" patients, because of the ease with which their repressive barriers broke down and because of the distortions in their ego structures and functions — manifested in severely regressive transference reactions and acting out — were perceived as presenting ego weakness. These patients could consciously experience primary-process material — primitive intrapsychic conflicts that would normally be deeply repressed — but seemed to lack the capacity for introspection, insight, and working through. This disparity was puzzling and could not be fully understood within the psychoanalytic models then prevailing.

Because these patients used the therapist ruthlessly as a transference object to gratify their needs and were unable to achieve object constancy (that is, to maintain a representation of the good object under the impact of being frustrated by it) their transferences were characterized as "narcissistic." The lack at that time of any clear concept of narcissism as a clinical entity, however, prevented further clarification of these transferences. Borderline patients were variously described as characterized by a primitive kind of megalomania, intense aggression, magical thinking, paranoid trends, severe mood swings, and a striking tendency to perceive significant

others as all good or all bad. Their weakened capacity for realistically evaluating either themselves or others raised questions regarding their reality testing, and this, together with their vague and
idiosyncratic thinking processes and the primitive nature of their
interactions with others, suggested that these patients might be
"prepsychotic." However, even to differentiate them from patients
presenting unmistakably psychotic reactions was difficult and led
some observers (Hoch and Polatin, 1949; Hoch and Cattell, 1959) to
consider them essentially psychotic.

The traditional psychoanalytic approach to development centered
on libidinal stages, and there was general agreement that these
patients presented "pregenital" fixations. Beyond that consensus,
however, was a puzzling awareness that, while these patients
evinced strong oral trends, they simultaneously also presented
strong aggressive tendencies related to all levels of psychosexual
development, and a particularly aggressive tinge in their oedipal
strivings. Borderline patients, in short, defied all efforts to hypothesize the origin of their psychopathology in the usual manner—
that is, by situating it along the line of libidinal development and its
stages. To make matters worse, although clinical observation
detected the presence of ego weakness, the examination of defense-
impulse constellations often afforded no clear delineation of which
agency within the tripartite structure (ego, superego, or id) was
defending against which impulse within which other agency.

The confusions regarding the psychological factors producing
borderline conditions were matched by the uncertainties regarding
their psychotherapeutic and psychoanalytic treatment. Clinical observations of treatment failure using unmodified psychoanalytic approaches in these cases accumulated through the nineteen-fifties and
led to Knight's (1954) recommendation that these patients be treated
with an essentially supportive approach that would contribute to
strengthening their ego functions and defenses. Even psychoanalysts
who attempted to maintain a strictly psychoanalytic technique began
to consider modifications, a trend that culminated in Eissler's (1953)
suggestion that "parameters" of technique be employed.

But the contradictions between those who preferred a purely supportive method and those who attempted to apply modified (or even
standard) psychoanalytic procedures could not be resolved as long

as clinical observations remained unintegrated with theoretical formulations.

NEW CLINICAL EVIDENCE AND THEORETICAL FORMULATIONS

The psychotherapy research project of the Menninger Foundation (Kernberg et al., 1972) permitted, for the first time, a study of both the effect of various treatment modalities on patients with "ego weakness" and (by providing the most detailed information available, session by session, on 42 patients who had undergone many months and years of psychoanalysis or psychotherapy) a clarification of the descriptive, psychodynamic, and structural intrapsychic characteristics of these patients. We found that patients with ego weakness who were treated with supportive (suppressive) psychotherapy— following the traditional conceptualization that such patients need to reinforce their defensive operations and that resolution of resistances by interpretation is therefore risky—did rather poorly. In contrast, many of the same category of patients treated with expressive (uncovering) psychotherapy did remarkably well, but, as predicted, did rather poorly with unmodified psychoanalysis. The study of the characteristics of expressive psychotherapy that were most effective with patients presenting ego weakness led me to gradually develop a treatment approach specifically geared to patients with borderline personality organization (Kernberg, 1975, 1976a, b). Regarding the intrapsychic structure and dynamic characteristics of these patients, I reached certain conclusions which, in turn, led me to further observations and conclusions (Kernberg 1975, 1977b, 1978b) outlined in what follows.

Splitting and Other Primitive Defenses

In the neurotic patient, the ego's defensive organization centers around repression and other advanced or high-level defensive operations, such as reaction formation, isolation, undoing, intellectualization, and rationalization, all of which protect the ego from intrapsychic conflicts by means of rejecting a drive derivative or its ideational representation, or both, from the conscious ego. In patients with ego weakness — that is, patients with borderline personality organization — in contrast, splitting and other related mechanisms, such as primitive idealization, primitive types of projection (particularly projective identification), denial, omnipotence, and devaluation, protect the ego from conflicts by means of dissociating or actively keeping apart contradictory experiences of the self and of significant others. These contradictory ego states are alternately activated, and, as long as they can be kept separate from each other, anxiety related to these conflicts is prevented or controlled. However, these defenses, although they protect borderline patients from intrapsychic conflicts, do so at the cost of weakening the patients' ego functioning, thereby reducing their adaptive effectiveness and flexibility. It should be stressed that, in practice, borderline patients present a clear predominance but not an exclusive presence of primitive defensive operations; one can also find occasional primitive defenses in neurotic patients, in the context of an overwhelming predominance of repression and related mechanisms.

These same primitive defensive operations are found in psychotic organization (particularly in patients with acute and chronic schizophrenic illness and during active stages of affective illness) and function to protect these patients from further disintegration of the boundaries between self and object. In other words, in psychotic organization, primitive defenses dilute or fragment intrapsychic conflicts so that patients' experiences of violent conflicts with others are reduced; in this process, the potential for fusing the self-experience with that of significant objects is also reduced. The work of Melanie Klein and of Fairbairn was helpful in clarifying the characteristics of primitive defensive operations and object relations; however, serious problems with Klein's and Fairbairn's underlying theories of early development and confusing aspects of their overlapping and yet contradictory terminology forced me to develop my own operational definition of splitting and other related defenses.

That the same defensive operations can be observed in borderline and psychotic patients and yet serve different functions is demonstrated by clinical evidence. When interpretation of splitting and other related mechanisms is made to patients with borderline personality organization, their ego integrates and their immediate functioning improves, whereas interpreting these defenses to psychotic patients brings about further (if only temporarily) regression in their functioning. This immediate shift into increased or decreased social adaptation and reality testing can be utilized for diagnostic purposes: whether the patient immediately improves or deteriorates under the effect of such interpretation contributes importantly to the diagnostic differentiation of borderline from psychotic organization.

The conception of an ego organization different from that of the neurotic patient, and the similarity of defense mechanisms to those found in psychotic patients suggested to me the hypothesis that the fixation and/or regression of borderline patients occupies a developmental intermediary position or level between that achieved by psychotic and neurotic patients. In itself, such a hypothesis might be considered trivial, but it becomes important if one considers that it permits us to sharpen the differential diagnosis between borderline conditions and the psychoses, and that the concept of ego weakness, although it continues to be useful in a descriptive sense, is now replaced by that of a different level of ego organization; ego weakness no longer stands for simply an "absence" or "weakness" of defensive operations and ego functioning.

However, these findings did not by themselves resolve the question whether ego organization of borderline patients represented an alternative model to that of neurotic and normal persons or whether it represented a fixation at and/or regression to a normally occurring stage of development. At issue here is a qualitative rather than quantitative difference. Another related question was whether an ego organization centering around splitting was indicative of an early normal developmental stage or an abnormal deviation. Further, if the fixation and/or regression of borderline patients reflects an early normal period of development, what are the normal time schedules for this developmental process and the conditions under which fixation and/or regression to it obtain? In searching for answers to these questions, I was led to another set of observations, namely, the qualitative characteristics of transferences of borderline patients and the implications of these for understanding the pathology of their internalized object relations.

Identity Diffusion

Patients with "ego weakness" who eventually were diagnosed as presenting borderline personality organization typically presented the syndrome of identity diffusion originally described by Erikson (1950, 1956). Identity diffusion is represented by a poorly integrated concept of the self and of significant others. It is manifested typically by a chronic subjective feeling of emptiness, contradictory self-perceptions, contradictory behavior that the patient cannot integrate in an emotionally meaningful way, and shallow, flat, impoverished perception of others.

Diagnostically, identity diffusion is detected by the patient's inability to convey to an interviewer the patient's significant interactions with others. The interviewer finds he cannot emotionally empathize with the patient's conception of himself and of others in such interactions (in contrast to his ability to detect clearly enough the primitive transference reactions in his current interaction with the patient). There are frequently such gross contradictions in the descriptions the patient gives of himself or of significant others that both he and other people sound more like caricatures than like real people.

By the same token, the quality of interpersonal relations of borderline patients is severely affected — the stability and depth as manifested by the warmth, dedication, concern, and tactfulness of the patient's relations with significant others. Additional qualitative aspects are his lack of empathy or understanding of others and his difficulties in maintaining a relationship when it is invaded by conflicts or frustration.

The quality of object relations is largely dependent on identity integration, which includes not only the degree of moment-to-moment integration, but also the temporal continuity of the patient's concept of himself and others. Normally, we experience ourselves consistently throughout time and under varying circumstances and with different people; and we experience conflict when contradictions in our self-concept emerge. The same applies to our experience of others. But in borderline personality organization this temporal continuity is lost, and these patients have little capacity for a realistic evaluation of others. The borderline patient's long-term relations with others, particularly those with whom he is most intimately related, are characterized by an increasingly distorted perception of them. He fails to achieve real empathy with others, his relations are chaotic or shallow, and intimate relations are usually contaminated by a typical condensation of genital and pregenital conflicts.

In contrast, patients with neurotic personality structure have a solid sense of self and an understanding in depth of significant others. The neurotic patient has the capacity for total object relations which reflect an integration of "good" and "bad" aspects of others, as well as an integration of such contradictory aspects in himself. In diagnostic interviews, such patients have a capacity to convey a live and real picture of themselves interacting with significant others so that the diagnostician can visualize their world: he gets to know people he has never seen.

The search for developmental antecedents for these characteristics in borderline patients at first brought about further confusion. To begin with, Erikson (1950, 1956) had gradually moved the timetable for the consolidation of ego identity to adolescence, thus confusing his own description of the differences between identity diffusion (a profound disturbance originating in early childhood) and identity crisis (a characteristic of adolescence), and raising the question to what extent borderline patients represent an abnormal solution to the developmental crises that emerge in adolescence.

Careful evaluation of identity diffusion in adolescence led me (1978b) to conclude—in agreement with Masterson's (1967) earlier work—that adolescent patients with various degrees of symptomatic neuroses and nonborderline character pathology do not present the syndrome of identity diffusion, and that, even when an adolescent patient presents a chaotic lifestyle or life situation, the diagnostic interview may produce evidence—severe neurotic conflicts with his environment notwithstanding—of a solid conception of himself and of significant others. In contrast, the syndrome of identity diffusion appears regularly in patients who present all other descriptive, structural, and dynamic characteristics of borderline conditions. In fact, a surprising finding has been how very normal adolescents without borderline personality organization are, and how strikingly different their developmental crises are from the chronic chaos and confusion that reflects the syndrome of identity diffusion (Offer, 1971, 1973; Kernberg, 1975, 1978b).

Beyond this finding, however, other questions remained: What is the relation of identity diffusion to the defensive organization of the ego characteristic of borderline patients? And what developmental stage, normal or abnormal, is involved? Three related findings seemed to clarify this issue: The first was the study of superego and ego pathology in borderline adolescent patients carried out by Jacobson (1964). Her findings led her to hypothesize a relation between lack of integration of ego and superego and the persistence of non-integrated internalized object relations as unintegrated components of ego and superego structures. The second finding was the clinical observation of the remarkable differences between the transferences of borderline and psychotic patients, in spite of their both presenting identity diffusion (Kernberg, 1975, 1976a, 1977a). The third was Mahler's description of the differences between the psychopathology of symbiotic psychosis and that of the stage of separation-individuation, particularly the rapprochement subphase (Mahler and Furer, 1968; Mahler, 1971, 1972b; Mahler et al., 1975).

My clinical observations indicated a constant relationship in psychotic patients between the loss of reality testing and the development of transferences in which fusion or merger phenomena appeared; a similar constant relationship emerged between the maintenance of reality testing, typical of borderline patients, and the absence of merger phenomena in the transference of these patients. To focus first on the merger phenomena: Psychotic patients, particularly at advanced stages of their psychotherapeutic treatment, present fusion experiences with the therapist, that is, they feel a common identity with him. For example, the psychotic patient may present a delusional conviction that the therapist experiences the same emotions or bodily processes as he does and may automatically assume that any idea expressed by the therapist is his own idea. This development creates a situation in the transference in which there seems to be a confusion between patient and therapist, an absence of any boundary between them, while, simultaneously, external reality seems to fade into the background or to become unavailable. This may be a confusing, disturbing, or painful experience for the therapist, especially if he is not prepared to enter into this kind of psychotherapeutic relationship with psychotic patients. The patient may experience intense rageful panic or messianic fulfillment at such times (Searles, 1965). In contrast, borderline patients, even when they regress to transference psychosis, do experience a boundary of some sort between themselves and the therapist: it is as if the patient maintained a sense of being different from the therapist at all times, but, alternatively, he and the therapist were interchanging aspects of their personalities. By the same token, a primitive "part-object" relationship is activated that can be diagnosed as a "nonmetabolized," dissociated aspect of a total object relation that has been defensively split into opposite components: There is a repetitive, alternating, sometimes quite chaotic "interchange" of personality attributes partly projected and partly enacted by the patient, but never a true experience of fusion or merger.

The clinical importance of this radical difference between the regressive transferences of borderline conditions and truly psychotic transference was not fully understood until the observations just mentioned, and until the analysis of symbiotic psychosis and abnormal outcome of the rapprochement subphase by Mahler (1972b), together with the clarification of "psychotic identification" by Jacobson (1964) could be integrated into a common frame, which then also clarified crucial questions regarding the developmental preconditions of borderline personality organization (see chapters 5 and 6).

Combining Mahler's and Jacobson's formulations with my own observations, I concluded (1975) that the early ego has to accomplish two tasks in rapid succession: it must differentiate self-representations from object representations, and it must integrate libidinally determined and aggressively determined self- and object representations. The first task is accomplished in part under the influence of the development of the apparatuses of primary autonomy; but it largely fails in the psychoses, because a pathological fusion or refusion of self- and object representations results in a failure in the differentiation of ego boundaries and, therefore, in the differentiation of self from nonself. In contrast, with the borderline personality organization, differentiation of self- from object representations has occurred to a sufficient degree to permit the establishment of ego boundaries and a concomitant differentiation of self from others. The second task, however—of integrating self- and object representations built up under the influence of libidinal drive derivatives and their related affects with their corresponding self- and object representations built up under the influence of aggressive drive derivatives and their related affects—fails to a great extent in borderline patients, mainly because of the pathological predominance of pregenital aggression. The resulting lack of synthesis of contradictory self- and object representations interferes with the integration of the self-concept and with establishing object constancy or "total" object relations.

The integrated self-concept and the related integrated representations of objects jointly constitute ego identity in its broadest sense. A stable ego identity, in turn, becomes a crucial determinant for the stability, integration, and flexibility of the ego, and also influences the full development of higher-level superego functions. This is typical of neurotic personality structure and normality. In contrast, failure to integrate the libidinally determined and the aggressively determined self- and object representations is the major cause for nonpsychotic ego disturbances, which, in turn, affect analyzability and the general treatment requirements for borderline patients. Although such a lack of integration derives from pathological predominance of aggressively determined self- and object representations and the related failure to establish a sufficiently strong ego core, these conditions contrast markedly with the psychoses, in which self-representations have not yet been differentiated from object representations.

In borderline conditions, there is at least sufficient differentiation between self- and object representations for firm ego boundaries and the related capacity for reality testing to become established. The problem is that the intensity of the aggression with which the mental representations are imbued and the intensity with which the all-good mental representations are defensively idealized make integration impossible. Bringing together diametrically opposed loving and hating images of the self, and of opposing images of significant others would trigger unbearable anxiety and guilt because of the implicit danger to the good internal and external object relations; therefore, there is an active defensive separation of such contradictory self- and object representations; in other words, primitive dissociation or splitting becomes a major defensive operation. As a consequence, splitting is used actively during rapprochement to separate contradictory ego states; the other defensive operations linked to splitting reinforce it and protect the ego from unbearable conflicts between love and hate by sacrificing its growing integration.

Further consequent to this development is a chronic overdependence on external objects (in an effort to achieve some continuity in interactions, thoughts, and feeling in relating to them) together with a failure to integrate the self-concept: the syndrome of identity diffusion. Moreover, contradictory character traits develop—for example, alternative ruthlessness and excessive guilt reactions, reflecting the contradictory self- and object representations, further creating chaos in the interpersonal relationships of the future borderline patient. Superego integration also suffers because the guiding function of an integrated ego identity is missing; contradictions between exaggerated, all-good, ideal-object representations and extremely sadistic, all-bad superego forerunners interfere with superego integration.

Therefore, superego functions which would normally facilitate ego integration are missing, and this reinforces the unchallenged persistence of contradictory character defenses and chaotic character traits. The lack of superego integration also causes excessive reprojection of superego nuclei in the form of paranoid trends. Furthermore, a lack of integration of object representations interferes with deepening of empathy with others as individuals in their own right, and lack of integration of the self-concept further interferes with full emotional understanding of other human beings. The end result is defective object constancy or an incapacity to establish total object relations.

Finally, because of the failure of ego and superego to integrate, nonspecific aspects of ego strength (anxiety tolerance, impulse control, the potential for sublimation) suffer. The overall outcome, which we see in borderline conditions, is the evolution of typical transferences that reflect contradictory ego states; these activate primitive internalized object relations within a psychic matrix that has not achieved a clear differentiation of ego, superego, and id.

Developmentally, then, the pathology of internalized object relations and the primitive organization of the ego around splitting appeared as related and as reflecting a stage of development preceding the establishment of object constancy but later than the symbiotic stage of development. Mahler's proposed timetable for the normal sequence of development thus permits us to link borderline pathology to a stage of development that covers, broadly speaking, the period from the first half of the second year to the second half of the third year of life (Mahler, 1971, 1972b; Mahler et al., 1975). This is somewhat later than I tentatively suggested in 1966 (see Kernberg, 1966, pp. 247–248; but see also Kernberg, 1976a, p. 37). Mahler's timetable also permits us to analyze the antecedents of borderline conditions in observable, behavioral, and developmental terms, as well as in terms of the assumed intrapsychic developments characteristic of these early stages.

The dimensions, then, of the predominant type of defensive organization of the ego (centering around splitting or around repression) and ego identity (identity diffusion or identity integration) differentiate borderline personality organization from neurotic organization and normality. In fact, for practical purposes, it is the presence or absence of identity diffusion that most clearly differentiates borderline from nonborderline conditions, for some patients may present a mixture of defensive operations, which reduces the reliability of this latter diagnostic criterion.

There are, however, exceptions to this statement: Narcissistic personalities, who have developed a pathological grandiose self that obscures their underlying identity diffusion, manifest predominantly a constellation of primitive defensive operations. Thus, the combination of an apparently solid (yet subtly grandiose) identity and the predominance of a constellation of primitive defensive operations centering around splitting facilitates the diagnosis of narcissistic personality, structurally related to borderline personality organization (although the nonspecific manifestations of ego weakness referred to before are absent in many narcissistic personalities).

In addition, to focus on primitive defensive operations in the interaction of the patient and the interviewer contributes to the diagnosis of reality testing, our next point.

Reality Testing

Reality testing is an ego function that permits the differential diagnosis of borderline personality organization from psychotic organization. It is a key element in differentiating atypical cases of chronic schizophrenic reaction from borderline personality organization, and represents an important contribution stemming from psychoanalytic exploration of the personality to descriptive diagnosis in psychiatry. Frosch's (1964) crucial work in differentiating reality testing from the subjective experience of reality and from the relationship to reality facilitated the descriptive analysis of this ego function, and made it possible to observe the constant relation between reality testing and the capacity to develop nonmerger transferences in the middle of severe transference regression. The constancy of this relationship led me to think of reality testing as a general structural characteristic of the ego rather than as a specific ego function.

Reality testing as I have defined it operationally on the basis of Frosch's work (Kernberg, 1977b) is the capacity to differentiate self from nonself, intrapsychic from external origins of perceptions and stimuli, and the capacity to evaluate realistically one's own affect, behavior, and thought content in terms of ordinary social norms. Clinically, reality testing is recognized by (1) the absence of hallucinations and delusions; (2) the absence of grossly inappropriate or bizarre affect, thought content, or behavior; (3) the patient's capacity to empathize with and clarify the diagnostician's observations of what to him seem inappropriate or puzzling aspects of the patient's affect, behavior, or thought content within the context of their immediate social interaction.

Reality testing thus defined needs to be differentiated from alterations in the subjective experience of reality, which may be present at some time in any patient with psychological distress, and from the alteration of the relation to reality that is present in all character pathology, as well as in more regressive, psychotic conditions, and is by itself of diagnostic value only in very extreme forms.

Jacobson (1964) was the first to suggest that the differentiation of self- from object representations is a structural intrapsychic precondition for the development of reality testing. The patient's potential for maintaining reality testing even in the middle of severe transference regression permits the therapist to maintain an analytic attitude and an essentially psychoanalytic approach to borderline patients. This approach requires that interpretations be carried out with these patients beginning with an examination of present reality testing and, if it seems weakened, with an interpretation of the primitive defensive operations that are affecting it. As mentioned earlier, interpretation of primitive defenses facilitates the restoration of reality testing in the treatment of borderline conditions, but in psychotic structure induces further loss of reality testing and the activation of merger phenomena in the transference.

Viewed in terms of development, the ability to test reality indicates that internalized object relations consisting of differentiated self- and object representations have been established; that is, the subject has developed beyond the symbiotic phase and into the phase of separation-individuation. Jointly, reality testing, identity diffusion, and the predominance of a defensive constellation centering around splitting characterize borderline personality organization. These three features are mutually related, and point to a definite period of intrapsychic development, namely, the rapprochement subphase of separation-individuation. Mahler's developmental studies (1971, 1972b) have shown that borderline structure is particularly related to pathological resolutions of the rapprochement subphase. The borderline personality is fixated at what constituted normal characteristics at an early stage of development; but pathological consequences derived from that fixation expressed in additional intrapsychic developments ("genetic" sequences in contrast to "developmental" sequences) codetermine the clinical characteristics of the final structural organization.

INTERNALIZED OBJECT RELATIONS AND
STRUCTURAL DEVELOPMENT

The analysis of the relationships between the structural characteristics of borderline personality organization and its developmental and genetic origins has led us to an object relations approach within a psychoanalytic framework. Object relations theory, a general term for this special approach within psychoanalysis, examines metapsychological and clinical issues in terms of the vicissitudes of internalized object relations. Object relations theory considers the psychic apparatus as originating in the earliest stage of a sequence of internalization of object relations.

The stages of development of internalized object relations — that is, the stages of infantile autism, symbiosis, separation-individuation, and of object constancy — reflect the earliest structures of the psychic apparatus. Discrete units of self-representation, object representation and an affect disposition linking them are the basic substructures of these early developmental stages, and will gradually evolve into more complex substructures (such as real-self and ideal-self, and real-object and ideal-object representations).

This process — which, roughly speaking, covers the first three years of life — includes the earliest substructures of the psychic apparatus that will gradually differentiate and eventually become integrated into ego, superego, and id.

In this context, Jacobson's, Mahler's, and my own conceptions have in common the assumption that the earliest internalization processes have dyadic features, that is, a self-object polarity, even when self- and object representations are not yet differentiated. By the same token, all future developmental steps also imply dyadic internalizations, that is, internalization not only of an object as an object representation, but of an interaction of the self with the object, which is why I consider units of self- and object representations (and the affect dispositions linking them) the basic building blocks on which further developments of internalized object and self-representations, and later on, the overall tripartite structure (ego, superego, and id) rest.

Psychoanalytic object relations theory, as defined, is an integral part of contemporary ego psychology. It is not an additional metapsychological viewpoint, nor is it opposed to the structural, development-genetic, dynamic, economic, and adaptive viewpoints; rather, it represents a special approach or focus within the structural viewpoint that links structure more closely with developmental, genetic, and dynamic aspects of mental functioning; it occupies an intermediary realm between psychoanalytic metapsychology, on the one hand, and direct clinical formulations in the psychoanalytic situation, on the other.

In the following chapters I review other object relations theories that have contributed to the exploration of normal and pathological development in the early years of life and their relevance for psychopathology, but, in my judgment, have fundamental shortcomings. Because of the valuable clinical contributions of Melanie Klein and Fairbairn and my efforts to incorporate some of their findings and formulations with my own approach, although I reject their basic theoretical underpinnings, I shall review them in some detail before expanding on the approaches of Jacobson, Mahler, and myself.

Chapter Two

Melanie Klein and Her Followers

The controversies that have surrounded the theoretical formulations of Melanie Klein and her school have been in part historically determined. In the nineteen-twenties and thirties, memories of previous splinter groups were still sharp and the psychoanalytic community reacted strongly to any set of theories that appeared to threaten the psychoanalytic mainstream. For the major part, however, these controversies were fostered by the categorical style and dogmatic flavor that characterized Melanie Klein's writings, and the development over the years of a Kleinian following which had a strongly disciplined, "monolithic," almost sectarian quality to it. As a result, a sharp division between psychoanalytic ego psychology and the Kleinian school developed in Great Britain and gradually spread to other countries. Efforts on the part of various theoreticians of the so-called Middle Group in Great Britain to select from within the Kleinian formulations clinically important contributions and to integrate them with the mainstream of psychoanalytic thinking did lead to a growing dialogue within the British — and, later on, the French and Latin American — psychoanalytic communities. But the "radicalization" of some subsequent Kleinian thinking (Meltzer, 1967, 1973, Meltzer et al., 1975; Bion, 1967, 1970, 1973,

1975) has increased the controversy, and has widened the gap separating the two schools of thought.

Because in my own work I have found Klein's writings to provide
important contributions to the understanding of borderline and psychotic conditions and to the understanding of early vicissitudes of
aggression, defense mechanisms, and object relations, it seemed
important to me to clearly differentiate these contributions from the
major body of her theories and technical approach which I reject.
Therefore, in what follows, I shall summarize the major aspects of
Klein's object relations theory and set forth my agreements and
disagreements with her formulations in the next chapter. The ideas
summarized here are drawn from her books (1932, 1948, 1957,
1961, 1963; Riviere, 1952), unless otherwise specified.

Although Klein's theories are centered upon a concept of internalized object relations and, as such, constitute the first development of
object relations theories in psychoanalysis after Freud, her heavy
emphasis on the influence of instinctual drives, particularly her
stress on the death instinct as the foundation of aggression throughout development, places her close to the psychoanalytic theorists
whose position is constitutionalist, instinct-oriented, as opposed to
the culturalists who stress the psychosocial determinants of intrapsychic conflict. Thus, paradoxically, the earliest object relations
approach within psychoanalysis is at the same time very far away
from the culturalist schools. Klein's theory of instincts is rooted in
traditional metapsychology rather than in contemporary neuro-
biology, which has led some critics rightly to point to its pseudobiological orientation. In fact, for a theoretical approach so insistent
on emphasizing the importance of instincts — particularly aggression
as an instinct — it is remarkable how little the Kleinian authors have
concerned themselves with the important developments in contemporary biological and ethological developments; their emphasis on
aggression, while based upon observations of the preeminence of
aggressive conflicts in severe psychopathology, conveys a dogmatic,
aprioristic quality.

In contrast, the approach of Fairbairn and his followers, while
closely related to that of Klein in many respects — Fairbairn and
Klein influenced each other in their theoretical and clinical thinking —

is much more attuned to scientific developments in other related fields. Fairbairn stressed even more than Klein the importance of internalized object relations as major organizers of the mind, and explicitly described his conceptualizations as an object relations theory; but he rejected what he considered Klein's unwarranted stress on inborn instincts as basic motivating factors. Jointly, the Kleinian and Fairbairnian approaches tend to be called the British school of psychoanalysis, as distinguished from the contemporary ego psychology approach of Anna Freud, Hartmann, Kris, and Loewenstein, and Rapaport.

INSTINCT THEORY AND OBJECT RELATIONS

Melanie Klein's efforts to apply a relatively nonmodified psychoanalytic technique to the psychoanalytic treatment of children, particularly by avoiding any supportive or reeducative measures in the preparatory stages of analysis (and, indeed, throughout the entire treatment) led her to observe intense anxieties colored by paranoid fantasies expressed in children's play as well as in their verbal communications. Similar efforts to apply psychoanalytic technique to a broad range of adult patients — including patients with severe character pathology and cases who nowadays probably would be considered borderline also revealed anxieties with a paranoid flavor, and characteristic oscillations between what Klein called "paranoid anxieties," that is, fears of external attack, and what she called "depressive anxieties" — intense guilt feelings over fantasied harm or destruction caused by the patient to loved objects.

The regularity with which these processes appeared permitted her to explore the underlying unconscious conflicts in terms of the vicissitudes of love and hate throughout early childhood and later development. She was impressed by the importance of the aggressive drive in codetermining internalized object relations from earliest childhood on, and described the combined vicissitudes of instinctual drives and early object relations in a concept of two early developmental stages or "positions," namely, the "paranoid-schizoid" and the "depressive" positions.

Klein's basic theoretical assumption was, in agreement with Freud's (1920) dual instinct—life and death—theory, that both death and life instincts are operant from birth on, and she particularly stressed the importance of inborn aggression as a manifestation of the death instinct. Both death and life instincts, she suggested, find mental expression in the form of unconscious fantasies, which, for Klein, exist from the beginning of life. Every instinctual impulse is represented by an unconscious fantasy which reflects the self (or ego—she used the two words interchangeably) and the object under the influence of crude, primitive emotions (the prototypes of what will evolve as love and hate).

The first manifestation of the death instinct is oral sadism. Cannibalistic wishes are projected outward from birth on in the form of persecutory fears linked to the first objects, and are experienced as fear of devouring objects, giving rise to the fantasies of a bad, destructive devouring breast (the "bad breast"). Oral sadism is reinforced by the trauma of birth and later fantasied as well as real frustrations stemming from mother. The principal emotions derived from oral aggression are envy and greed. Envy is expressed by the prototypical fantasy that the frustrating object, originally the breast, willfully withholds its supplies; oral envy expresses the hatred of this withholding object and the wish to spoil it in order to eliminate envy.

Klein implied that the absence of the breast when it is needed was not simply experienced as a lack, but as an active, willful aggressive withholding by a sadistic object. Thus, frustration evolves into paranoid, persecutory fantasies. Envy gives rise to greed and reinforces greed; oral envy also underpins later envy of the penis and the other sex in general. Envy eventually evolves into the envy of creativity in others and into a particular kind of guilt over one's own creativity because of the fear of the envy attributed to others. This unconscious guilt over creativity also predisposes to later types of oedipal guilt. Jealousy is a later emotional development, characteristic of triadic oedipal situations. The child hates a third person because he sees that person as depriving him of love supplied by the desired object.

The life instinct (libido) is also expressed from the start of life in pleasurable contacts with gratifying objects, primarily the "good breast." These objects are invested with libido and introjected as internal objects infused with emotions representing the earliest manifestations of love. Fantasies about the good, gratifying breast are introjected as the core ego identification or good inner object. The projection of the good inner object into (Kleinians prefer "into" to "onto") new objects emerging in the perceptual field constitutes the basis of trust, the wish to explore reality, and learning and knowledge. Gratifying experiences reinforce basic trust, shape the expression of libido, and influence the relative balance of life and death instincts. Cycles of projection and reintrojection of good objects foster psychic growth, and good inner objects promote ego synthesis.

The principal emotion linked with the expression of libido is gratitude, which expresses libido directed to external good objects that are also good internal objects. Implicitly, Klein rejected the assumption that, in the earliest stages of development, the child is incapable of responding in a loving way to gratifying objects, and she saw what to the observer might appear as purely "need-gratifying relations" as the expression of a struggle between envy and gratitude. Gratitude, she affirmed, is closely connected with the emotion of trust based upon the secure enjoyment of the good breast. Gratitude decreases greed (while envy increases it) because gratitude leads to satisfaction with what is received, whereas envy tends to spoil it. Gratitude is the origin of authentic generosity, as distinct from reactive generosity (a defense against envy), which eventuates in the feeling of being robbed. Guilt, a significant emotion in later stages of development, reinforces feelings of gratitude, but is not its source.

Both life and death instincts are intimately linked with object relations: this is a key concept of Melanie Klein's. In contrast to Freud's (1914) concept of an initial autoerotic phase followed by a narcissistic phase, and finally, by a phase of object investment, Klein thought that autoeroticism is based upon gratifying experiences with mother (on the first object relation, therefore) and that narcissism represents an identification with the good object. She saw Freud's hallucinatory wish fulfillment as introjective fantasies of the good inner object (breast). Similarly, although the death instinct in her theory is originally largely projected in terms of paranoid fears, part of it is fused with libido, giving rise to the development of masochistic tendencies.

In general terms, external stimuli invested with libido or aggression become primitive objects. Objects are at first part objects (this is characteristic of the paranoid-schizoid position), and only later become total or whole objects (characteristic of the depressive position). Klein uses the term part object in two senses: as partial aspects of real persons — such as the breast — that are perceived by the infant as if they were the object with whom he is relating, and also as either a part of or total persons perceived in a distorted, unrealistic way under the influence of the projection of pure libido or aggression, so that these objects are either all good or all bad. The good and bad breast are the first (part) objects involved in the earliest unconscious fantasies representing, respectively, libido and aggression. Klein stressed the importance of very early internal object relations in determining the vicissitudes of instincts, intrapsychic conflicts, and psychic structures; she also stressed the importance of pregenital aggression, especially oral sadism, in determining the quality of primitive internal objects. The bad and the good internal objects, in short, are a direct reflection of the vicissitudes of inborn aggression and libido.

THE EARLY EGO AND ITS DEFENSES

In agreement with Freud (1923), Klein thought that the ego originates from a common matrix of ego and id in an effort to deal with reality. She considered the ego to start with the beginning of life and described as its basic functions — also originating with the beginning of life — the experience of and defenses against anxiety, processes of introjection and projection, object relations, and functions of integration and synthesis.

Anxiety, she proposed, constitutes the ego's response to the expression of the death instinct; it is reinforced by the separation caused by birth and by the frustration of bodily needs. Anxiety becomes fear of persecutory objects, and later, through reintrojection of aggression in the form of internalized bad objects, the fear of outer and inner persecutors. The content of persecutory anxiety or paranoid fears varies according to the level of psychosexual development. There are, first, oral fears of being devoured, then anal fears of being controlled and poisoned; these early contents later shift into oedipal fears of castration. Basically, these fears represent aggressive wishes toward and fantasies about the mother, particularly about the contents of her body. These primitive persecutory fears constitute the basis of persecutory delusions in schizophrenia and paranoid psychoses. Klein thought that constitutional factors determined the degree of anxiety tolerance. She also considered these persecutory fears the origin of primitive superego anxiety (superego functions start with the internalization of the bad objects as part of the integrative functions of the depressive position).

Introjection and projection, Klein proposed, are primary processes determining ego growth as well as defensive operations of the ego: they constitute, together with splitting, the basic defenses against anxiety. By their operation, introjection and projection foster the integration of the ego and the neutralization of the death instinct. Both good and bad experiences are projected. The projection of inner tension states (reflecting basically the death instinct) and of painful external stimuli constitutes the origin of paranoid fears, but the projection of pleasurable states (reflecting basically the life instinct) gives rise to basic trust. Good internal objects, derived from the introjection of good experiences, constitute basic stimuli for ego growth. In the earliest stage of development, the paranoid-schizoid position, all aggression is projected outside; in the later depressive position, projection of aggression is only partially successful, and there is a reintrojection and tolerance of bad external objects as internal persecutors which now constitute the early superego. At this stage of development, introjection and projection determine a variety of good and bad external and internal objects.

The tendency to perceive objects as either ideal (all good) or persecutory (all bad) is the consequence of the early defensive operation of splitting. Splitting is the active separation of good from bad experiences, perceptions, and emotions linked to objects. Only at later stages of development, when splitting mechanisms decrease, is a synthesis of good and bad aspects of objects possible and the coming into existence of ambivalence toward whole objects.

DEVELOPMENTAL POSITIONS

Klein assigned the paranoid-schizoid position to the first half and the depressive position to the second half of the first year of life, but capable of being reconstituted at various times or even in moment-to-moment developments in the course of life. Thus, both persecutory and depressive anxieties and mechanisms are involved in conflicts related to all psychosexual levels. This is another of her key concepts: paranoid-schizoid and depressive anxieties and defenses constitute a sequence activated in all clinical conditions where unconscious intrapsychic conflict triggers heightened defensive operations and anxieties in the ego. These "positions" are therefore not only developmental stages but also what might be called synchronic (in contrast to diachronic) characteristics of ego functioning—relatively stable, dialectically related ego organizations which have to be interpreted as part of the working through of conflicts at all levels of development.

For practical purposes, Kleinian authors often stress the importance of first working through paranoid defenses related to any particular conflict in order to strengthen the ego's capacity to enter the depressive position, in which depressive anxieties predominate and can be worked through. A premature focus on depressive anxieties may drive the underlying paranoid-schizoid defenses and anxieties underground. Here the observations of Klein and Fairbairn overlap: both had found that the working through of unconscious guilt and depressive anxieties uncovered an earlier or more fundamental level of schizoid defenses (Fairbairn) or paranoid-schizoid defenses and anxieties (Klein).

The paranoid-schizoid position is characterized by the predominance of splitting and other related mechanisms, part-object relations, and a basic fear concerning the preservation or survival of the ego; this fear takes the form of persecutory anxiety. Persecutory fears stem from oral and anal sadistic impulses, which, within certain limits of intensity are a normal characteristic of the earliest phase of development and, if not excessive, allow the infant to pass into the depressive position. Excessive persecutory fears, however, determine a pathological strengthening and fixation at this level and underlie the development of schizophrenia and paranoid psychoses. The principal defensive mechanisms of the paranoid-schizoid position are splitting (a concept Klein adopted and developed from Fairbairn's observations), projective identification (first described by herself), stifling and artificiality of emotions (again influenced by Fairbairn), and the mechanisms described earlier in the psychoanalytic literature of idealization and denial of internal and external reality.

Splitting occupies a central position in this constellation; Klein stressed that both object and impulses are split, so that good and bad objects are maintained separately. Splitting is linked with the mechanism of projection in that, in the context of the paranoid-schizoid position, good objects are totally introjected, and bad objects are totally projected. Projective identification, in contrast to projection, consists of the projection into another person of split-off parts of the ego or self or of an internal object. Rather than simply dissociating itself from that projected part, the ego, under the effects of projective identification, aims to forcefully enter into the external object and control it.

Both splitting and projective identification deal principally with the projection of bad inner objects and bad parts of the self—in short, with primitive aggression. Excessive aggression results in excessive splitting mechanisms in order to protect the good internal and external objects from contamination with badness. When aggression is particularly strong and bad objects predominate, there may be secondary splitting of bad objects into fragments and these fragments may be projected into multiple external objects, thus giving rise to multiple persecutors. Bion (1967) has described the development of "bizarre objects" representing minute fragments of pathologically split and projected bad internal objects. The need to control the object under the impact of projective identification expresses simultaneously the defense against persecutors and the acting out of primitive sadism in relation to the object.

Splitting mechanisms are also related to stifling and artificiality of emotions. Excessive splitting mechanisms or their pathological persistence may determine a general fragmentation of the affective experiences of the ego, leading to the subjective experience of depersonalization or to general affective shallowness. Here,

Fairbairn's work on the schizoid personality clearly influenced Klein. The stifling of emotions and emotional artificiality protect the ego from awareness of its own aggression and persecutory anxiety. Splitting mechanisms are also connected with denial of inner and external reality. Bion (1967) has described splitting processes that affect cognitive links and result in a disorganization of formal thought processes, which fosters loss of the relationship to reality and of reality testing and is characteristic of schizophrenia. Denial of internal aggression and of the bad aspects of needed objects also implies denial of reality aspects of the ego and of the external world, so that splitting and denial reinforce each other and lead to a general impoverishment of reality testing.

Splitting is also linked with idealization, an exaggeration of the good qualities of internal and external objects, together with a denial and splitting off of contradictory evidence regarding the object's real characteristics. Idealization of external objects also satisfies fantasies of unlimited gratification from them (Klein's prototypical fantasy of "the inexhaustible breast") and serves as a protection against the possibility of frustration-derived increments of aggression. Idealized external objects protect against persecutory objects, and the predominance of aggression over libido results in an excessive development of idealization.

All these defensive operations may abnormally prevail beyond the original paranoid-schizoid position in the first few months of life, leading to pathological fixation at this constellation and various types of psychopathology. The flight toward an idealized inner object may serve to protect the person against an unbearable reality, but at the cost of loss of the capacity for reality testing, and may give rise to exalted or messianic states, typical of psychoses. Excessive development of projective identification (within an overall atmosphere of reduced reality testing linked to the operation of the entire constellation of paranoid-schizoid mechanisms) may bring about the delusional thought that all power is vested in external objects, in contrast to the self's being perceived as impoverished and weak. Fantasies and delusions of being externally controlled, characteristic of paranoid conditions, also stem from the pathological activation of this mechanism. Whereas in paranoid conditions the prevailing fears are of external persecutors, hypochondriacal symptoms result from the projection of persecutory fears into the patient's own body zones, organs, and functions. Fear of poisoning and of pathological control from the outside may be an expression of persecutory fears of a paranoid and hypochondriacal nature.

Klein's contributions to the psychopathology of various types of character formation focused particularly on the schizoid personality; her conclusions regarding the prevalence of splitting mechanisms and their consequences for external and internal object relations were similar to Fairbairn's. She proposed that obsessive traits may reflect a secondary defense against fears of external control by taking over control in dealing with external reality. She described personalities with narcissistic and excessively dependent features as being dependent on idealized external objects; their flight into overinvolvements and sexual promiscuity was a constant turning from an object contaminated with badness to another object that is idealized. Her analysis of patients' unconscious envy of the analyst as the representation of the needed and frustrating mother as a basic source of negative therapeutic reaction was developed further in Rosenfeld's contributions to the study of pathological narcissism (1964b).

Klein proposed that the infant's developing cognitive functions permit him (or force him) to become aware that the good and bad external objects are really one, and that mother as a whole object has good and bad parts, thus resulting in a move from the paranoid-schizoid to the depressive position. The infant now also begins to realize that he harbors aggressive feelings toward the good object and recognizes the good aspects of the object he attacked and perceived—at such times of attack—as bad. The full projection of aggression characteristic of the paranoid-schizoid position is no longer operant, projection is only partially successful now, and the persecutory fears characteristic of the paranoid-schizoid position are replaced by the new fear of harming the good internal and external objects. Depressive anxiety or guilt is expressed in the concern that it is now more important to preserve good objects of the ego than the ego itself. One defensive mechanism that persists with a change in function is idealization, which evolves, during the depressive position, into an idealization of the good object, based no longer on splitting but on a defense against guilt feelings toward the object. The internal aggression toward the good object is acknowledged rather than split off or projected, and the object is idealized so it will not be destroyed by this aggression. This depressive kind of idealization leads to overdependence on others.

Other new defense mechanisms characteristic of the depressive position now make their appearance and normally permit the working through of the anxieties of this position. A fundamental difference exists regarding the two positions: While external factors (cognitive maturation, decrease of the fear over one's own aggression, and good experiences with mother—all of which reassure against the danger of aggressive contamination of good object relations) foster the resolution of paranoid-schizoid defenses, the very mechanisms of the depressive position tend to resolve depressive anxieties. The depressive position, therefore, unlike the paranoid-schizoid position, has a growth potential.

The predominant defensive operations of the depressive position are reparation, ambivalence, and gratitude. These mechanisms are mutually linked and reinforce each other. Reparation consists in an effort to reduce the guilt over having attacked the good object by trying to repair the damage, express love and gratitude to the object, and preserve it internally and externally. Reparation is the origin of sublimation. Gratitude, originally an expression of the libidinal investment of good objects from the beginning of life on, now also reinforces the love of the object, which is feared to be harmed or damaged by the aggression expressed toward it. Guilt, in other words, reinforces gratitude, and gratitude and reparation reinforce each other and increase the capacity for trusting others and the self's capacity to give and receive love.

Ambivalence is a general expression of emotional growth rather than a specific defense per se; the infant's awareness of love and hate toward the same object fosters a deepening of his understanding about himself and of others. The tolerance of ambivalence implies a predominance of love over hate in relation to whole objects. In more general terms, the integration of love and hate brings about deepening of emotions and emotional growth, deepening self-awareness and capacity for empathic perception of others, and the capacity for further differentiation between objects — thus initiating the differentiation along sexual lines characteristic of triadic oedipal relations.

MOURNING

Klein stressed the importance of the unconscious fantasies characteristic of the depressive position: that the good mother has been lost or destroyed because of the infant's greed and destructive fantasies. The sorrow and concern over mother and other objects contained in these fantasies represents the earliest processes of grief and mourning, which Klein considered to be a crucial part of development in the second half of the first year of life. Actual experiences of weaning from the breast and the related implicit loss of mother foster such mourning processes, while the satisfactory experiences with the real, good external mother who continues to be alive and available reassures the infant as to his inability to destroy his object and confirms the dominance of love over hate. Mourning processes increase the awareness of reality and reality testing, and the availability of the good mother strengthens the infant's confidence in his inner goodness and his capacity to love.

Failure of this normal outcome of the depressive position is reflected in either pathological mourning or the reactive development of what Klein described as "manic defenses." In pathological mourning, reparation fails to reassure the infant regarding his own goodness, ambivalence leads to despair at the predominance of hatred over love, and typical fantasies develop regarding the loss of the good external and internal objects caused by their fantasied destruction by the hatred directed toward them. The death of both the external and internal good objects is perceived as a consequence of excessive sadism. The internalized bad objects that would normally become integrated with the good internal objects to reflect whole (in contrast to part) object relations condense instead as an early sadistic superego characterized by cruelty, demands for perfection, and hatred of instincts.

Klein proposed that the superego normally derives from the reintrojected bad objects that had been split off and projected earlier in the paranoid-schizoid position; processes of synthesis of bad with good internalized objects normally mitigate that early superego and differentiate it from the excessively sadistic superego characteristic of pathological mourning. She described the self-reproaches of the depressed patient as directed not against the object but against the self and internal impulses; she considered suicide to correspond to the unconscious fantasy of destroying the bad self in order to preserve and protect the good object from it. She saw depressive psychosis as the clinical expression of pathological mourning and interpreted hypochondriacal delusions as related to unconscious fantasies of a total destruction of the objects of the inner world; fantasies of destruction of the external world would reflect projection of the fantasied destruction of the internal world; delusions of internal emptiness and destruction of the world at large also reflect pathological depressive fantasies.

Thus, depressive psychosis and manic-depressive illness in general, in Klein's thinking, reflect the failure to establish securely a good inner object in infancy; patients of this type have not been able to work through the infantile depressive position. Normal mourning repeats and works through the processes of the depressive position and reinforces the synthetic processes of the ego by which bad and good part-objects are integrated into whole objects. Although neurotic depression occupies an intermediary place in psychopathology between normal mourning and the pathological mourning characteristic of depressive psychosis, Klein did not clearly spell out differentiating features for these intermediary conditions. She links depressive psychosis with paranoid psychotic elements in that, in a general regressive defense against intolerable mourning, there may be a reinforcement of earlier paranoid-schizoid mechanisms, in other words, of paranoid fears as a defense against pathological guilt and depression.

An alternative defensive constellation to pathological mourning which reflects the incapacity to work through the depressive position is that of manic defenses. These defenses include, once more, idealization, here used in the service of the protection of an extremely idealized self against guilt and contamination by aggression by means of purified exalted states reflecting fantasies of merging of the self with good, unrealistically idealized objects. Another manic defense is manic triumph, a sense of triumph over the lost object reflecting the death wishes against the object, which may be reflected clinically, in extreme cases, as conscious triumph over the world, an exciting experience of power over an otherwise dead or dying universe. Klein considered manic triumph to be present—though subtly—in normal mourning as well, causing here an increase in unconscious guilt.

Other manic defenses are omnipotence, contempt, compulsive introjection, and identification with the superego. Again, all these defenses are linked with each other and reinforce each other. Omnipotence is based on the identification with an idealized and powerful good object and consists in the denial of other aspects of internal and external reality—such as the patient's vulnerability, the need for objects, and the need for dependency on objects. The denial of the need for objects also permits denial of aggression expressed toward them. Omnipotence is related to projective identification in that it includes a tendency to exert control and mastery of external objects, a control providing reassurance that they are not in danger and not dangerous. Contempt experienced or expressed toward objects often accompanies omnipotence. Such contempt is also expressed in compulsive introjection, a pathological development of compulsive relationships with objects, which implies the fantasy that since there are so many objects a few less do not matter. Manic patients' primitive fantasies of a cannibalistic feast are typical of the activation of this mechanism. Klein characterized identification with the superego, originally described by Freud (1917) and Rado (1928), as an identification with the sadistic superego. As part of the activation of this defensive operation, depressive guilt and aggression are both denied and projected into external objects, which in consequence are considered and treated as the hated, depreciated, bad self.

Clinically, the pathological predominance of manic defenses is reflected in hypomanic psychosis; when less severe, the clinical picture is that of the hypomanic personality. Hypomanic personalities tend both to admire and devalue others excessively, to think in large numbers, and to neglect details—that is, to neglect the real objects, regarding whom there is denial of guilt. Klein linked these characteristics of hypomanic personalities with narcissistic object relations, in which the flight into multiple relationships with external objects implies the denial of unconscious guilt toward them. Riviere (1936) and Rosenfeld (1964b) have developed this concept in their studies of the narcissistic personality. According to the Kleinian concept, the narcissistic personality combines the psychopathology of envy (related to oral aggression and primitive types of negative therapeutic reaction) with the personality characteristics reflecting manic defenses.

SUPEREGO DEVELOPMENT AND OEDIPAL CONFLICT

The psychoanalysis of children, using her play technique from the onset of language development, convinced Melanie Klein of two regular findings: that oedipal conflicts in her child analytical patients started much earlier than had been assumed in the past, and that superego functions could be observed from the second and third year of life on. Each of these findings seemed to be in contradiction to Freud's assumption regarding the origin of the superego at the height of the Oedipus complex, and his timing of the development of the oedipal complex. Paradoxically, however, these two findings in combination permitted Klein to agree with Freud that oedipal fears and prohibitions contribute importantly to superego development. Klein first (1932) postulated that oral frustration brings about a premature oedipal development, which she placed in the third year of life. Later, however, she stated that oedipal problems, molded under the primacy of oral drives, were active from the first year of life and that these early stages of oedipal development were the basis of the later classical oedipal constellation.

She saw the origin of the superego as related to the depressive position—actually codetermining this developmental phase—and proposed that the superego derives from the reintrojected bad objects that earlier (in the paranoid-schizoid position) had been split-off and projected, a reintrojection made possible by the mitigation of bad objects because of the introjection of whole objects as part of the depressive position. Hence, guilt derives from the reintrojection of projected sadism, and the superego is the synthesis of bad inner objects with a demand aspect reflecting introjected whole objects.

Under normal circumstances, as part of the depressive position, the predominance of love over hate and the subsequent internalization of predominantly good, demanding whole objects into the superego neutralize the bad inner objects. However, even under ideal circumstances, there is a certain contamination of the good objects by the bad objects in the superego, thus increasing internalized demands for perfection. Under less than optimal circumstances, such demands for perfection deteriorate into the unremitting harshness of infantile and childhood unconscious morality.

Under clearly pathological conditions (which I referred to before when describing pathological mourning and the pathology of the depressive position) a pathological, excessively cruel, demanding, and perfectionistic superego determines an incapacity to work through the depressive position and brings about severe depression or a regression to an earlier paranoid-schizoid constellation. Under these conditions a reprojection of the sadistic superego may occur as part of an effort to deflect intolerable guilt outside — which reinforces persecutory in contrast to depressive fears — and a transformation of the original sadism into the superego's hatred of the id.

In contrast, under normal circumstances, the superego's realistic demands for improvement and reinforcement of the ego's reparative and sublimatory trends contribute to the working through of the depressive position, to the experience of the crucial need to preserve the good inner objects, and regulate ego functions by depressive anxieties reflecting the guilt over dangers to the good internal objects.

Klein believed that oedipal developments start in early infancy, under the primacy of oral drives and conflicts, so that oral and genital conflicts overlap. She based her theory on the observation of condensed oral and genital conflicts in the second and third years of life, and assumed that this condensation already existed during the preverbal stages of development. In her later years, Klein assumed an inborn knowledge of the genitals of both sexes, thus explaining how primitive oral and genital fantasies characterized experiences and

conflicts from the first year of life on. She described intricate connections between libidinal and aggressive oral longings and fears and
their oedipal counterparts in children of both sexes. The longing for
oral dependency on the mother is displaced onto the father, which
originates the negative Oedipus complex (the first "feminine position") in boys and positive oedipal strivings in girls. Pathological
exaggeration of these trends is an important determinant of homosexuality in men and fosters premature oedipal strivings in girls
which predispose to hysterical developments.

The displacement of oral aggressive fantasies in both sexes determines the projection of sadistic fantasies onto the primal scene and
distorts the sexual relations in terms of primitive aggressive oral fantasies. This contributes, in boys, to the development of castration
anxiety, transforms the oedipal mother into a dangerous figure, and
interferes with a positive oedipal identification with father. In girls,
such predominance of oral aggression condenses preoedipal and
oedipal fears of mother and interferes with the positive oedipal relationship. For Klein, oral aggression in girls, displaced from mother
to father, is a crucial determinant of penis envy. In addition, in both
sexes, premature flight into the oedipal stages as a defense against
preoedipal conflicts may bring about a defensive sexual promiscuity
and flight from depth in object relations in general. Klein stressed
the envy of the opposite sex in both sexes, tracing it to oral
aggressive sources.

For practical purposes, the Kleinian description of the condensation of preoedipal and oedipal conflicts provides explanatory formulations for frequent unconscious fantasies such as of combined
father/mother images — and the related lack of sexual differentiation
in severely regressed conditions, the image of a devouring phallic
mother representing regressive castration fears in boys as well as one
type of combined father/mother image, and the fantasy of vagina
dentata and of the destructiveness of genital penetration. By the
same token, the superego prohibitions against oedipal sexuality
derive largely from the sadistic quality of the primitive superego, a
consequence in turn of primitive unconscious fantasies reflecting
oral sadism.

THE PROBLEM OF DEFINING A
KLEINIAN PSYCHOANALYTIC TECHNIQUE

Melanie Klein assumed that she was following Freud's classical psychoanalytic technique and, in fact, considered her method of treating adult patients much closer to the Freudian model than that of the ego psychologists. It is perhaps for this reason that she never wrote an overview of her technique and that her references to technique are dispersed in her clinical case material and only one of her books (Klein, 1961). Hanna Segals's book (1964) includes, together with a general outline of Klein's theories, clinical case material illustrating the Kleinian technical approach; Segal (1967) has also written a brief summary of Klein's technique.

Kleinian psychoanalysts adhere strictly to the classical psychoanalytic setting and deal with the patients' material exclusively by means of interpretation. Interpretations are for the most part transference interpretations, and, in contrast to the ego psychology approach — which stresses the importance of interpretation from surface to depth of the material, from the analysis of defenses to the analysis of content — Kleinian analysts underline the importance of analyzing unconscious intrapsychic conflicts at the level of the patient's currently deepest activated anxieties. Interpreting at the level of the patient's maximum unconscious anxiety means, for the Kleinians, both very early interpretation of deeply unconscious material and formulation of interpretations in terms of the earliest assumed nucleus of an entire genetic series of related unconscious conflicts and contents. In practice, this means interpretation of primitive fantasies and defenses related to the two early developmental positions from the beginning of treatment. It follows from Klein's belief that all the anxiety situations a child goes through will reactivate persecutory and depressive anxieties that primitive defenses, contents, and fears will appear in the transference.

Because Kleinian theory connects, by means of the psychopathology of the paranoid-schizoid and the depressive positions, the clinical syndromes of the neuroses, character pathologies, and the major psychoses, Kleinian authors consider the deepest level of unconscious anxiety to represent "psychotic anxieties" in all cases. In other words, the unconscious conflicts, defenses, and anxieties characterizing schizophrenia, paranoia, and manic-depressive illness are present in all cases. Bion (1967.), for example, stresses the universal existence of psychotic and nonpsychotic aspects in the personality. This concept of psychopathology has motivated Kleinian psychoanalysts to apply the same psychoanalytic technique to patients at all levels of severity of psychopathology (with the exclusion of organic cases) and to disregard, for practical purposes, considerations regarding contraindications for psychoanalysis in terms of levels of severity of psychopathology.

The application of nonmodified psychoanalytic technique to severe types of character pathology, borderline cases, and psychoses has provided Kleinian psychoanalysts with clinical material that, in their opinion, confirms their general theoretical conceptions regarding the relation between the two earliest developmental stages and all kinds of psychopathology.

I mentioned earlier that, generally speaking, Kleinians tend to interpret paranoid-schizoid features before depressive features; Kleinians stress the importance of interpretation of both negative and positive aspects of the transference in terms of both of these developmental constellations. Klein (1950) also stressed the importance of carefully exploring very early defenses and conflicts in the initial and termination stages of psychoanalysis and underlined the importance of sufficient working through of the two developmental positions as a precondition for successful termination of psychoanalysis.

In condensing her formulations, I have tried to stay as close as possible to Klein's own terms and have particularly stressed the internal connections among various aspects of her thinking. In the next chapter, I examine these theories and their clinical implications critically, and separate those contributions which seem to me important in the development of an ego psychology object relations theory from other, highly questionable theoretical assertions and problematic technical approaches.

Chapter Three

An Ego Psychology Critique
of the Kleinian School

I have already alluded to some of my misgivings about certain aspects of Kleinian theory. Nonetheless, other aspects of Melanie Klein's theoretical formulations have advanced my understanding of clinical phenomena presented by patients suffering from severe character pathology. I refer particularly to Klein's observations on primitive defensive operations, such as splitting and projective identification; her description of primitive fears and fantasies, such as highly unrealistic condensation of oedipal and preoedipal material under the overriding influence of aggression; her formulations about primitive object relations, such as the activation of part-object relations in the transference, which combine bizarre features with a dissociated quality — very different from the childhood experiences usually recovered or reconstructed in ordinary analysis.

While many of these puzzling clinical phenomena had also been described by writers not related — and even strongly opposed — to the Kleinian school, the specific definition of defense mechanisms predating the establishment of repression carried out by Klein, and of the nature of part-object relations connected with them, was helpful in clarifying the clinical material of patients in severe regression or with chronic chaotic developments in the transference.

However, while the internal connections between defenses, object relations, and fantasies in Klein's formulations seemed clinically relevant, the overall theoretical frame into which she and her followers organized these observations, and the psychoanalytic technique implemented by the Kleinian group—labeled "classical," but, in my opinion, introducing important distortions into the psychoanalytic situation—seemed to me highly questionable. In addition, Klein's doctrinaire style of exposition, her systematic ignoring of alternative ways of looking at the same clinical phenomena and of considering alternative theoretical formulations, and, finally, the semantic confusion caused by the introduction of new, and the new use of old, terminology, all caused me to question the Kleinian approach to theory and treatment.

The problem was how to utilize the important clinical findings of Melanie Klein and some of her co-workers within a theoretical and clinical context that would do justice both to these clinical observations and to the scientific developments brought about by psychoanalytic ego psychology in the realm of development, psychopathology, and technique. One important bridge to an ego psychology approach was provided by Fairbairn's criticism of the lack of structural considerations in Klein's theories; but, while Fairbairn's clinical observations and his analyses of vicissitudes of internalized object relations clarified some of the problems created by Klein's failure to differentiate the self from the object components of internalized object relations, his formulations created additional problems (to which I refer in the next chapter).

In contrast, Jacobson's analysis of object relations in terms of ego psychology and Mahler's developmental observations from the same stance provided a theoretical frame that permitted me to integrate within it selected Kleinian observations and formulations. The result is a linking of developmental aspects of structure formation with various types of defensive organization, object relations, and instinctual developments within a more comprehensive psychoanalytic frame. Regarding the clinical applications of this ego psychology object relations approach, my technical formulations on how to interpret primitive defensive operations and object relations in the transference (which I spell out in Chapters 9 and 10) are in sharp opposition to Kleinian technique. Many years ago (1969) I reviewed the critiques of Melanie Klein's theories stemming from ego psychology. It is time that I update and expand that critique.

THEORETICAL ISSUES

The concepts of an inborn death instinct and of the death instinct as the crucial—and earliest—determinant of anxiety are unwarranted extensions of Freud's speculative hypothesis regarding a death instinct and are unfortified by convincing evidence. The principal exponents of Kleinian theory (Bion, 1967; Rosenfeld, 1971; Segal, 1973) have nevertheless continued to adhere to these concepts, and their failure to respond to criticisms of these concepts bespeaks either their inability to do so or their dogmatism.

Klein's concept of an innate knowledge of the genitals of both sexes and of sexual intercourse is, as many others have pointed out, in striking contradiction to the cognitive capabilities of the infant in the first few weeks and months of life. Bion (1962, 1963) further elaborated on this idea by postulating an innate preconception of the Oedipus myth as part of the ego's equipment for dealing with reality. Bion's idea of inborn preconceptions, "thoughts" which require the development of an "apparatus for thinking," is part of a highly idiosyncratic theory of earliest development of cognitive processes, occasionally illustrated by clinical observations dealing with psychotic patients, but without direct evidence of either analytic or other observational material from normal or psychologically disturbed children. Thus, it seems fair to state that Bion simply translates Klein's formulation in this regard into a new concept, reaffirming the inborn knowledge of the genitals, sexual intercourse, and the oedipal conflict.

The "pushing back" of intrapsychic development—especially that of complex relationships between oedipal and preoedipal conflicts—into the first few months of life appears unjustifiable in view of the clinical evidence presented. The cases of children analyzed from the

age of two years and older in which early oedipal material and relationships between pregenital and genital conflicts can be found may
present a regressive pregenital expression of genital conflicts or a
"retroactive" coloring of early experiences by later material, and cannot be used, I think, as evidence for processes assumed to occur in
the preverbal stages, particularly the first few months of life. Direct
observation of children in the first year of life provides evidence
regarding a capacity for anxiety and cognitive processes of a more
complex nature than was suspected years ago, and probably allows
for fantasy formation, which, however, cannot be categorically
affirmed nor, on the basis of present knowledge, be assumed to be of
the complexity and kind which Kleinian authors accept as fact.

In talking about a hungry, raging infant who, on being offered the
breast, turns away from it, and who may have the fantasy of having
attacked and destroyed the breast which is then felt to have turned
bad and to be attacking in its turn, Segal (1973, p. 14) states: "Some
analysts think that these fantasies arise later and are retrospectively
projected into babyhood. This is surely an unnecessary additional
hypothesis, especially as there is a marked consistency between what
we can observe in infants' behaviour, in phantasies which are actually expressed once the stage of play and speech have been reached
and the analytic material in the consulting room." Segal's statement
illustrates insufficient consideration of actual developmental factors
in the first year of life, of the clinical evidence pointing to retrospec-
tive falsification of memories and to reinterpretation of the past,
and, in more general terms, of the importance of differentiating the
organization of fantasy as an intrapsychic structure from the genetic
origins of that fantasy.

Klein neglects the developmental aspects of structural differentiation within both ego and superego formation, and never explains
how "internal objects" are integrated into ego and superego, how
later developments differ from earlier ones, or how progression, fixation, and regression determine an individual history of psychological
development. Bion (1962, 1963) and Segal (1973) have attempted
to meet the criticism of Kleinian theory regarding its neglect of structural considerations. Bion has presented a complex system of cognitive development based on the Kleinian theories of splitting and

projective identification, of transition from the paranoid-schizoid to the depressive position, and of symbol formation. Insofar as he has presented the hypothesis of a hierarchy of intellectual processes ranging from the most primitive to the most abstract capacity for mathematical thinking, his system reflects, indeed, a structural development—at least regarding cognitive structures—within Kleinian theory. Unfortunately, however, his theory of the development of thinking appears quite divorced from other available knowledge regarding the development of perception and cognition in the child. Bion's failure to supply sufficient supporting evidence which might be utilized to contrast his constructions with other structural formulations makes it very difficult to evaluate his theory of cognitive development. His is a structural theory developing within the Kleinian orientation, but, in my understanding, it is difficult to see how these structural formulations might relate to the more usual structural concepts of psychoanalytic theory.

Segal's structural analysis (1973), while closer to the standard concepts and language of psychoanalytic metapsychology than Bion's, still appears to leave open some questions regarding psychic structure raised by Klein's theory of internal objects. Segal's glossary defines internal objects as objects introjected into the ego; the ego identifies with some of these objects, which thus become assimilated into the ego, contributing to its growth and characteristics. Other objects remain separate internal objects, and the ego maintains a relationship with them. Segal states that the superego is such an object—thus equating, it seems to me, what in ego psychology terms might be described as object representations with so complex a structure as the superego. Segal conveys the impression that the tripartite structure is but one instance of the development of relationships between internal objects and the ego, with the additional confusing implication that objects are both included in the ego and relate to it at the same time. Even granting that some of the problems of these conceptualizations are semantic (for example, derived from the lack of differentiating, in Kleinian thinking, the ego from the self) the inescapable conclusion is that the earliest internalized objects are treated as equal to highly complex intrapsychic structures: this implies a collapse of all developmental stages into one and a serious neglect of a developmental view of psychic-structure formation. All of which is in striking contrast to Jacobson's careful distinction between early and later stages of ego and superego formation, and her explanation of the extent to which internalized object relations are assimilated into later, more integrated, structures.

There is a remarkable disregard of structural differences between various types of psychopathology throughout Klein's own writings and those of her followers. The impression is conveyed in numerous cases that the same dynamic constellations apply to all kinds of patients, and, in fact, for many years this neglect of differential psychopathology was reflected in the Kleinian tendency to apply the same treatment technique to all patients along the entire spectrum of psychological illness. While the descriptions of paranoid-schizoid defensive operations, manic defenses, and the psychopathology of the depressive position point to different dynamic, genetic, and structural characteristics of manic-depressive illness, schizophrenia, and paranoid and schizoid personality structures, in practice, all these formulations are applied equally to all patients. It is thus not at all clear why different patients have different types of psychopathology, and whether differences in dynamics have any relevance for treatment indication, technique, and prognosis. Rosenfeld's papers on the psychopathology and treatment of narcissistic personalities (1964b, 1971, 1975, 1978) constitute an important departure from this tradition, the first effort to link Kleinian thinking with descriptive and structural aspects of a specific type of psychopathology.

The vagueness and ambiguity of Kleinian terminology is a major stumbling block to fully clarifying Kleinian theory itself, internal inconsistencies within that theory, and the possible relationships between that theory and the mainstream of psychoanalysis. Efforts by Kleinian authors to bring more precision into their terminology and to relate it to other psychoanalytic approaches are illustrated in Segal's glossary (1973), and in Rosenfeld's paper on depression (1959). In fact, Segal's summary of Kleinian theory (1973) is a most lucid overview of Melanie Klein from within her school, and Segal's effort to illustrate theoretical concepts clinically makes this an eminently readable book. Her brief surveys of Kleinian psychoanalytic technique (1962, 1967), and her brief summary of Kleinian contributions to psychoanalysis (1977) define the essentials of Kleinian psychoanalysis today and permit the non-Kleinian reader to grasp this approach more clearly than was possible in the past. Rosenfeld (1959), in comparing studies of depression made by writers from various psychoanalytic orientations and in attempting to relate Kleinian concepts and terminology to corresponding developments in ego psychology, also contributes to clarifying somewhat the ambiguity of Kleinian terminology.

However, ambiguity of terminology — a problem ubiquitous in psychoanalysis — is especially troublesome in some areas of Kleinian formulations. There are shifts in the way the terms ego and self are used throughout Kleinian literature, which makes it difficult to grasp the exact meaning of such important concepts as projective identification. Klein (1946) described projective identification as the projection of split-off parts of the self into another person. One aim of this process is to forcefully enter into the object and control the object by parts of the self. Here she used the concept of ego and self interchangeably. Elsewhere (1963), however, she described the ego, referring to Freud, as the organized part of the self, while "the self is used to cover the whole of the personality, which includes not only the ego but the instinctual life which Freud called the id" (p. 4). Rosenfeld (1964a) described projective identification as "not only a term referring to the taking over or identification with an envied role or function but it also implies a projection of unwanted parts of the self into another object causing this object to be identified with the projected parts of the self" (p. 61). Here the concept of projective identification is broadened to include the reaction of the object, that is, an interpersonal process is described as part of an intrapsychic mechanism. While I think many analysts working with borderline and psychotic patients would agree with the clinical phenomena described by Rosenfeld (see, for example, Searles, 1963), the shift in the definition of the underlying concept creates clinical as well as theoretical problems when one attempts to relate projective identification to other defensive ego functions. Segal (1973) has provided yet another, somewhat different definition of projective identification.

The definition of "splitting," as important in Kleinian terminology as projective identification, may serve as another example of shifting meanings attached to the same term. Although throughout much of her work Klein described splitting as an early mechanism related to the paranoid-schizoid position, to be replaced largely at a later stage by other defenses, such as repression, at one point she practically equated splitting and repression (1952b). The Kleinians' broad use of the term splitting, as evidenced in their published clinical material, further illustrates the general difficulty presented by their terminology when efforts are made to integrate it with the mainstream of psychoanalytic thinking. It was this terminological difficulty that moved me to redefine operationally, on the basis of my clinical observations, the constellation of primitive defensive operations I observed as predominant in borderline personality organization.

TECHNIQUE

The application of the same, unmodified psychoanalytic technique to patients with all levels of severity of illness, from neurotics to psychopaths and schizophrenics (Segal, 1967), in itself the consequence of the neglect of descriptive psychopathology by Kleinian authors, seem to me highly questionable. I think overwhelming clinical evidence exists indicating that psychotic patients and a majority of borderline conditions, not to speak of antisocial personality structures, do not respond well to an unmodified psychoanalytic approach. Clinical case illustrations in the Kleinian literature include patients with any of these conditions (with the exclusion only of organic brain syndromes) and do not refer to any limitations to analyzability dependent on the severity of psychopathology. Nor do Kleinians write about treatment failures. The only exception to this statement that I have been able to find is Rosenfeld's paper on borderline conditions with narcissistic features (1978). In describing a patient who developed a transference psychosis, and the need, when disruption of the treatment process was imminent, to sit the patient up and discuss with him the immediate reality of all his complaints and suspicions about the analyst, Rosenfeld seems to acknowledge the need for what we call setting up parameters of technique.

The published clinical case material from Klein and other members of her group conveys the feeling that they overemphasize or overextend the importance of transference as contrasted with the impingement of the patient's external reality in the psychoanalytic situation. This tendency reflects, at the clinical level, a corresponding tendency to underemphasize the importance of environmental factors — in contrast to that of assumed inborn intensity of drives (particularly aggression).

Kleinian authors seem to pay little attention to the patient's defensive organization, especially the natural structuring of defense mechanisms of the ego and character defenses in the early phases of analysis. The premature, "deep" interpretations of unconscious fantasy and transference manifestations, by-passing the defensive structure, create the danger of intellectually indoctrinating patients, rather than allowing deep unconscious material to emerge naturally and gradually when the defenses against it are resolved through interpretation. I have not found Kleinian case material to provide evidence that the analytic relationship deepens over time; it conveys the impression that the same constellation of primitive conflicts is interpreted again and again from the very beginning of the analysis and that no significant shifts occur in the nature of the transference. It is true that in many cases, one can follow the shift between paranoid-schizoid and depressive and/or manic defensive constellations, but the absence of significant changes in the overall climate of the psychoanalytic situation over a long period of time is still striking. Genetic reconstructions are offered at any point in the analysis, often referring to assumed developments in the first year or even months of life, without indicating that the patient's awareness of his intrapsychic past has deepened.

The overriding importance Kleinian analysts give to the interpretation of the primitive defenses, relating them to early conflicts and primitive object relations, is associated with their relative neglect of interpreting later defenses of the ego centering around repression, and especially character defenses. The omission of character analysis in Kleinian technique is, in my opinion, an important shortcoming, and a result of the theoretical underemphasis of the ego's structural development. The issue of premature, "deep" interpretations in the early analytic hours is also related to the problem of failing to diagnose character defenses in the analytic situation.

Segal (1967), in defending the Kleinian early interpretation of the transference, gave an example of a candidate-analysand who started the first session by declaring his determination to be qualified in the minimum time, and who spoke in the same session about his digestive troubles and, in another context, of cows. The analyst interpreted this as implying that she was the cow, like the mother who breast-fed him, and that he felt that he was going to empty her greedily, as fast as possible, of all her "analysis-milk." Segal stated that this interpretation immediately brought out material about his guilt over exhausting and exploiting his mother. The fact that oral greediness was implied in the patient's associations is probably true. One might wonder, however, to what extent this "eager" patient-candidate would accept such a "deep" interpretation as part of his wishes to learn the new magical language of the analyst, and to what extent such "learning" would feed into related defenses of intellectualization and rationalization, including the intellectual acceptance of transference interpretation. The patient's greediness might also reflect a narcissistic character structure; the extent to which such character defenses might later interfere with deepening of the transference should be clarified by exploring that defensive structure further, rather than gratifying the very eagerness by a "direct interpretation" of the possible ultimate source of this trait.

In other words, deeper levels of the defensive organization, especially of the patient's character structure, may be seriously overlooked by this approach, the defensive organization going underground with possible serious complications at later stages of the analysis. Kleinians often talk about the analysis of the "deepest" sources of anxiety: proceeding from the surface to depth does not apply merely to the depth of the content but to the depth of the defensive organization. The natural ordering of the material may be seriously interfered with by interpretations that, while seemingly "in depth," actually by-pass important defenses along the road leading from present developments in the transference through the structural organization of the predominant fantasies to their genetic antecedents.

An additional example may illustrate this point. Joseph (1960), another leading Kleinian analyst, in describing an analytic hour of a patient with antisocial behavior, summarized her interpretation of the unconscious meaning that was implied in the patient's reaction to his losing his job. The patient said that he did not know why he lost his job and said that he thought his boss was a crook. Later in the hour the patient talked about tears coming into his eyes when watching a film of a plane crash in which fourteen people were killed. The analyst felt that these were "strikingly sincere" depressive feelings. It turned out, however, that the patient had lost his job for stealing (he told the analyst this three days after the session in question). The analyst saw the stealing as "not just an acting out of greedy impulses, but a more complex method of avoiding the deeper guilt and anxiety about stealing by the spoiling of his good object — at depth the mother's breast" (p. 530). What is interesting is the analyst's failure to focus on the patient's lying to her; one might wonder what additional meaning the analyst's interpretations in depth have for the patient when the patient knows that these interpretations are based on obviously incomplete information of the patient's reality. Rather than speculating about deep conflicts around the avoidance of guilt, the first question one might ask oneself here is whether or not there was any conscious guilt that the patient experienced about lying to the analyst, and what reaction the patient would have when confronted with his lying: guilt or anger? fear or indifference? In other words, guilt and defenses against it operate throughout a complex layer of defense-impulse configurations, and the interpretation of such configurations only at their "ultimate" depth is highly unreliable without considering all other aspects involved.

One may wonder to what extent a patient with severe character pathology who undergoes a Kleinian analysis may surprise the analyst many months or years after the beginning of the treatment with a completely unexpected misuse or distortion of all the analytic understanding that has been conveyed to him. Perhaps the awareness of this problem is what has prompted Bion (1963) to discuss the "reversed perspective," to describe the situation in which the patient and analyst apparently agree on an interpretation, when actually the patient seizes on an ambiguity in the analyst's phrasing or intonation to give his interpretation a slant the analyst does not intend.

Rosenfeld (1965) acknowledged that "the intelligent narcissist often uses his intellectual insight to agree verbally with the analyst and recapitulates in his own words what has been analyzed in previous sessions. . . . The patient uses the analytic interpretations but deprives them quickly of life and meaning, so that only meaningless words are left. These words are then felt to be the patient's own possession, which he idealizes and which gives him a sense of superiority" (p. 177). Rosenfeld's thinking here seems to be different from that of other Kleinian authors regarding character defenses.

The combination of a peculiar use of terms related to infantile development, the consistently active behavior of the analyst, the atmosphere of certainty within which interpretations are given, all lend a special quality to the psychoanalytic situation in typical Kleinian analyses wherein the patient submits his productions and language to an indoctrinating effect, thus seeming to confirm the analyst's theories by associations centering on those theories and the language associated with them. Kleinian analysts freely use the terms of breast, milk, feeding, as well as similar terms regarding early excretory functions in such ways that a metaphorical statement interpreting the predominant transference situation and a concrete reference to its genetic antecedents are condensed into one. This tendency blurs the patient's capacity to make a distinction between thoughts that emerge in association to the analyst's interpretations, thoughts that are secondary-process elaborations of these interpretations, and more primitive material that might spontaneously emerge as a representation of unconscious fantasy linked to early development. The tendency to condense metaphor and direct reference to earliest experience reaches a maximum intensity in the interpretations by Meltzer (1967, 1973; Meltzer et al., 1975), another leading Kleinian, whose direct interpretation of children's play in terms of unconscious fantasies of a most primitive kind seems to become an overriding, almost idiosyncratic concern. Similarly, Meltzer's reporting of interpretations of the manifest contents of dreams of adult patients with only minimal information about the patients' associations and general clinical developments, and his interpretations of practically all unconscious fantasies as if they directly reflected contents of the first two years of life, convey the impression that, with this indoctrinating utilization of a language that condenses the theoretical and the concrete, he has carried Klein's approach to an extreme.

Kleinian clinical material shows an overemphasis on primitive conflicts and mechanisms which again reflects a neglect of the different characteristics of patients with different types of psychopathology. There is a certain ambiguity in the Kleinian linkage of paranoid-schizoid, depressive, and manic defenses to their respective "positions," positions reflecting very primitive or early conflicts derived from predominantly pregenital factors: Although Kleinian authors insist that these early mechanisms may be used as well as defensive operations in later developmental stages (implicitly acknowledging that the content related to such defenses may be entirely different in the typical neurotic case from what it is in a borderline patient), in practice, their clinical material invariably links these defenses to very early conflicts, so that a practical if not a theoretical contradiction remains.

It is as if in this area Kleinian authors were paying lip service to their own theoretical flexibility, as stated, for example, by Klein herself. She stresses (1950) that persecutory anxiety (relating to dangers felt to threaten the ego) and depressive anxiety (relating to dangers felt to threaten the loved object) may appear connected with all anxiety situations a child goes through: "Thus, the fear of being devoured, of being poisoned, of being castrated, the fears of attack on the 'inside' of the body come under the heading of persecutory anxiety, whereas all anxieties related to loved objects are depressive in nature" (p. 79). Even without considering at this point the issue of normal versus pathological interrelationships between pregenital and genital conflicts, the question remains why these early mechanisms are so pervasively interpreted at an early level in patients whose instinctual development and ego structure is of a much higher level than that of borderline or psychotic cases and in whom, presumably, shifts to later defensive operations and conflicts have taken place.

In other words, either the Kleinian mechanisms are linked to early conflicts and would thus come to the forefront only in certain cases, or they are not linked to such early conflicts and should be interpreted in the context of later genital or oedipal developments. The importance of this issue lies in the need to relate the patient's defensive operations with other defenses and contents according to the stage of development with which the conflict under focus is connected. For example, manic defenses may have become integrated into the character structure, acquired the function of a reaction formation, and be utilized as such against impulse configurations distant from those which originally brought these manic defenses into existence. A patient using manic mechanisms may reflect the activation of a character defense in the transference, directed, for example, against fear of punishment for incestuous strivings. One frequently sees defenses against envy linked not only with oral conflicts but with oedipal rivalry and as part of narcissistic character defenses.

The general neglect of analysis of defense in contrast to the analysis of content is a major problem with Kleinian technique. Segal (1967) has attempted to deal with this criticism, formulated by many ego psychologists in the sense that the Kleinian analysts interpret the content of unconscious fantasies and pay insufficient attention to the analysis of defenses. She quoted Isaacs' (1948) statement, "Thus phantasy is the link between the id impulse and the ego mechanism, the means by which the one is transmitted into the other" (p. 92), and added (Segal, 1967, p. 171), "This applies to all mental mechanisms, even when they are specifically used as defenses." The implication is that defensive mechanisms are manifestations of unconscious fantasies, so that the interpretation of unconscious fantasies serves at the same time the purpose of interpreting defense and content. For example (Segal, 1973), the mechanisms of introjection and projection are related to fantasies of incorporations and ejection, and Segal suggests not interpreting mechanisms to the patient but helping him relive the fantasies contained in these mechanisms.

The description of mechanisms such as introjection and projection as closely related to fantasies of an ejecting or incorporating kind seems clinically justifiable, although one would still wonder to what extent such a relationship holds true for later forms of projective mechanisms. The generalization, however, to the effect that all defensive operations are expressed by fantasies is questionable. Repression, intellectualization, and isolation are defenses in which it is much more difficult to accept concrete unconscious fantasies as representing these mechanisms. Defense mechanisms usually have multiple functions and are structurally linked with different conflicts—and fantasies—as well as more or less autonomous ego functions. Segal's effort to justify the Kleinian technique of "deep" interpretation of unconscious fantasy, in stating that these fantasies represent at the same time the defensive operations involved, does not, in my opinion, answer the criticism from ego psychologists regarding the neglect of defense analysis.

The neglect of defense analysis merges with the general neglect of character analysis in Kleinian technique already mentioned. If we add to this the neglect of sufficient clarification of external reality in the early stages of analysis, the failure to systematically work through character defenses may cause an unnecessary prolongation of the analysis by driving character defenses underground, by fostering submission to the analyst's theories, and by losing the extremely important function of monitoring the development of the patient's capacity for introspection and self-analysis. Greenson (1974) has written a related review, summary, and critique of the management of the transference in Kleinian psychoanalysis.

RECENT DEVELOPMENTS

Melanie Klein has contributed significantly to highlighting the importance of early object relations in normal and pathological development, a generally accepted psychoanalytic concept at this time. The importance of aggression in early development, the evidence that superego formation occurs earlier than was originally assumed, and the importance of studying the relation between genital and pregenital conflicts have been accepted by many non-Kleinians. The application of classical technique to the psychoanalysis of children is one of Klein's (1927) generally acknowledged major contributions. The understanding of primitive defense mechanisms has helped in psychoanalytic and modified psychoanalytic approaches to severe types of character pathology, particularly narcissistic character structure, the treatment of borderline conditions, and psychoanalytic psychotherapy with psychotic patients. The paradox is that, while having contributed to the treatment approaches of these patients, the Kleinian group itself has remained so rigidly closed to any examination of modifications of the standard technique, of the indications and limitations of psychoanalysis to various types of psychopathology.

It is probably fair to consider Segal, Rosenfeld, Meltzer, and Bion representative of the Kleinian school at this time. Segal and Rosenfeld have been engaged in major efforts to relate Kleinian thinking to the mainstream of psychoanalysis, Segal by means of her summary of Kleinian theory and technique and Rosenfeld in his review of depression and his articles on narcissism. Rosenfeld, in contrast to the majority of Kleinian authors, has been referring to non-Kleinian psychoanalytic literature in his recent writings; both he and Segal are concerned with exploring Kleinian theories from a more structural and developmental viewpoint, and Rosenfeld has explicitly acknowledged environmental factors (1978) to a far greater extent than other Kleinians.

At the same time, Meltzer and Bion have moved into areas that appear even more distant from ego psychology and from the mainstream of psychoanalysis in general. I have already described Meltzer's work. It is my impression that there is a widening gap between the work of Segal and Rosenfeld, on the one hand, and of Meltzer's, on the other. Although Bion's writings are perhaps even more difficult to follow than Meltzer's, he presents a logically cohesive argument that evolves into a series of extremely condensed, at times strange, yet evocative writings. In his recent work (1970, 1974, 1975, 1977a, b) he has expressed, even if indirectly, a sharp criticism of the authoritative style with which traditional Kleinian psychoanalysts seem to formulate their interpretations. He now stresses the essential unavailability of the ultimate knowledge about any patient's (or person's) intrapsychic processes, and the need to acknowledge that the understanding reached by means of interpretation is at most an approximation of the ultimate truth of an intrapsychic experience. His recommendation to approach each session with a patient "without memory or desire" (that is, without preconceived theories or wishes to influence the patient in any direction), is in direct opposition to Meltzer's categorical interpretations of primitive mental content, and, in his most recent writings, may represent a potential departure from the traditional Kleinian approach. While psychoanalysts working with borderline and schizophrenic patients may find his earlier clinical observations intriguing and stimulating—his notions, for example, of "containing" functions in the transference, of fragmentation as an extreme manifestation of splitting, of bizarre objects as a consequence of pathological projective identification plus fragmentation, and the notion of "reversed perspective"—in his latest writings (1974, 1975, 1977a, b) there has been a new shift into an emotionally charged attitude, an almost mystical atmosphere, which seems uncomfortably directed against a scientific approach to the study of personality.

Chapter Four

Fairbairn's Theory and Challenge

Among the psychoanalytic theoreticians who have made object relations theory a major focus of their work, W. Ronald D. Fairbairn stands out because of his consistent effort to formulate a developmental model based upon the internalization of object relations, and also to establish a comprehensive object relations theory which would replace traditional metapsychology, particularly instinct theory.

In spite of his geographic isolation in Edinburgh, Fairbairn's ideas were intensively debated in the British psychoanalytic community. The originality of his clinical contributions regarding schizoid personalities and the relation between schizoid processes and hysterical dissociation, as well as his frontal attacks on Freud's dual-instinct theory made his work controversial, controversy further complicated by Melanie Klein's influence on him and by his radical rejection of the death-instinct theory. Indeed, fortunately for us, because he and the Kleinian group used similar terminology to cover very different concepts and because he revised some of his ideas, Fairbairn was several times prompted to restate his basic contributions. These overviews (1949, 1951, 1963) present an integrated and consistent viewpoint with broad theoretical and clinical implications.

Fairbairn remained relatively unknown to the American psycho-analytic community and the non-English speaking psychoanalytic societies throughout the nineteen-forties and fifties. It was Guntrip's book *Personality Structure and Human Interaction* (1961) with its detailed exposition of Fairbairn's views and almost fervent defense of these views against various criticisms which had been raised about them that made Fairbairn's views more widely known both in Great Britain and the United States. In fact, Guntrip's analysis of Fairbairn's work includes not only a detailed review of his major contributions, but an explicit outline of Fairbairn's theoretical system, its origins and relations to other formulations, and a passionate yet lucid support of Fairbairn's views. To this day, Guntrip's presentation of Fairbairn's theories is the most comprehensive we have.

In my opinion, however, Guntrip's presentation suffers from important shortcomings. He seems to me to have uncritically idealized Fairbairn's theories and at the same time to have subtly distorted them. Chiefly by means of emphasis, Guntrip makes it appear that Fairbairn is supporting Guntrip's own theoretical biases. In addition, Guntrip, by sharply attacking instinct theory and metapsychology, stretches Fairbairn's critique to accommodate his own views.

For example, Fairbairn stressed that libido was intrinsically object-seeking, and that the pleasure connected with good object relations corresponded to the "reality principle" in its most profound sense (in contrast to a "pleasure principle" unrelated to reality). But Guntrip implied that for Fairbairn the pleasurable aspects of satisfactory object relations were a consequence of them and not a primary motive for the libidinal approach to objects. Also, Guntrip fails to mention that Fairbairn adhered closely to classical psychoanalytic technique. Fairbairn proposed that, in addition to the analysis of the transference, the qualities of the personal relationship between the analyst and the patient were a crucial therapeutic factor in bringing about therapeutic change, but this view did not imply a retreat from a systematic analysis of the transference. Guntrip's blurring of the distinction between psychoanalytic and psychotherapeutic technique does not correspond to Fairbairn's clear delimitation of psychoanalytic treatment. Also, in order to highlight his own battle cry against traditional metapsychology, Guntrip fails to explore a number of significant theoretical issues wherein Fairbairn's thinking was potentially congruous with Freud's genetic and structural viewpoints and even with formulations of contemporary ego psychology regarding energic deployments in early development.

It is true that Fairbairn was inclined to emphasize his areas of disagreements with Freud, but this trend is softened by his thoughtful and profound understanding and acknowledgment of Freud's theoretical and clinical contributions, particularly Freud's clarification of neurotic psychopathology and his development of psychoanalytic technique as a basic psychological research instrument. In this regard, one might say that Guntrip, while idealizing Fairbairn, also places greater stress on what, from a less partisan viewpoint, may appear the more problematic aspects of Fairbairn's contributions.

Furthermore, in his effort to replace traditional metapsychology by a "complete object relations theory of the personality," Guntrip (1961), although he reviews Fairbairn's theories in great detail, is much less systematic in reviewing his clinical contributions, such as the characteristics of the schizoid personality and of various types of psychopathology. Guntrip thereby significantly impoverishes the impression one gets of Fairbairn's contributions (this is particularly regrettable since the space given over to Fairbairn in Guntrip's book exceeds the length of Fairbairn's own theoretical statements).

The impression that Guntrip's summary of Fairbairn does not do justice to the richness of Fairbairn's thinking is supported by an article Guntrip wrote (1975) in which he describes his own psychoanalysis with Fairbairn (and subsequently with Winnicott). He criticizes Fairbairn for not deviating from standard technique and candidly admits that he selected Fairbairn as his analyst in the first place because he thought Fairbairn agreed with his own thinking and there would hence be no problem with theoretical discussions (!). While it would ordinarily not be appropriate to evaluate one man's personal motives for writing about another man's work, Guntrip's inclusion in his discussion of Fairbairn of his personal analysis with him (Guntrip wrote his book while he was being analyzed by Fairbairn) seems to me to justify the conclusion that Guntrip's idealization of Fairbairn was not devoid of significant ambivalence, an ambivalence that is reflected in his summary of Fairbairn's work.

Glatzer and Evans (1977) and Anzieu et al. (1977) have also written about Guntrip vis-à-vis Fairbairn and Winnicott.

Sutherland's (1963, 1965, 1979) reviews of Fairbairn's work and Wisdom's (1962, 1963, 1971) comparative studies of the contributions of Fairbairn and Melanie Klein are also basically sympathetic, yet—in contrast to Guntrip—not uncritically partisan. In spite of the brevity of Sutherland's and Wisdom's articles, they jointly convey a more comprehensive idea of Fairbairn's basic contributions to psychoanalysis, in my opinion, than the reader is left with after an exhausting study of Guntrip's book.

Because some of Fairbairn's ideas have contributed to my own thinking and because I suspect they are not as well known as they might be and in order to correct certain impressions left by Guntrip, I am offering a summary and critique of Fairbairn's contributions — including what others have said about his theory—and describing how his work relates to contemporary ego psychology.

FAIRBAIRN'S CONTRIBUTIONS

Basic Theory: Schizoid Position

Fairbairn's core contributions include one clinical (1931) and five theoretical papers (1936, 1941, 1943, 1944—with a 1951 addendum— and 1946). All these papers are included in Fairbairn's book (1954a), in addition to other clinical and miscellaneous papers and two of the overviews (1949, 1951) previously mentioned. Although several of Fairbairn's later publications (1954b, 1955, 1957, 1958, 1963) further clarified his theoretical thinking, and add significant clinical information in the process, in my opinion, the main body of his work lies in the earlier theoretical papers and in the clinical paper of 1931. This latter demonstrates the subtlety and acuity of Fairbairn's clinical understanding, his highly sophisticated treatment of an enormously difficult and complicated case.

Although Fairbairn possessed a truly elegant style of writing, it is not easy to extract his theory from a reading of his papers. Fairbairn himself, in his introduction (p. ix), explains why: ". . . this series of papers represents, *not the elaboration of an already established point of view, but the progressive development of a line of thought.* In other words, the series embodies the actual working out of a point of view, step by step." The raw material came from Fairbairn's consulting room; the point of view that emerged came from his analysis of clinical data — especially of dreams and transference phenomena.

In analyzing his patients' dreams, Fairbairn paid particular attention to the symbolic meanings attached to all the persons — real and fantastic, including various images of the same person and of the dreamer himself — in these dreams. He found in these "personifications" a remarkably stable organization.

Fairbairn at first saw personifications of objects (what I would call object representations) and the related personifications of aspects of the ego (or self) in dreams as the expression of intersystemic conflict, with each personification standing for the superego, the id, or the ego. Gradually, however, he reached the conclusion that the most precise and clinically most relevant formulation to account for these characteristics of dreams was a conception of the patient's ego as divided into a preconscious or conscious ego that related to a conscious or preconscious idealized internal object, in contrast to two repressed, unconscious, subsidiary ego segments that related to a prohibitive or rejecting "antilibidinal" object, and an exciting, gratifying "libidinal" object. All personifications in dreams could be sorted into representatives of these three self and object series.

Fairbairn proposed that this universal characteristic of dreams reflected a "schizoid" operation, namely, a splitting of the ego in the service of defense, with a consonant splitting of a fundamental, core object that was libidinally invested and yet frustrating at the same time. The frustrating aspect of the object was repressed as a "bad internal object" (the antilibidinal object) and the exciting aspect of the object as the unavailable repressed libidinal object. The segments of the ego relating to these two split-off and repressed aspects of the object constituted the "antilibidinal ego" and the "libidinal ego." (Fairbairn originally designated the antilibidinal ego as the "internal saboteur," but replaced this term later.)

Fairbairn described clinical connections between these universally "schizoid" tendencies of dreams and the unconscious meaning of hysterical conversion symptoms, dissociative episodes, and multiple personalities.

In contrast to these personifications which reflected the latent meaning of hysterical symptoms, the patient's conscious and preconscious ego was devoid of both primitive libidinal aspirations of a sexual and pregenital kind, and of the identifications with sadistic prohibitions and needs reflected by the antilibidinal ego in relating to the antilibidinal object. This relatively impoverished "central" ego was related, in turn, to an "ideal object" reflecting the remnants of those internalized aspects of the external object that were shorn of the split-off, frustrating, and exciting aspects of it.

In the transference, Fairbairn now perceived the gradual enactment of a sequence of internalized object relations, beginning with the initial relation of the conscious "central" ego to the analyst as an "ideal" object. This initial relationship was tenaciously maintained by the patient in order to avoid the eruption of the bad internal object and the corresponding unconscious need for a submissive, clinging, masochistic dependency on a sadistic, persecutory object projected onto the analyst (the relation between the antilibidinal object and the antilibidinal ego); beyond that relationship, patients tried to avoid the even more threatening activation of the libidinal ego in relating to the libidinal object. To the obvious question, why would the activation of the libidinal object-libidinal ego relationship appear as dangerous? (other than because of superego or "antilibidinal object plus antilibidinal ego" prohibitions) Fairbairn developed clinical and theoretical answers which stemmed from his study of patients with schizoid personalities.

Fairbairn was struck by the similarity between the chronically detached, withdrawn, emotionally apparently superficial attitude of schizoid patients and the central ego attitude of hysterical patients during periods of depersonalization and dissociative states, and also the impoverishment of the dominant ego segment of patients with multiple personalities. He was particularly impressed by what seemed to him a fascinating continuum in the psychopathology of hysteria and that of schizoid personalities. In fact, it was the intensive psychoanalytic study of patients with schizoid personalities that led him to formulate answers to the general questions of the origin of splitting processes within the ego, the causes and mechanisms involved in the splitting of internalized objects, the nature of the conflicts involved, and the primary and secondary defensive operations characteristic of various types of psychopathology.

The finding that careful analysis of superego pathology in schizoid patients often did not lead to resolving unconscious guilt, but to a worsening of the patients' detachment in the transference led Fairbairn to search for causes of this active process of detachment and ego splitting, and to conflicts that predated the Oedipus complex and the consolidation of the superego. He regularly found that schizoid personalities, in attempting to withdraw within the transference, were defending against a dreaded activation of a basic relationship in the transference characterized by a libidinal investment of the analyst experienced as a preoedipal, particularly oral, mother. This libidinal investment seemed a major threat to these patients, a threat derived from the fear that their love of the object would be devastatingly destructive to the object.

In analyzing this fear, Fairbairn found a typical constellation of feelings and fantasies, in essence reflecting the patient's conviction that mother could not love him, that his own love for mother had exhausting, emptying-out qualities which were destructive to her and at the same time threatened the patient with a fundamental feeling of futility, a sense of depletion related to the wasting of his own love without a receptive, responsive object. These patients' experience of deprivation had the effect not only of intensifying their oral needs but also of imparting an aggressive quality to such needs. By the same token, the patient's frustration derived from his perception of mother's lack of love made the patient experience his own love as demanding and aggressive. Therefore, the patient had to withdraw, not only because of the sense of futility and fear over the aggressive qualities of his own love, but also because of the projectively motivated feeling that mother's lack of response indicated her aggression toward him.

For all these reasons, the patient had to maintain a carefully guarded isolation and detachment in the transference, thus protecting the remaining "ideal" relationship with the analyst (the relation between the residual, "central" ego and the ideal object), while dissociating all his love and hate in the split-off, repressed relations of segments of his ego (self) to bad and exciting inner objects.

Fairbairn linked the chronic subjective experience of artificiality and of emotional detachment of schizoid personalities with these patients' attitude of omnipotence, objective isolation and detachment, and marked preoccupation with inner reality. He interpreted schizoid patients' "introversion" as a replacement of the relation with the external object by relations with their internal ones. He described schizoid overvaluation of intellectual pursuits as an expression of detachment and a displacement from repressed internal object relations to the intellectual sphere: he saw in this development the schizoid basis of subsequent complicating obsessive intellectualization linked to anal conflicts. Schizoid omnipotence reflected the patient's secret superiority over external objects—particularly the analyst—derived from the patient's sense of control and manipulation of his internal world, and his related sense of freedom and independence from the external world. Schizoid patients also developed the capacity for carrying out superficial social roles, thus protecting from the invasion of libidinal demands both residual object relations in reality and the secrecy of the patient's internal world.

Fairbairn concluded that, because of a deep fear that their needs to love and be loved would be frustrated, schizoid individuals unconsciously struggle against a true investment of others and regress to and/or are fixated at an essentially receptive, demanding stage of object relations in which they experience themselves as only on the taking side and carefully avoid having to give of themselves. Giving becomes equivalent to being emptied out, a catastrophic reminder of the sense of depletion derived from libidinal investment not responded to.

A regression in relating from persons to "part objects," such as the surge to gratify sexual impulses, particularly perverse sexual needs in replacement of adult genitality, is another schizoid process Fairbairn describes. Efforts to avoid "giving" may reinforce the need to repress all affects to avoid affective investment. In order to avoid a sense of loss, the patient may curtail his links with his own artistic products, stifle his creativity, and take active measures to drive away those who potentially threaten him with love (thus triggering the danger of the destructive effects of the patient's own love).

Fairbairn saw schizoid patients' sense of being wasted, their sense of unreality, their intense self-consciousness and constant self-observation as consequences of the impoverishment of their central ego by excessive splitting. He also observed that, as an effect of the libidinal withdrawing from external objects, further splitting processes occurred; the end point of ego impoverishment reflected not simply a deficit state but an active ongoing defensive process.

The study of transference developments of schizoid patients provided Fairbairn with evidence that there was an active "de-emotionalization" of object relations resulting in the patients' characteristic detachment in the relations with external objects, side by side with an intense preoccupation with internal reality. This internal reality seemed to consist of the same split-off and repressed object relations that Fairbairn had already found in hysterical pathology and as a universal characteristic in dreams.

Like others of that era, Fairbairn occasionally uses *self* as equivalent to *ego*, but mostly refers to *ego aspects* or *ego fragments* to describe what we call self-representations. And, as already mentioned, he uses *internal objects* or *personifications* for what we would call object representations. It was the variety of personifications appearing in a patient's dreams that contributed to Fairbairn's dissatisfaction with Freud's tripartite structure of the mind and to propose the existence of other functional units.

The final synopsis of his point of view, occupying less than a page of the *International Journal of Psycho-Analysis* (1963, p. 224), facilitates the presentation of a brief outline of his object relations theory. He starts off succinctly: An ego, he says, "is present from birth. Libido is a function of the ego. There is no death instinct; and aggression is a reaction to frustration or deprivation." Hence, he adds, "there is no such thing as an 'id.' The ego, and therefore libido, is fundamentally object-seeking." This ego present at birth is a "pristine" ego, that is, a whole ego which has as a key function the libidinal search for infantile dependence on a gratifying object. Erotogenic zones are not themselves primary determinants of libidinal aims but only channels mediating the primary object-seeking aims of the ego. Libido, there-fore, in contrast to Freud's assumption that it originally follows the pleasure principle (or is "primarily pleasure seeking") is essentially reality oriented and fulfills the reality principle in promoting attach-ment to the earliest objects, first, mother's breast, and later, mother as a total person. In fact, in Fairbairn's thinking, an excessive dependence on the breast as a "part object" may signal the deteriora-tion of the relation to mother as a total object and its regressive replacement by a part-object relation.

Insofar as Fairbairn rejects aggression as an instinct, he comes close to the culturalists; but insofar as he stresses the importance of "endopsychic structures," that is, of an internal world of object rela-tions, as the central focus of analytic work, he is very far from directly equating the intrapsychic with the interpersonal, prevalent in culturalists' approaches. In presenting an instinct theory centering exclusively upon (an object-seeking) libido and rejecting aggression as an instinct, Fairbairn would seem to come close to Jung, a corre-spondence strengthened by Fairbairn's focus on introversion and the schizoid personality's replacement of external by internal, fantastic object relations. However, for Fairbairn, introversion is determined by a defensive withdrawal from threatening object relations and not by constitution, and clinically he is totally identified with a Freudian model of psychoanalytic psychopathology, diagnosis, and treatment technique. In a sharply critical yet elegant reply to Abenheimer's (1955) Jungian critique of his writings, Fairbairn (1955) clarifies that, for him, internal objects are not simply "images," but endo-psychic structures. They are not, therefore, "inborn" images. He also states that, in contrast to Jung, he agrees with Freud "in regard-ing aggression as incapable of being resolved into libido"; and although he rejects Freud's dual-instinct theory, he continues "to accept Freud's view that libido and aggression constitute the two primary dynamic factors in mental life" (1955, p. 145).

I would here raise a question about rejecting aggression as an instinct. Fairbairn stresses the importance of conceiving the ego as a dynamic structure, that is, a structure that energizes, primarily, object relations and, secondarily, the intrapsychic function of internalized objects. He also underlines the importance of conceiving of structure and function as two aspects of the same dynamic whole. While I see this as an eminently reasonable suggestion, Fairbairn creates an artificial dichotomy between inborn dispositions to certain behaviors and external experiences as originating other behaviors; he then arbitrarily assigns libido to the inborn disposition (to object relations), while equally arbitrarily assigning aggression to the effects of frustrating object relations. One cannot, however, escape the conclusion that what frustrating object relations evoke are inborn behavioral dispositions to aggression and corresponding painful affect states. Similarly, it is the presence of a gratifying object that evokes inborn capabilities for pleasurable affects and behavior dispositions toward attachment to objects. Thus, aggressive behavior reflects an inborn disposition activated by certain experiences with objects, and the same complementarity of inborn disposition and experiences with objects obtains for libido as well. In Fairbairn's thinking, it is the pleasurable experience at the breast that immediately activates the libidinal attachment of the pristine ego. I find arbitrary the assignment to libido of a primary instinctive quality, while aggression is denied that quality.

Given the history of the development of Fairbairn's ideas, and the influence of Kleinian thinking on his developmental model, it may well be that Fairbairn, in an effort to differentiate his views from those of Melanie Klein (1952a, b), stressed the difference with her in terms of his concept of aggression, while maintaining her telescoping of early development into the first few months of life, with all the problems and internal contradictions that implied.

The earliest and original form of anxiety, Fairbairn suggests, is separation anxiety, activated when frustrations, including, basically, temporary separations from mother occur. These frustrations bring about the internalization of the object and also the development of ambivalence toward it. As Fairbairn himself puts it, "Two aspects of the internalized object, viz. its exciting and its frustrating aspects, are split off from the main core of the object and repressed by the ego" (1963, p. 224). Fairbairn calls the exciting, gratifying aspects the libidinal object and the frustrating, rejecting, prohibiting aspect the antilibidinal object. "Thus," he continues, "there come to be constituted two repressed internal objects, viz. the exciting (or libidinal) and the rejecting (or antilibidinal) object." He describes the main core of the internalized object, which is not repressed, as the ideal object or ego ideal. The resulting internal situation represents the basic schizoid position, antedating, in Fairbairn's view, the depressive position Melanie Klein describes.

All three ego structures as well as their respective internal objects have energic properties. Because the libidinal and antilibidinal objects are "cathected by the original ego, these objects carry into repression with them parts of the ego by which they are cathected," leaving the central ego unrepressed, "but acting as the agent of repression." Hence, "the original ego is split into three egos — a central (conscious) ego attached to the ideal object (ego-ideal), a repressed libidinal ego attached to the exciting (or libidinal) object, and a repressed antilibidinal ego attached to the rejecting (or antilibidinal) object" (1963, p. 224). This tripartite structure differs from Freud's in that, not only is there no id, but all three structures are fundamentally ego structures, so that Freud's ego represents only one segment of the original pristine ego.

Following Freud, Fairbairn considered anxiety the most direct symptom of unconscious intrapsychic conflict. It was aggression directed by the antilibidinal ego against the libidinal ego that transformed pleasurable excitement into painful anxiety. Fairbairn thus came close to Freud's first theory of anxiety — the assumption that anxiety reflected dammed-up libido (or rather, dammed-up libidinal needs reflecting the repressed relation between libidinal ego and libidinal object). In agreeing with Freud that oedipal conflicts were central in the psychopathology of hysteria, he explained the origin of oedipal conflicts, however, as derived from the earlier struggle with the ambivalently loved and needed mother of the earliest oral period of development.

In the light of his analysis of the relationship between oedipal conflicts and intrapsychic structures, Fairbairn saw his endopsychic structures as constituted by successive fusions and condensations of internalized objects and corresponding ego segments from successive stages of development. He was aware that the organization of all internalized object relations that he proposed remained remarkably close to Freud's tripartite structure. Fairbairn stated, however, that Freud's superego included not only Fairbairn's antilibidinal ego and antilibidinal object, but also Fairbairn's ideal object, and that it corresponded to a later and more complex stage of development than the psychic structures based upon schizoid processes in the pre-oedipal period. He also objected, on principle, to the analogy of his "tripartite" structure with Freud's: in contrast to Freud, Fairbairn, as previously mentioned, considered all three structures as representing *ego* structures, and as provided with energic functions derived from the libidinal investments in all three of them.

Fairbairn thus conceives of endopsychic structures as not rigid, impersonal, frozen molds but actively maintained and dynamically interacting object-relations-determined. He differentiates the establishment of the schizoid position, and the related consolidation of endopsychic structures, from the pathological fixation at this stage of development reflected by schizoid factors in the personality—which he considers quite universal—and from the schizoid personality proper (the prototypical psychopathology of the schizoid position).

Fairbairn conceptualized penis envy, castration anxiety, and genital longings for both parents in the positive and negative oedipal situation as an expression of deterioration of the object relations to the parents resulting from the repression of major affective libidinal needs. In other words, Fairbairn considered the longing for genital relations with the oedipal objects and the corresponding fears and prohibitions a consequence of the regression from total, integrated, to part-object relations with the oedipal parents. He defined adult, mature heterosexual relations as total-object relations which permit mutual dependency and the expression of libidinal needs through predominantly, but not exclusively, genital channels. For Fairbairn, the various erotogenic zones represented not the origin of libidinal stimuli but the channels available for expression of libidinal needs directed to objects. He (1955) defined anal and phallic conflicts not in terms of libidinal stages, but as particular "techniques" activated in a sequence directed primarily by the nature of interactions and conflicts with parental objects as the child moves from infantile dependence to mature independence.

It is difficult to clearly relate Fairbairn's thinking to that of
Melanie Klein, in spite — or because — of their attaching different
meanings to the same terms. Klein (1946), under the influence of
Fairbairn's contributions to the understanding of schizoid personality characteristics and defenses, decided to rename the earliest
stage of development the "paranoid-schizoid position," rather than
"paranoid position," and she agreed with Fairbairn in that this position predated the development of the depressive position. Klein also
agreed with the particular emphasis Fairbairn laid on the inherent
relation between hysteria and schizophrenia. She strongly dis-
agreed, however, with Fairbairn's revision of the theory of mental
structure and instincts, with his view that only the bad object is
internalized, and with his underrating of the role aggression and
hate play from the beginning of life. Fairbairn originally proposed
that only bad object relations induced internalization and splitting
mechanisms. A gradual shift away from this early view led him to his
final proposal that the original internalization is that of the actually
experienced mother as a consequence of the infant's efforts to deal
with the unavoidably frustrating aspects of this first love object.

Other clinical differences between the two British theorists derived
from these theoretical differences: Klein's stress on the need
to systematically analyze the positive and negative transference
from a position of technical neutrality contrasts with Fairbairn's
assumption that the reality aspects of the analyst's personality are
the most important therapeutic factor. Fairbairn criticized Klein's
overemphasis on aggression, and Kleinian authors think that
Fairbairn (as well as Balint and Winnicott) underemphasized the
importance of aggression, particularly regarding severe and early
psychopathology.

Fairbairn formulated the specific danger situations characteristic of
the schizoid and the depressive positions. The most devastating and
basic experiences were those of ego fragmentation, of loss of a sense
of oneness, and a conviction of futility (characteristic of the schizoid
position) under the impact of the fear of the destructiveness of one's
love. The principal danger of the depressive position, he proposed —
here agreeing with Klein — was the devastating loneliness he derived
from the loss of the loved object destroyed by one's own aggression.

In exploring the unconscious guilt feelings generally characteristic of superego functioning and the abnormally intense expression of guilt in depression, in particular, Fairbairn differed from Freud. He called the defense of the superego a "moral defence." It reflected an effort to maintain the good object relation with bad objects by reinforcing the internalization of the split-off, bad (frustrating and exciting) object. In depression, this reinforced internalization was an effort to transform the "unconditional badness" of the object into a "conditional" one, that is, the development of the fantasy that it was the child's own badness that brought about frustration or attack from the good object. Hence, the sadistic self-accusations of the depressed patient reflected not only the object's aggression directed against the ego, but the antilibidinal ego's effort to protect the good relation with the ideal object by attacking the libidinal ego as if it were bad, as having caused the frustration from the object.

The theoretical consequences of this explanation of the schizoid and depressive positions led Fairbairn to increasingly stress the primary nature of libidinal relations, the secondary nature of aggression as derived from frustration of the infant's libidinal needs by mother, and the primarily object-directed quality of libido. On the clinical side, however, Fairbairn stressed the crucial importance of internalized bad objects and bad object relations and the need to interpretively resolve the defensive function of the activation in the transference of the central ego-ideal object relation. Only the full activation of the bad internalized object (in both its frustrating and gratifying aspects) in the transference permitted the reduction of splitting of the endopsychic structure and an increase in the depth and scope of the central ego so that it could develop fully satisfactory libidinal relations with external objects.

Fairbairn felt that, because Freud had developed his structural model, particularly his concept of the superego, under the influence of his study of mourning and melancholia, he had overestimated both the importance of aggression in psychopathology and the conflicts between later stages of the superego and the ego, and had neglected the underlying characteristics of schizoid developments. Nevertheless, Fairbairn acknowledged repeatedly that it was Freud's description of the superego as an internalized structure having the capacity for repressive action and reflecting the internalization of the parental images of the oedipal conflict that had first stimulated Fairbairn to formulate endopsychic structure in terms of internalized object relations. Fairbairn felt that he had taken a step that evolved from Freud's structural theory.

Internalized Object Relations in Psychopathology

Fairbairn also explored the relation between the characteristics of the schizoid personality and other psychopathological conditions, particularly narcissism, repetition compulsion, negative therapeutic reaction, and the relation between the dynamics of schizoid and depressive psychopathology.

While he described hysterical psychopathology as the prototype of all psychopathology, illustrating the dynamic organization of endopsychic structure based upon schizoid processes (that is, splitting of an original, pristine ego into three subsidiary ones with their respective internalized object relations), Fairbairn considered the schizoid personality proper a most severe type of psychopathology. In the schizoid personality, a self-perpetuating splitting of the central ego occurred as a consequence and expression of extremely severe fears of any libidinal object relationship. The schizoid personality is characterized by an impoverished central ego relating to objects mostly stripped of their aggressive and libidinal characteristics, a general impoverishment of the affective capabilities of the central ego, and a withdrawal into an internal world of fantasy which permits the gratification of libidinal and aggressive needs intrapsychically and is reflected in detachment, secrecy, and subtle superiority in the relation with external objects. This condition represented, for Fairbairn, a highly pathological fixation at or regression to the basic intrapsychic organization elaborated into a specific clinical syndrome. In the transference, the schizoid patient's detachment from the analyst, his withdrawal into fantasies drained of emotion, the sense of emptiness and futility the patient conveys about himself and also induces in the analyst, have to be explored as a very active consequence of defensive splitting of the patient's total emotional relation with the analyst. Split-off segments of that relation emerge in dissociated emotional experiences, in the activation of fleeting, nonintegrated, nonverbal aspects of the patient's behavior, in displacements toward other objects, and in the patient's dreams. The analysis of all this material permits the gradual transformation of the initial "ideal," friendly but distant relation to the analyst.

In a broad sense, Fairbairn differentiated a psychopathology of "infantile dependence" (both of the early oral and the late oral stage), namely, the schizoid and depressive positions, from the psychopathology of the "quasi-independent" or "transitional" stage of development of later childhood, characterized by various ways of dealing with internal and external objects that included what he called the phobic, hysterical, paranoid, and obsessive "techniques." The final stage of development, following the infantile dependent and the transitional one, was the stage of "mature dependence," characterized by whole object relations and genital primacy. At one point, Fairbairn (1946, p. 175) explicitly defines his term *primary identification* "to signify the cathexis of an object which has not yet been differentiated (or has been only partly differentiated) from himself by the cathecting subject." I find it hard to reconcile this statement with the repeated affirmation that a pristine (that is, integrated and therefore differentiated) ego exists from birth on, and that a search for object relations exists when there is not yet any differentiation between the ego (or self) and the object.

Fairbairn criticized Abraham's (1924) effort to devise an organized scheme of psychopathology on the basis of fixation and/or regression to certain stages of libidinal development. He agreed with Abraham's description of the first two stages of development — the earliest oral stage characterized by sucking and the later oral stage characterized by biting. He rejected, however, Abraham's relating subsequent developmental stages to various types of psychopathology. Fairbairn suggested that the major neurotic syndromes — phobic neurosis, hysteria, obsession, and paranoid personality — reflected alternative methods of dealing with the same intrapsychic conflicts that gave rise to the schizoid and depressive positions.

Fairbairn saw the development of masochistic tendencies as a key manifestation of the activation of previously split-off bad internalized object relations in the transference. In the masochistic relation there is a desperate attempt not only to activate the relation between the antilibidinal ego and the antilibidinal object (a relation which, in itself, illustrates the libidinal ties between these two endopsychic structures) but also to modify the antilibidinal object and to transform its hatred into love. In a general sense, the desperate search for libidinal gratification on the part of the libidinal ego in relating to the libidinal object is condensed with the activation of the bad object relation in order to bring about the gradual mitigation of the latter and its consolidation with the good one in the same relationship.

According to Fairbairn, the child takes onto himself the badness of his frustrating, persecuting objects and also internalizes his good objects, which then combine in assuming a superego role. In explaining the internalizing of the bad object, he remarks, "It is better to be a sinner in a world ruled by God than to live in a world ruled by the Devil" (1943, p. 66). Paraphrasing this, in light of his concept of the "conditionally bad object," we might say that the Devil is internalized in an effort to transform him into an irate God, and later condensed with the ideal God in order to maintain the hope for an eventual redemption in God's world. This hope lies hidden in the activation of masochistic object relations in the transference.

Masochistic needs thus reflected, for Fairbairn, a key phase in the resolution of pathological schizoid states, and he saw the need to reactivate these split-off and repressed object relations as the basic explanation of repetition compulsion as well. In fact, Fairbairn stressed that the psychoanalytic resolution of unconscious guilt feelings might, if anything, bring about an intensification of the patient's resistances and of negative therapeutic reactions because the patient then would be faced with coming to terms with his libidinal attachment to bad, ambivalently loved objects. Fairbairn also linked the masochistic components of hysteria with underlying schizoid features.

Fairbairn pointed to the internal relationships of hypomanic, psychopathic, and narcissistic defenses against deeply repressed, denied, and split-off dependent needs. He stressed the connections between schizoid psychopathology, narcissistic features, and psychopathic tendencies, but he did not actually differentiate narcissistic pathology or clarify to what extent the psychopathic personality reflected complicating developments within an essentially schizoid psychopathology. Although he gives a comparative description of the defenses (he calls them techniques) characteristic of hysterical, phobic, obsessive, and paranoid psychopathology, Fairbairn had relatively little to say about these various types of "transitional" psychopathology and conveys the impression that his outline is essentially an answer to Abraham's schema of psychopathology. In this connection, it is of interest to note how little Fairbairn has to say about the psychoses, particularly schizophrenia. This stems, I suspect, from his tendency to remain close to the clinical base.

Psychoanalytic Technique

Fairbairn has written little on psychoanalytic technique. He maintained a standard technique during most of his professional years and rejected the abandonment of both the historical and genetic approach of the existential and the culturalist psychoanalytic approaches (he explicitly rejected the interpretation in the "here and now" *only*). He stressed the importance of the interpretation of resistances, the central nature of the interpretation of the transference, but expressed his concern that a combination of technical neutrality plus interpretations in terms of what he called "impulse psychology" only (in contrast to interpretation in terms of the reactivation of repressed object relations) might convey to the patient an excessive distance on the part of the analyst (1957). There is some irony in the protest Guntrip (1975) expressed at Fairbairn's adherence to classical psychoanalytic technique — implying distance and lack of personal involvement — in contrast to Guntrip's experience with his second analyst, Winnicott. In my opinion, Guntrip's criticism here speaks for Fairbairn.

Fairbairn stressed however, that therapeutic effects do not derive only from the analyst's interpretations — particularly from the interpretations of the transference — but also, and fundamentally, from the analyst's capacity to provide, by means of his real interest and concern, the necessary counterbalance to the activation of bad repressed object relations in the transference.

Later in his professional life, Fairbairn (1958) raised questions regarding the validity of the requirement that the patient should

lie on a couch with the analyst out of view. Although he did not favor
the face-to-face interviews advocated by the Sullivanians, he eventually adopted an arrangement in which, while patient and analyst
were not ordinarily looking at one another, they were sitting within
each other's potential field of vision. He stressed that the relationship
of the patient to the analyst was the decisive therapeutic factor
upon which the other therapeutic factors — insight, recall of infantile
memories, and catharsis — rested.

Fairbairn saw as the primary aim of psychoanalytic treatment to
bring about a synthesis of the personality by reducing "that triple
splitting of the pristine ego which occurs to some degree in every
individual, but in some individuals to a greater degree than others"
(1958). He considered the chief resistance to change as stemming
from the unconscious effort to maintain the internal world of object
relations as a "closed system," within which, in subtle expressions in
fantasies and dreams, in symptoms and avoided relations with external objects, the patient attempts to maintain the libidinal ties between the split-off and repressed bad objects and their corresponding
split-off and repressed parts of the ego.

CRITIQUE

In 1953, Winnicott and Khan in an extensive review of Fairbairn's book, criticized sharply — and, in my opinion, appropriately —
Fairbairn's claims that his theory supplants that of Freud. The
strong need, whatever its origin, to differentiate his theoretical
formulations from Freud's has done poor service to Fairbairn's
presentation of his theories and created what seems to me, in agreement with Winnicott and Khan, a largely unnecessary polemic
atmosphere around Fairbairn's work. Guntrip's enthusiastic, uncrit-
ical, and distorting presentation of Fairbairn's views, to which I have
already referred, has only exacerbated this tendency.

Winnicott and Khan (1953) pointed out that Fairbairn cannot
consistently maintain a view in which the infant is always a separate
entity, seeking an object that is distinct and yet emerges from within
the infant's own entity. They agreed with Fairbairn's stress that at

the root of the schizoid personality is the infant's failure to feel that the mother loves him in his own right, but pointed to the difficulty of finding out whether Fairbairn considers this the mother's failure or the result of the child's projection onto her of his own hate. They suggested that, in contrast to Fairbairn's own statement to the contrary, there is much in his book to indicate that it is the child's projection onto mother of his own hate that is importantly involved.

Winnicott and Khan (p. 331) also criticized the hopelessness of trying to correlate Fairbairn's statements with Klein's, "since Klein's work has been set down with great clarity, and Fairbairn's discoveries seemed to run criss-cross with those of Klein."

Another of their major criticisms derives from the problem created by Fairbairn's assumption that a primary identification with the object is compatible with a primary conception of an independent object. They state (p. 332) "Now if the object is not differentiated it cannot operate as an object. What Fairbairn is referring to then is an infant with needs, but with no 'mechanism' by which to implement them, an infant with needs not 'seeking' an object, but seeking detension, libido seeking satisfaction, instinct tension seeking a return to a state of rest or un-excitement; which brings us back to Freud." They feel that "Fairbairn's clinical intuitive sense brings him all the way while his theory gets bogged down a few miles in the rear."

Balint (1956a, b), in agreement with Winnicott and Khan's views, affirms the need for a consideration of pure pleasure-seeking along with the central importance of object relations. Zetzel (1955) also criticizes Fairbairn's underemphasis of the importance of aggression, and points to the similarity of Balint's and Fairbairn's position in this regard. Wisdom (1962, 1963, 1971), in comparing Fairbairn's and Klein's approaches, has probably clarified more than anybody else where implicit areas of agreement and disagreement lie, particularly regarding their concepts of introjection and projection, the psychopathology of hysteria and depression, and some of the philosophical implications of their work.

Sutherland (1963, 1965, 1979) has introduced important modifications into Fairbairn's model which have permitted him to establish bridges between Fairbairn's thinking and certain aspects of an ego psychology approach. Sutherland reintroduces the concept of instincts into Fairbairn's clinical observations by pointing to the ethological studies on attachment and to Bowlby's (1969) work, and by connecting Fairbairn's endopsychic structures with a concept of split-off affect states.

Sutherland (1963) made an important addition to the concept of the division of the pristine ego into substructures, stressing that each of them contains "a) a part of the ego, b) the object that characterizes the related relationships, and c) the affects of the latter." Sutherland stressed that the split-off ego structures of Fairbairn's model should be conceived as (p. 115)

> interrelated dynamic psychological systems, constantly in active relationship with each other and with the outer world. Each structure has a great complexity and depth into which is built its history. The particular experiences of the person will contribute many subsystems which could, for instance, be precipitates of repressed relations at the oral, anal or phallic phases of classical theory; but there is a tendency for these constituent subsystems to group or to assume a hierarchical order around the image of one person, even if only loosely. The first manifestation of a bad object relationship in the course of analysis may therefore center around one or other of these subsystems, but as the analysis proceeds all the components come to the surface.

Sutherland also focuses on the potential relations between Erikson's (1950) developmental model and Fairbairn's approach.

Referring to Fairbairn's technical approach, Sutherland stresses that "the repressed not only returns, but it tends to return to the representative of the more comprehensive relationship from which it was originally split off." Sutherland (1979) points out that, for Fairbairn, "impulses" are related to reality from the start, and the pleasure principle is an accompaniment of relationships with objects in reality and a guide to them.

Sutherland (1979) considers the self—his term for Fairbairn's ego—an overall system integrated by subsystems represented by the split-off self components described by Fairbairn, and suggests that the self may be considered "a supraordinate structure of great flexibility and perhaps in the nature of a 'field force,' its primary function [being] the container of motives from all the subsystems which have differentiated from it. Subsystems such as the behavioral systems of the ethologists, or the higher level organizations we call the subegos and internal objects all fall within its influence." He goes on to suggest that the value of the "self," conceptualized as "the overall dynamic structural matrix," is that "we can give underpinning to the personal level of action as 'I' and yet allow for the self to be dominated at different times and in different situations by any of its subsystems such as the superego, the antilibidinal ego, the exciting object, etc. etc."

By focusing on the intimate connection between object and self-structures in intrapsychic subsystems, Sutherland approaches, I think, Jacobson's concept of the build-up of internalized object relations in terms of self- and object representations. This relation of Fairbairn's to Jacobson's thinking can also be considered in Sutherland's stress on the affect components of internalized object relations. It is a paradox that Fairbairn, so vehemently in protest against Freud's instinct theory, consistently uses terms such as libidinal and aggressive cathexes or investment to refer to the dynamic qualities of endopsychic structures. In fact, to consider such libidinal and aggressive investments of self- and object representations as affective investments, and to consider these investments as the basic drive derivatives indissolubly linked to self- and object representations, offer a new perspective to the relation between ego psychology and object relations theory. Fairbairn, writing his central theoretical papers in the nineteen-forties, tended to ignore the writings of contemporary ego psychologists, particularly those in the United States. Jacobson's paper "The Self and the Object World" was published in 1954, and it was only in 1963 that Sutherland's reformulation of Fairbairn's statements on endopsychic structures permitted this relationship between Fairbairn and Jacobson to become apparent.

I agree with Sutherland (1979) that Fairbairn emerges as the theoretically most profound, consistent, and provocative writer of the British "middle group," including here particularly Balint, Winnicott, and Guntrip. Fairbairn was able to transform into a theoretical statement what analysts had long sensed before—and after—him, namely, that in all clinical situations we never find pure drives, but always an activation of affects reflecting such drives in the context of internalized object relations reenacted in the transference. I think Fairbairn was right in feeling that this concept was already implicit in Freud and required just one step further for fundamental reexploration of metapsychology; but I totally disagree with his assumption that this view requires an abandonment of Freud's metapsychology.

Our current knowledge about inborn motor, perceptive, and affective patterns which mature rapidly in the first few weeks and months of life and are reflected in early attachment behavior confirms, I believe—in agreement with Sutherland—Fairbairn's concept that libido is always object-seeking and does not exist independently from object-seeking. However, this statement also ignores the contemporary instinct theory that instincts are the hierarchical organization of inborn behavior patterns under the influence of the environment. In psychological terms, pleasurable, rewarding early object relations develop into an organized drive—or supraordinate motivational system, for which the concept of libido seems to me adequate and convincing in the light of Freud's theory of the continuity between early and later object-related instinctual aims.

Fairbairn's observation that libido emerges in the context of object relations and cannot be observed outside that context is perfectly consistent with my concept of the organization of libidinal drive throughout development (1976a, Chapter 3). By the same token, while Fairbairn is correct, it seems to me, in observing that aggression emerges as a response to frustration, he, as well as many behaviorists and culturalists, neglects the fact that there are inborn affective, perceptual, and behavior patterns that activate aggressive behavior, thus contributing for aggression the same maturational and developmental conditions as for libido.

Aggression as a drive is the supraordinate integration of aggressively invested object-relations into an overall hierarchically supraordinate motivational system. This concept of aggression is in fact clinically in harmony both with Fairbairn's stress on the crucial importance of the activation of aggressive internalized object relations in the transference, and with Sutherland's (1979) warning against simplistic deficit theories of psychopathology that neglect the enormous importance of dissociated envy and aggression in early development.

Regarding the relation between Fairbairn's model and ego psychology object relations theory, it seems to me that an impressive contribution of Fairbairn's theory resides in his proposal, at least ten years before the related work of Jacobson (1964) and of Mahler (1972a), that the internal world of object relations starts out as a dyadic, internalized relation between a self-component and an object component, what we would now call a self-representation and an object representation. In fact, I think the structural units of self- and object representations linked by determined affect dispositions, first described by Fairbairn and then elaborated by Sutherland, are the basic constituents of the id or dynamic unconscious. I have never understood why Fairbairn felt that such a concept of the id (the repressed exciting object and the libidinal ego related to it) is necessarily in contradiction to Freud's concept of the id. It is true that Fairbairn was not alone in assuming such an incompatibility; a good many traditional ego psychologists in this country, particularly Rapaport, would probably agree on the mutual incompatibility of these two models.

However, I think that Jacobson's and Mahler's developmental concepts, and beyond that, Hartmann's (1939) elaboration of the concept of an original ego-id matrix that predates the id as a discrete, organized system, points to the compatibility of Freud's and Fairbairn's model in this area. Fairbairn's protest against the relation between his tripartite model and that of Freud is weak not only in terms of his ignoring Hartmann's concept (in harmony with Freud's) of a primary undifferentiated ego-id. Fairbairn, in defining Freud's superego in terms of his own endopsychic structures, fails to note that in the tinking of contemporary ego psychology not all guiding value systems are incorporated in the superego, and, insofar as the superego reflects the infantile, sadistically infiltrated, childhood-derived morality that is essentially repressed and irrational, it corresponds much more closely to Fairbairn's antilibidinal object and antilibidinal ego than to his "ego-ideal."

In short, I see Fairbairn as having alerted us to the fact that, in contrast to the older concept of the id as a "reservoir" of "impulses," all three systems, ego, superego, and id, originate from the organization of internalized object relations, and I consider this concept compatible with the contemporary ego psychology approach that maintains Freud's structural theory and his dual-instinct theory linked to a developmental model centering on internalized object relations.

Fairbairn, in following Melanie Klein, ignored or neglected the lack of differentiation between self- and object representations that characterizes earliest development. Fairbairn, therefore, failed to consider early developmental stages that predate the differentiated self- and object components of his "schizoid position," which he saw as the fundamental endopsychic structure, as the earliest intrapsychic structural development. In contrast, Jacobson and Mahler's concept of earliest experience as reflecting a fused self-object representation — the original, undifferentiated, libidinally invested mother-infant dyad out of which both the internal world of object relations and the conception of the self gradually emerge — is, it seems to me, a better way of formulating the gradual origin of subjective awareness derived from intrasystemic early conflicts and of the conscious-self concept as related to the dynamic underpinning of the tripartite system.

A major problem with Fairbairn's theory of endopsychic structure is similiar to that of the Kleinian approach: the telescoping of all developments into an assumed extremely early sequence of schizoid and depressive "positions," thus neglecting the important connections between structural developments in the preoedipal stages of life and the consolidation of the tripartite structure under the influence of oedipal conflicts. Both Klein and Fairbairn had important contributions to make to the understanding of the connections between preoedipal and oedipal conflicts, but, because of the strange telescoping of development into the earliest months of life, both missed the boat. Winnicott avoided this collapse of early developmental stages. He assumed an earliest stage of undifferentiation (predating self and object differentiation) and described the pathology of early differentiation as related to excessive intrusion or impingement by mother with the subsequent consolidation of a "false self." Winnicott, however, did not formulate a fully integrated developmental model. The schizoid dynamics described by Fairbairn and Winnicott — as well as, presumably, Klein's paranoid-schizoid operations — would correspond, broadly, to Mahler's period of separation-individuation, with Fairbairn's schizoid defenses probably ranging from early differentiation to the rapprochement stage.

One more problem derived from Fairbairn's collapse of early development is his failure to differentiate splitting from repression proper. While I agree with his idea of the continuity of early splitting mechanisms, the later dissociative ego defenses leading to hysterical dissociative states and, finally, repression proper, there are developmental transformations involved in these increasingly complex processes that Fairbairn misses completely. Particularly striking is his failure to mention the clinical differences between splitting mechanisms and repressive mechanisms in adult patients.

And yet, Fairbairn's concept of "dynamic structures" in referring to the stable organization of internalized object relations constitutes a potentially powerful link between the early ego substructures that enter into self- and object representations and the tripartite structure and the emerging self. Although Fairbairn himself wrongly, I believe, thought that his viewpoint was in opposition to the dual-instinct theory, he rightly objected to the mystical and mechanical, impersonal qualities of instinct as reflected in the concept of a death instinct and the general use of aggression as conceptualized by Klein.

While starting out with Klein's description of multiple internal objects in his formulations, Fairbairn transcended her lack of structural thinking, the "free floating" internal objects in her theories, and he also brought back the real relation with mother, which was strongly underemphasized in the pseudobiological orientation of the Kleinian school.

The gradual integration of the self-components of early internalized object relations permits the concept of an emerging self that does not stem from impersonal instincts per se but from the organization of the self-representations, part of a world of internal object relations which is activated in the context of activation of inborn instinctive patterns and gradually leads to the simultaneous organization of drives and internalized object relations to form the tripartite structure. Bowlby, who originally developed his formulations under the influence of the British middle group, traced the organization of drives from primary inborn attachment behavior. However, he grossly neglected the organizing importance of intrapsychic structures reflecting object relations enacted under the impact of loving and hating affect states. My own efforts to integrate Bowlby's and Fairbairn's findings with the more recent and sophisticated developmental models of Jacobson and Mahler seem to me to do justice to clinical psychoanalytic findings, and to relate naturally the psychoanalytic concept of the self and the object world to the structural properties of the psychic apparatus.

Fairbairn's consistent stress on the link between particular self- and object components as dynamic units (in the context of what I would prefer, in agreement with Sutherland, to describe as an affective investment of such units) represents the earliest effort to link with metapsychology the clinical observation that we never see pure drives but always object relations under the effect of drive derivatives. Fairbairn's stress on considering endopsychic structure both a structure and an energy system seems to me, in the light of contemporary biological thinking as well as clinical evidence, a more sophisticated basis for updating psychoanalytic metapsychology than the numerous efforts to altogether eliminate energy concepts from psychoanalytic thinking because older, "hydraulic" energy models no longer seem satisfactory.

Chapter Five

The Contributions of Edith Jacobson

Because of the profound influence she has had on my thinking and because, to date, there have been only two overviews of her work — one dealing exclusively with her writings on depression (Mendelson, 1974), the other focusing chiefly on developmental aspects (Blanck and Blanck, 1974), I should like to offer a summary of Edith Jacobson's contributions.

To start, a few words about the impact Jacobson's work has had on the psychoanalytic field in general. The ideas contained in her writings are complex and highly elaborate. Her original proposals are imbedded in a careful analysis of the implications of her findings for psychoanalytic theory and technique, and she deals most respectfully and carefully with potential objections and alternative formulations. All this makes the study of her work difficult and militates against being able to extract from it an "exportable," simple scheme. Jacobson was never one of those fashionable figures who from time to time arise transitorily within the psychoanalytic field and seem to clarify all intricate issues by means of a few simple generalizations. However, by the same token, her influence on psychoanalytic theory formation has been profound and definite, and is still growing.

Perhaps the most important contribution Jacobson has made to psychoanalysis is her comprehensive developmental and psycho-structural model, which includes object relations theory, a sophisticated model which provides a clearly circumscribed and yet broad frame of reference for the psychoanalytic understanding of the entire spectrum of psychopathology and of normal development.

Starting out in 1937 with the exploration of superego formation in women, Jacobson analyzed the relation of depressive syndromes to ego and superego formation and the relation between normal and pathological affects, on the one hand, and structural development, on the other (Jacobson, 1943, 1946, 1952, 1953a, b, 1954a, b, d). In 1954, she formulated her ideas on the development of self- and object representations in her classic paper "The Self and the Object World" (1954c). Throughout the following ten years, she systematically explored depressive syndromes in the light of the influences on the ego and superego of normal and pathological object-relations-derived structures, mapped out the vicissitudes of depressive affects and moods in this context, applied her model to the study of normal and abnormal adolescence, and clarified an entire constellation of early defense mechanisms intimately connected with the vicissitudes of self- and object differentiation, mechanisms predating the definite integration of the psychic structures ego, superego, and id (1956, 1957a, b, 1959, 1961). Her book *The Self and the Object World,* published in 1964, summarizes her main propositions and discusses carefully, point by point, her theoretical contributions, which have expanded the boundaries of metapsychology and have proved clinically invaluable. After further clarifying her evolving concepts regarding psychosis (1966), and the treatment of psychotic disorders (in her 1967 Freud Anniversary Lecture and Monograph, *Psychotic Conflict and Reality*), Jacobson updated all her work on depression in her book *Depression* (1971).

AFFECT THEORY

Jacobson took as her point of departure the long-standing psycho-analytic debate: Are affects discharge processes (Freud's [1915] second theory of affects and Rapaport's [1953] firm conviction) or are affects central subjective states potentially including but not identical with discharge phenomena (Freud's [1894] first theory of affects and Brierley's [1937] assumption)? Jacobson (1953a) concluded that affects had to be considered discharge processes, but also as dispositions originating within each of the psychic structures (thus combining Freud's second theory of affects with his third and last theory [1926], which considered at least some affects as originating within the ego and not only the id). However, Jacobson herself soon felt that this effort to preserve Freud's second and third theories led to unsatisfactory classifications of affects, and, while temporarily leaving aside the ultimate question of the relation between instinctual drives and affects, she rapidly moved into a study of the development of affects and their clinical characteristics.

She first clarified that a theory of affects as discharge processes should not be confused with the concept of affects as processes of tension reduction (Jacobson, 1953a). On the contrary, she suggested, there are pleasurable tensions as well as unpleasurable discharge phenomena, and the function of the pleasure-unpleasure principle is to produce an optimal oscillation between the polarities of tension and relief, thus contributing to the constancy principle by means of an ever-changing, dynamically maintained optimal tension. Accordingly, discharge processes encompass both mounting and falling tensions, and affects are to be conceived as both tension states and discharge processes. The reality principle influences the pleasure-unpleasure axis with the ultimate objective of maintaining an optimal tension state in the face of external reality. Jacobson observed, however, that certain pathological structures within the ego and the superego, related to self- and object representations, might bring about such a severe distortion in this regulatory process, that— particularly in psychotic depression—the pleasure principle might have to be sacrificed entirely to adjust, by means of a pathological "optimal" tension, to a distorted intrapsychic reality. This observation contributed to drawing her attention to the relation between affect theory and self- and object representations.

Another of Jacobson's major observations was that, even if one considers affects discharge processes, the discharge of affects that is so prominent in the case of primitive affect states becomes a much less conspicuous phenomenon in the case of complex, higher level, sophisticated affects, which may combine aggressive and libidinal drive derivatives in various proportions. Feelings are more than discharge states; they represent drive investments in self- and object representations as well as in external objects; they constitute an obvious enrichment of mental life and should not be viewed merely as excessive or insufficient tension to be regulated. Self-esteem, for example—a crucial and complex libidinal affect investment of the self—cannot be considered simply a drive-determined, affective discharge process.

The most definite finding that anchored her clinical theories of affect to the vicissitudes of self- and object representations was the study of moods (1957b). Moods, she proposed, are diffuse, temporarily fixed affect states that involve the entire world of self- and object representations and are both regulated and regulating. They reflect a major impact on intrapsychic life of a sudden influx of libidinal or aggressive drive derivatives. Moods are general affective colorings of the entire experience of the self and the world of objects; they are a potential protection from disorderly discharge processes and a potential danger for severe distortion of all psychic experience. Jacobson described normal mood processes in the phenomenon of falling in love, she described the diffuse elation after overcoming a danger or unexpectedly resolving a tension state, and the sadness and grief of normal mourning.

Jacobson differentiated normal moods from pathological ones, particularly those of neurotic and psychotic depression, by pointing to the predominance of aggressive drive derivatives in the case of pathological depression, and the effects of primitive, pathological, exaggerated superego control in the form of violent mood swings that replace the more focused, cognitively delimited, and circumscribed self-criticism emanating from more mature levels of superego functioning. In drawing attention to these differences she clarified the fundamental role of affect control vested in the superego.

In addition, she differentiated neurotic from psychotic depression (1953b, 1971, Chapter 6). In the latter, a pathological refusion of self- and object representations takes place within the ego and within the superego, thus bringing about the classical attack of a highly pathological, idealized, yet sadistic superego onto a devalued and fused self-object representation in the ego. She concluded that, at all levels of depression, in addition to the qualitative aspects of the affects involved (and the drive cathexes represented by such affective processes), the normality or pathology of the affect and its impact on the entire psychic system depend on the structural arrangements of self- and object representations within the ego and superego. Sadness, for example, a component of grief, reflects the mourning for a loved, realistically or neurotically lost object; in severe depression, the capacity for sadness is lost because the pathological devaluation of the object and its psychic representation (which has been fused with a devalued self-representation) interfere with the experience of normal longing for the loved and unavailable object. It is only when psychotic depressed patients begin to improve that some of them are again able to feel not only depressed but sad.

In summary, Jacobson evolved a conceptualization of affective processes that explained their fundamental intrapsychic regulatory functions by means of their investment in self- and object representations, and she clarified the mutual relationships between affective discharge and intrapsychic tension, on the one hand, and the vicissitudes of ego and superego structures, particularly their constituent self- and object representations, on the other. She drew our attention to the intimate connections between affect differentiation, the vicissitudes of intrapsychic self- and object representations, and of ego and superego differentiation insofar as they integrate affects in the context of object relations.

On the basis of Jacobson's findings—but, I think, in contrast to her view—I now conceive of affects as deriving from constitutionally determined pleasurable and unpleasurable subjective states that first arise in the undifferentiated psychophysiological self, are then integrated and differentiated in the context of internalized "good" and "bad" object relations, and, eventually are the most important contributors to the differentiation of instinctual drives into libido and aggression (Kernberg, 1976a, Chapter 3).

Loewald (1978) has suggested a related conclusion: that the psychic apparatus originates from an interactional field in which both instincts and the psychic apparatus gradually differentiate within the dyadic matrix of early object relations.

DEPRESSION

Jacobson's study of depression starts out with a critical assessment of Bibring's (1953) formulations. She agrees with Bibring that depression originates as an intrasystemic affect state of the ego, that it reflects the discrepancy between a real and a wished-for or ideal self-image: in other words, depression arises as an affect state indicative of narcissistic frustration. However, on the basis of her own observations of depressed adolescent and adult patients, and of the study of normal and pathological affects and moods during the subphases of separation-individuation described by Mahler (1952; Mahler and Furer, 1968), Jacobson (1953b, 1961, 1971) concludes that the origin of depression within the ego does not preclude the existence of conflicts prior to such narcissistic frustration and deflation of self-esteem. She stresses the normal reaction to frustration of oral-dependent needs from mother in terms of the mobilization of hostile and demanding affects: she also points out that clinically one never sees a depressive affect in which there is not an involvement of both libidinal and aggressive drive derivatives and an interaction between real and ideal self-representations and real and idealized object representations, in addition to relationships with actual objects.

Jacobson stresses that the vicissitudes of affects cannot be separated from the vicissitudes of drive derivatives and object relations. Thus, she proposes an ego psychological theory of depression that assumes the origin of depressive affects within the ego; but, insofar as these affects are invested in self- and object representations, they will eventually become integrated with superego as well as with ego functions, and they will provide the superego with its important control function over the ego by means of mood swings. Jacobson then goes on to examine the clinical manifestations and the underlying psychodynamic implications of neurotic, borderline, and psychotic depressions, and differentiates depression in manic-depressive or affective illness from schizophrenic depression.

On the basis of extensive clinical observations, she reconfirmed Freud's (1917) and Abraham's (1911, 1916, 1924) conclusions regarding the predominance of early oral and sadistic conflicts in depressed patients and the abnormally intense dependence on ambivalently loved, idealized, and hated objects that are feared to be frustrating and rejecting. She described various stages in the development of psychotic depression, stages that permitted her to identify the predominant object relations and defensive operations involved: she thereby contributed significantly to the clinical understanding and the metapsychology of the crucial stages in the development and resolution of psychotic depression.

The beginning stage is the growing sense of narcissistic frustration derived from partly real and partly fantasied frustrations from real objects. Jacobson proposed that the principal anxieties and conflicts in depression are related to the fear of abandonment by the object, and to a related fear resulting from the development of aggression against the needed and frustrating object (1943, 1946, 1953b, 1954b). The main initial defensive mechanisms activated are an increasing idealization of the needed object and an effort to partially identify with that object by self-idealization achieved in closeness with it. The denial of the object's frustrating and aggressive aspects is part of this idealization, and the patient's denial of his own aggression and frustration also tends to reinforce the idealization.

The failure of these mechanisms leads to a catastrophic devaluation of the object and its representations. Jacobson described the defensive mechanism of devaluation as usually linked to preoedipal aggression. At best, such a devaluation is partial and temporary and contributes to a hostile self-affirmation and, indirectly, to increased autonomy. At worst, the devaluation reflects such an aggressive destruction of investment in the object and the object representation, that it leads immediately to an impoverishment of the self. This impoverishment reflects the loss of both the idealized object and the protective functions of the corresponding intrapsychic object representation. Here begins the distinction between neurotic and psychotic depression.

In neurotic depression, with relatively minor tendencies toward denial and idealization, with stability of self- and object representations,

and with the maintenance of some reality testing and object investments in other areas, the sense of loneliness and abandonment,
perhaps even the sense of unconscious guilt reflecting superego pressures, are relatively tolerable and do not progressively increase the
destruction of the object world.

In psychotic depression, however, further defensive mechanisms
and restitutive efforts develop which lead to more devastating
deterioration in internalized object relations. First the patient masochistically renews his efforts to idealize the love object and to sadistically extract love and narcissistic supplies from it; at the same time,
he projects aggression onto the object, making it all at once strong
and powerful and potentially dangerous and bad; the tendency
toward masochistic behavior and self-devaluation, together with
angry demands directed at the powerful, bad, although potentially
ideal, object complement each other.

But because this defensive posture threatens the patient with
the open expression of aggression in the context of a sadomasochistic
relationship with the ambivalently loved object, additional defenses
are brought into play that are typically psychotic. There is a renewed
devaluation of the object and a pathognomonic double introjection
of it into the superego and into the ego. Jacobson here utilizes Rado's
(1928) observation that the depressed patient attempts to recover the
ambivalently loved object by introjecting it in the form of an ideal,
powerful, and sadistic object into the superego, with the implication
that the ego's submission to the superego is also an effort to regain
the love of the lost object. But, she stresses, this introjection into
the ego and superego brings about pathological fusion processes in
both structures.

The internalization of the object into the ego is represented by the
devalued, deflated aspect of the object, first reflected in a deflated
object representation and, later, in the refusion of the deflated self-
and object representations. The internalization of the object into the
superego is followed by the fusion of that idealized, yet sadistic,
object with sadistic superego forerunners, so that an ideal, yet sadistic, primitive ego ideal attacks from the superego the devalued, fused
self-object representation. It is this double refusion within ego and
superego, typical for psychotic depression, that interferes with the

maintenance of ordinary ego boundaries and reality testing, thus reinforcing the distorting effects upon reality testing derived from the depressive mood triggered by the superego as an expression of its sadistic attacks on the ego.

Thus, in psychotic depression, the superego-ego boundary is still maintained, but reality testing is lost, and a psychotic transformation of all psychic experience takes place, together with a total loss of the real object. In schizophrenic depression (Jacobson, 1954b, d, 1966) — including both schizoaffective illness and depressed moods in schizophrenia proper — the process of refusion of self- and object representations proceeds further. This refusion includes additional fragmentation and fusion of such representations, with the reconstruction of primitive, pathological new units which reflect unrealistic combinations of real and ideal, self- and object fragments. At the same time, the dissolution of the constituent identifications of ego and superego bring about a loss of ego and superego differentiation.

In borderline conditions, however — an intermediary situation between that of psychotic depression and neurotic depression — the intermediary stages of this chain of events are, paradoxically, stronger and prevent the final psychotic regression. The reason is that the prevalence of denial, sadomasochistic tendencies, idealization, devaluation, and contradictory object relations of borderline patients, together with their relative lack of superego integration, permit repetitive cycles of idealization and devaluation, sadomasochistic interactions, a clinging search for new objects, and depressive episodes to go on in an endless, "unstable stability."

In addition to idealization, denial, and devaluation, Jacobson (1957a, 1959, 1964) also focused on depersonalization, introjection, and projection as typical defensive operations in borderline conditions. Depersonalization is actually a result of ego regression rather than a specific defensive mechanism; it depends upon the denial of mutually contradictory self-representations, particularly the need to deny segments of the self-experience that are in radical opposition or contrast to a person's core identity. (It is well known that Jacobson first conceptualized this process as a result of her experiences with co-prisoners in German concentration camps; her pointing to the intimate connection between intrapsychic and external reality in maintaining normal ego identity is another important aspect of this formulation.) Introjection refers to the modification of the self-representation after the object representation, projection refers to the modification of the object representation after the self-representation. Introjection and projection thus reflect early mechanisms employed to restore the unity between self and object lost with separation-individuation; early global imitation of the object is later followed by partial, selective identifications with it, within the context of an overall ego identity.

One further defense mechanism — or rather, complex set of expressions of all these defenses in the patient's interaction with the environment — is the attempt, in early stages of refusion of self- and object representations in psychotic depression, and, even more so, in schizophrenic illness, to forcefully engage in real although highly pathological interactions with objects in the external world in a final effort to control internal object relations and their vicissitudes under the effects of excessive ambivalence, aggression, and chaotic alternations of idealization, devaluation, projection, and introjection. The withdrawal from external reality is not a preliminary step of psychotic regression, but an indication of the failure of the first line of psychotic defenses.

Jacobson utilized all these discoveries and formulations in proposals regarding the psychoanalytic approach to the treatment of depression in borderline and psychotic depressed patients (1954d, 1956, 1966). She stressed the need to warn the patient tactfully, when idealization was prominent, of its potential negative consequences and defensive functions. At a later stage, when sadomasochistic transferences predominate, the interpretations of these resistances must be matched by the analyst's careful monitoring of his countertransference, the need to maintain warmth and dedication to the patient when he is desperately trying to induce the analyst to behave sadistically. When the patient is obviously in a psychotic regression and is completely devaluating the analyst, the ongoing availability of the analyst, even the possibility of establishing parameters of technique to underline the analyst's continuing aliveness and dedication to the patient, may be important aspects of an essentially interpretive approach. The analyst must also clarify ego boundaries and reality when reality testing is lost. A very important contribution to the understanding and interpretation of the patient's reality is the analysis of the complex interactions of manic-depressive patients with their — often surprisingly similar — spouses.

OBJECT RELATIONS THEORY

Jacobson, combining her findings in the treatment of patients with affective disorders and of adolescents with severe identity problems (narcissistic conflicts in particular) with Mahler's findings regarding autistic and symbiotic psychosis in childhood and normal and pathological separation-individuation (Mahler, 1952, 1957, 1958; Mahler and Furer, 1968) — findings that Mahler, in turn, had interpreted in the light of Jacobson's formulations — integrated them into a comprehensive developmental framework. Starting from the metapsychological contributions of Hartmann, Kris, and Loewenstein (Hartmann, 1948, 1950, 1952, 1955; Hartmann et al., 1946, 1949; Hartmann and Loewenstein, 1962), particularly from Hartmann's clarification of the differences between the ego and the self, Jacobson then related her developmental model to psychoanalytic metapsychology. Her developmental schemata represent an "intermediary language" between theoretical and clinical psychoanalysis. What follows is a summary of that developmental frame (Jacobson, 1954c, 1964).

Intrapsychic life starts out as a primary psychophysiological self within which ego and id are not yet differentiated and within which aggressive and libidinal drives are undifferentiated as well. The first intrapsychic structure is a fused self-object representation which evolves gradually under the impact of the relationship between mother and infant. The first few weeks of life, before such a primary self-object representation is consolidated, constitutes the earliest, presymbiotic — or, to use Mahler's term, autistic — phase of development. Pleasurable affects are the first emerging manifestations of the differentiating libidinal drive, and their investment in the fused self-object representation represents the first intrapsychic libidinal investment. Insofar as that fused structure represents the origin of both self- and object representations, libidinal investment in the self and in objects is originally one process.

The symbiotic phase of development comes to an end with a gradual differentiation of the self-representation from the object representation, which contributes importantly to the differentiation of the self from the external world. When differentiation begins, two processes make their appearance: (1) the defensive refusion of libidinally invested self- and object representations as the earliest protection against painful experiences, giving rise, when this process is excessively or pathologically maintained, to what will later become psychotic identifications characteristic of symbiotic psychosis of childhood and of affective psychoses and schizophrenia in adulthood (1954a, b, c, 1957a, 1964, 1966, 1967, 1971), and (2) the differentiation of painful experiences into aggressively invested self- and object representations as an early effort to separate and deny the frustrating interactions between self and mother and their intrapsychic representations. A fused, undifferentiated self- object representation invested with aggressive drive derivatives becomes the counterpart of the libidinally invested one, so that, at a certain point, the intrapsychic world of object relations consists of "good" and "bad" self-representations and similarly "good" and "bad" object representations.

Efforts to restore the ideal, symbiotic relationship with mother now give rise to processes of introjection and projection, geared to replace refusion in fantasy with a mutual modeling of self- and object representations, in order to maintain good or ideal relations between self- and object representations and to deny and project bad ones: these bad self- and object representations will become the sadistic superego forerunners, the first layer of superego development. The stage of separation-individuation is thus characterized by multiple differentiated, but not integrated, good and bad, self- and object representations.

The next stage of development consists in the gradual, more realistic integration of good and bad self-representations into real self-representations, and the integration of good and bad object representations into real object representations. In this process, partial aspects of self- and object representations become total self- and object representations. The completion of the separation-individuation phase and the establishment of object constancy marks, precisely, the accomplishment of this developmental task (Mahler et al., 1975).

An additional set of ideal self- and object representations develops throughout all this time, particularly during the second and third years of life. As self- and object representations become more realistic, the child becomes aware of his own shortcomings as well as of shortcomings and frustrations that stem from the good mother. He builds up ideal self-representations reflecting aspired-for changes in himself which would restore the ideal relationship with mother that existed during the symbiotic phase, such ideal self-representations being complemented by ideal object representations, namely, the good or ideal mother lost when the child acquired a more realistic assessment of the relation between himself and the mother. The early reaction formations against instinctual, particularly anal, drive derivatives in the second year of life are controlled by the aspirations and demands incorporated into such ideal self- and object representations. It needs to be stressed that, in contrast to the earlier good and bad self- and object representations, these later, ideal mental representations are based, not on the denial of their respective opposites, but on the realistic integration of good and bad self- and object representations; they reflect a more mature and sophisticated form of idealization.

The normal development of idealization processes must be examined, however, in the context of the simultaneous development, throughout all this time, of processes of devaluation which complicate the picture. Efforts to deny and to devalue the bad aspects of mother and of object representations—and, by the same token, the bad aspects of self-representations—lead the child to reject certain aspects of frustrating or dangerous closeness with mother, foster autonomy, and further differentiate self from objects. Also, in order to protect the good relationship with mother, compensating idealizations are built up which reinforce ideal object representations and, by means of introjection, ideal self-representations. Miscarriage of all these processes leads to the development of the depressive psychopathology described earlier.

The next stage of development, which starts with object constancy, takes place throughout the fourth and fifth years and is completed with the passing of the Oedipus complex and the beginning of latency. During this phase, ideal self- and ideal object representations are integrated into the ego ideal and the ego ideal is incorporated as part of the superego. It is only now that a clear differentiation between ego and superego occurs, thus completing the establishment of the tripartite structure which was initiated with the separation of ego and id when repression began to prevail over the earlier primitive defense mechanisms of introjection, projection, denial, idealization, and devaluation. In addition, the delimitation of ego boundaries initiated by the differentiation of self- and object representations has gradually consolidated the ego boundaries with external reality as well as with the id. It is the refusion of self- and object representations under pathological conditions that precipitates the breakdown of ego boundaries and loss of reality testing.

Jacobson, in the most comprehensive exploration of the superego in psychoanalytic literature, described three broad layers of superego formation (1954c, 1964). The first and deepest layer is represented by the sadistic forerunners that reflect the internalization of fantastic, sadistically prohibitive, and punitive object representations or, rather, "bad," fused self- and object representations that the infant projected onto the frustrating mother and other objects as part of an effort to deny and project the aggressively invested object relations. A second layer is constituted by the integration of the ego ideal on the basis of the fusion of ideal self- representations and ideal object representations; this represents the child's final efforts to reconstitute the original libidinally invested symbiotic relation with mother at a higher level of intrapsychic aspirations and demands. Under optimal circumstances, a mutual toning down of the earliest sadistic and the later idealized superego forerunners occurs, repeating within the evolving superego the processes of integration of good and bad object relations which occurred earlier within the ego. Jacobson described how such integration and toning down permit, in turn, the internalization of a third layer of superego determinants, namely, the realistic, demanding, and prohibitive aspects of the parents that characterize the later stages and completion of the Oedipus complex and bring about the final constitution of the superego as an integrated structure.

Once this has been achieved, the superego takes over the important functions of protecting the libidinal investment of the self and of regulating self-esteem by means of mood swings. Throughout the next stage of development, latency, such dispositions toward mood swings gradually decrease, and processes of depersonification, abstraction, and individualization occur in the superego, bringing about regulation of self-esteem by more focused, delimited, cognitively differentiated affects and demands. Specific guilt feelings and self-criticism reflect a sophisticated developmental elaboration of depressed moods under the influences of superego integration. The mature superego is characterized by control exerted through mild or modulated mood swings, guilt feelings, and a growing sense of autonomy, whereas a pathological, excessively aggressive and primitive superego is characterized by the predominance of severe depressive mood swings. In addition, feelings of inferiority and shame now reflect the participation of the ego ideal in superego regulation of the ego; the greater the defect in superego integration, the more do feelings of inferiority and shame predominate over the capacity for experiencing modulated depressed affects (such as sadness) and differentiated guilt feelings.

At the same time, throughout the oedipal period and latency, the integration of the self-representations into an organized self-concept proceeds, and ego identity, originally stemming from the integration of good and bad self-representations at the time object constancy is established, is further consolidated. Jacobson (1964) criticized Erikson (1956) for his excessively broad use of the term ego identity, and for his deemphasis of infantile stages of identity formation. She nevertheless considered his concept of "identity formation" valuable, provided it included processes of organization within all structures of the psychic apparatus. She suggested that the objective process of normal identity formation is reflected in the normal subjective feeling of identity. The integration of the self-concept within the ego strongly influences the integration of superego forerunners and, in turn, superego integration strongly reinforces the integration of the ego, particularly of the self-concept.

Jacobson described the partial repersonification, reprojection, and redissolution of the superego that occurs as a key aspect of the adolescent task to reinforce infantile prohibitions against oedipal strivings, while at the same time, the adolescent needs to identify with an adult model of sexual behavior and to integrate the tender and erotic aspects of sexual drives. Here, the careful study of the nature and extent to which such partial redissolution and reprojection of the superego occurs and the extent to which normal ego identity is still maintained differentiate normal and neurotic adolescents from their borderline and narcissistic counterparts (Jacobson, 1954c, 1961, 1964). Severe identity conflicts in adolescence reflect failure in the stage of development in which good and bad self-representations are integrated into a total self-concept, as well as the derived failure to integrate idealized and sadistic forerunners of the superego. Under these circumstances, the internalization of the third superego layer of realistic parental images also fails and parental images are distorted by powerful projective processes, reactivating a chaotic world of all-good and all-bad self- and object representations. These failures also foster the continuation of primitive defensive mechanisms and intefere with the integration of the superego, thus creating a vicious circle of lack of differentiation and integration of the tripartite structural system. This is characteristic of borderline conditions and narcissistic psychopathology, and Jacobson studied the effects of such developments on the characteristics of depression in these personality structures. In contrast, the successful integration of the superego and the consequent reconfirmation of ego identity creates the background of neurotic psychopathology and normality.

IMPLICATIONS AND CRITIQUE

I think that Jacobson's developmental model includes the only comprehensive psychoanalytic object relations theory that links earliest development in the realm of affect differentiation, object relations, early defensive mechanisms, and vicissitudes of early instinctual development with the structural model of the tripartite psychic apparatus, and thus provides a developmental frame for psychoanalysis. Her close collaboration with Mahler provided Mahler with a frame of reference which was vital to her study of autistic and symbiotic psychosis and separation-individuation; in turn, Mahler's revolutionary findings provided strong supportive material for the development of Jacobson's model. The clinical and metapsychological studies of depressive reactions in normal, neurotic, borderline, and psychotic patients provided Jacobson with the clinical evidence which stimulated her theoretical formulations regarding relatively advanced levels of development and the harmonious linkage between early development and that following the consolidation of the tripartite structure.

Several other major efforts to develop an integrated object relations theory seem to me to have important and self-defeating shortcomings. Sullivan's (1953) efforts to develop a concept of the psychic apparatus that reflects interpersonal interactions failed to provide any structural model of development, could not integrate drive theory, and generally underestimated the complexity of unconscious, intrapsychic development. Erikson (1950, 1956, 1963), within an ego psychology frame, attempted to trace the development of ego identity and, in studying the sequence of processes of introjection, identification, and ego identity, arrived at his developmental model of stages of psychosexual development. However, as Jacobson herself pointed out (1964, Chapter 2), he underestimated the importance of early determinants of identity formation, overestimated the importance of adolescent conflicts in determining the vicissitudes of ego identity, and never evolved a complete developmental outline which would simultaneously spell out the vicissitudes of drive derivatives, affects, object relations, structure formation, and defensive organization.

I have already stated what I consider the shortcomings of Fairbairn's and Melanie Klein's object relation theories (see also Kernberg, 1976a, Chapter 4). I shall merely add here that Jacobson (1964) pointed out that Melanie Klein failed in not differentiating self- from object representations and their development, arbitrarily pushed intrapsychic developments into the first half of the first year of life, and neglected almost totally the relation between normal and abnormal early development, on the one hand, and the consolidation of the definite tripartite structure, on the other (see also Kernberg, 1976a, Chapter 4).

Against this background of failure in alternative attempts to establish a satisfactory object relations theory, Jacobson's work stands out as a unique metapsychological contribution to integrating internalized object relations with the structural theory, extending the work of Hartmann, Kris, and Loewenstein.

Jacobson's work has implications for psychopathology that are equally important. Her contributions and those of others related to her general theoretical frame, particularly Mahler's, have already had a definite impact on the applications of psychoanalytic theory and technique to various psychopathological conditions and to psychiatric theory generally. Let us review these contributions briefly, following Jacobson's developmental line.

The first stage of development, preceding the establishment of the fused self- object representation, is reflected—when prolonged or permanent—in the autistic syndromes of childhood. It may well be that organic factors are important in codetermining the failure to establish the original fused self- and object representation as an intrapsychic structure in many cases, and that a regressive destruction or deterioration of such intrapsychic structure may determine or codetermine an autistic syndrome in other cases. Object relations theory thus offers a common final pathway for organically and psychologically determined early pathology: Mahler's contributions in this area are well known (Mahler and Furer, 1968).

Regarding the second stage of development, an excessive prolongation of the symbiotic phase or a defensive regression in terms of a refusion of self- and object representations (what Jacobson has called psychotic identification) characterizes symbiotic childhood psychosis and schizophrenia in adulthood. In addition to Mahler's fundamental work in this area, Searles' contributions (1965) regarding schizophrenic transferences, Lewin's (1950) study of elation, and Jacobson's own work on depressive psychosis illustrate how the refusion of self- and object representations determines loss of reality testing and typically psychotic interactions in the transference.

Jacobson has explored the diagnostic and therapeutic implications of pathological refusion of self- and object representations in depressive psychosis and schizophrenia (1954d, 1956, 1966, 1967, 1971). She has pointed out that in schizophrenia, fragments of self- and object representations are re-fused and pathologically reorganized into new units, while the tripartite psychic structure completely disintegrates and all higher-level internalized object relations disintegrate as well. Therefore, the schizophrenic patient assumes new, partial, pathological identity fragments. In contrast, in depressive psychosis, the refusion of self- and object representations occurs within the ego and within the superego, without a dissolution of an integrated superego structure as such. This has fundamental consequences for maintaining certain aspects of the relation with reality, and for the enactment in the transference of a primitive object relation between an all-powerful, sadistic, fused self- object representation in the superego and a deflated, devalued, fused self- object representation in the ego.

Proceeding to the next stage of development, when self- and object representations are differentiated from each other but not yet integrated into total object representations and a comprehensive self-concept, the spectrum of pathology of borderline personality organization becomes predominant. Here, Mahler (1971, 1972a) has described the relation between abnormal separation-individuation, particularly of an abnormal rapprochement subphase, and the pathological development of splitting mechanisms and primitive object relations that characterize the borderline conditions. This is also the area in which I have applied Jacobson's work in great detail (Kernberg, 1975, 1977b) and attempted to describe systematically the constellation of primitive defensive operations, primitive object relations, and particular condensations of pregenital and genital conflicts under the overriding influence of aggression characteristic of these cases. My own theoretical frame of reference and, in fact, my theory of technique and actual therapeutic strategy with borderline cases and narcissistic pathology (1976a, b) derive from Jacobson's work. Her findings have particular relevance to the clinical situation in that, by a careful analysis of primitive dissociated part-object relations in the transference, one can foster, by interpretive means, the integration of contradictory, conflictual self-representations into an integrated self and of conflictual, contradictory object representations into integrated conception of objects.

In broader terms, Jacobson's formulations permit us to understand why patients may have sharply defined intrapsychic conflicts and defenses and stable, highly pathological ego structures without presenting an integrated tripartite structure, and how, in these cases, the interpretation of impulse and defense is an interpretation of mutually contradictory and conflictual internalized object relations.

It needs to be stressed that many of the clinical manifestations of borderline conditions in the psychoanalytic situation: the understanding of the borderline patients' pathological object relations, their severely narcissistic conflicts, and disintegrated or dissociated identifications, and the vicissitudes of their reality testing were clarified by the pioneering contributions of Stone (1954), Frosch (1964, 1970, 1971), and Greenson (1954, 1958). I think that Jacobson's formulations have provided an integrated frame for these observations and a theoretical and clinical set of tools for further clarifications and treatment of these conditions.

The next stage in Jacobson's developmental line is represented by the full integration and consolidation of the superego, and the consequent further integration of the ego and reinforcement of the repressive barrier with the id. Here, neurotic conditions and non-borderline character disorders represent the main psychopathology. Classical psychoanalytic theory and its enrichment with modern ego psychology have provided the basic theoretical, clinical, and technical understanding in this area.

To conclude: Jacobson's contributions demonstrate, in my view, the vitality that psychoanalysis offers today and promises for the future. I am convinced that her object relations theory has been one of the fundamental lines of progress in psychoanalytic theory and technique.

Chapter Six

Mahler's Developmental Theory:
A Correlation

The stages of development which in earlier work (1972; 1976a, Chapter 2) I called stages 1 through 5 correspond very closely to the stages of early development described by Margaret Mahler, namely, the autistic, symbiotic, separation-individuation, and "on the road to object constancy" developmental phases. Indeed, the sequences of psychic development Mahler postulated on the basis of her work with children presenting autistic and infantile symbiotic psychosis, and her developmental studies of normal and abnormal features of separation-individuation show a remarkable correspondence with the developmental hypotheses I arrived at on the basis of the psycho-analytic and psychotherapeutic exploration of adolescent and adult patients with borderline personality organization.

This correspondence strengthens significantly, it seems to me, our respective conclusions. Mahler's findings regarding the chronology of phase sequences within her developmental framework provide fundamental evidence regarding the timetable of points of fixation and regression that were much more difficult, if not impossible, to determine on the basis of psychoanalytic work with adult patients suffering from borderline personality organization. By the same token, my findings regarding the multiple interrelationships of descriptive, dynamic, and structural features of certain transference developments in borderline patients that correspond to the main themes of the rapprochement subphase of separation-individuation provide, I think, a psychoanalytic dimension from adulthood that reinforces Mahler's assumptions about intrapsychic correlates of developmental observations in early childhood. Particularly, the predominance of splitting operations in borderline patients and their transferences — which reveal lack of integration of self- and object representations of "good" and "bad" kinds but no fusion of self- with object representations — reflect structurally the developmental stage of separation-individuation that follows symbiosis and precedes object constancy. It is probably no coincidence that both Mahler and I have found Jacobson's (1964, 1971) theory of the development of internalized object relations and their integration into ego and superego structures a crucial theoretical tool.

The application of Mahler's theoretical formulations to the psychotherapeutic treatment of borderline children and adults and to psychoanalytic technique in general (Mahler and Kaplan, 1977; Furer, 1977; Kramer, 1979) has added another dimension to treatment technique and should permit further study of similarities and differences of our approaches to these patients.

Because Mahler's theory is so well known and so easily available, I shall assume the reader's familiarity with it and confine myself in what follows to spelling out the principal areas of agreement between her conceptualizations and mine, and those aspects of both theory and treatment technique where I see disagreements or differences in approach.

THEORETICAL ISSUES

I have already described Jacobson's concept of the earliest phases of development, and how her formulations and Mahler's meshed. Mahler (Mahler and Gosliner, 1955; Mahler and Furer, 1968; Mahler et al., 1975) is in general agreement with Jacobson's formulations, but conveys the impression that "bad" fused self-object representations remain at the periphery of the core self and are less crucial in organizing intrapsychic experience than I have suggested. Thus, while Mahler (1971), in agreement with me, suggests that the painful "bad" quality of experience may be the first basis of later splitting mechanisms, she does not stress, as I would, the continuity of the originally fused, "bad" self-object representation of the symbiotic phase with the later splitting of "good" and "bad" mother and "good" and "bad" self of the rapprochement subphase. The difference here seems to be largely one of emphasis.

Also, while the differentiation of "good" and "bad" affects — in the context of the "good" and "bad" undifferentiated self- and object representations — constitutes, in my view, the earliest manifestation of the organization of drives into libido and aggression and, by the same token, the simultaneous investment of these earliest drive manifestations into the earliest internalized object relations, Mahler is much less explicit regarding the relation between the earliest "good" and "bad" experiences as primitive affect states and whether they actually represent differentiation of aggression and libido. Mahler here agrees with Jacobson (1964) in maintaining the concept of primary narcissism, that is, the investment of the primary undifferentiated self with undifferentiated drive energy, in contrast to my assumption (and Jacobson's [1954c] earlier assumption) that, insofar as the earliest manifestations of libidinal investment are into a fused self-object representation, "primary" narcissism and "secondary" narcissism (that is, narcissism related to the vicissitudes of object investments) are equivalent. If, as I think, the earliest libidinal investment is in a self and object that are not yet differentiated, the concept of primary narcissism (and, by implication, of primary masochism) is no longer warranted.

The difference in emphasis that I mentioned has relevance for the psychoanalytic psychotherapy of psychotic states: In my opinion, the analysis of intensely aggressive object relations of psychotic patients, within which self and object are not differentiated, illustrates the enormous importance of the structures governed by fused, "bad" self- and object representations.

In addition, whether the earliest affect states are representations of the beginning stage of drive differentiation or constitute in themselves the first manifestations of differentiating drives has theoretical implications. I have reached the conclusion that drives constitute overall motivational systems which stem from the hierarchical organization of affect states into a libidinal and an aggressive constellation. The linkage between biological instincts and psychic drives would be represented by inborn affect dispositions that are integrated as "good" and "bad" affect states into object relations, thus determining an overall hierarchical organization of drive systems, or libido and aggression in the broadest sense. As I have proposed before (1976a), I conceive of aggression and libido as the basic motivational systems that incorporate in their organization both affects and object relations. I think that drives stem from biologically determined inborn affect dispositions, which, together with inborn perceptual and behavior patterns, are activated as affect states in the context of early object relations.

Internalized object relations, in turn, are organized on the basis of units of self- and object representations related to each other in the context of a dominant affect state. This affect state represents the "signal" of the respective drive reflected in this particular object relation. These basic object relations units determine, as they develop, the integration of the tripartite structure. The affect states activated in the context of object relations are either positive, rewarding, gratifying, or negative, aversive, frustrating: this will give to their respective object relations a basic quality of "good" or "bad."

Jacobson, Mahler, and I agree that the differentiation of self- from object representations permits the consolidation of ego boundaries, reflects the end of the symbiotic stage of development, but does not yet signify an integrated ego (or, rather, an integrated self) or an integrated conception of objects. To the contrary, between the symbiotic phase and the attainment of object constancy and the related consolidation of the tripartite psychic apparatus, an intermediary developmental structure must be assumed, wherein differentiation of self from objects, and lack of integration of the self and of the conceptions of objects are key features. This is one of Mahler's crucial contributions: the enrichment of her early concept of this developmental stage into a solid body of evidence, culminating in her description of separation-individuation and its subphases.

In addition to providing the developmental and clinical evidence that was linked up with Jacobson's theoretical formulations and clinical observations of narcissistic and borderline pathology of adolescence, Mahler also provided more general clinical evidence for the ego psychology approach to structural development, as opposed to the British schools'—particularly the Kleinians'— assumption of highly sophisticated, complex intrapsychic structuring in the first year of life (which implies a full differentiation of self from object, as well as the capacity for an integration of the conception of the self and of objects in the second part of the first year of life). Mahler's evidence here prompted me to reconsider my previous, tentative, assumptions about the timetable of earliest development (Kernberg, 1972, 1976a, Chapter 2), alluded to earlier.

Mahler's description of the subphases of separation-individuation (differentiation, practicing, and rapprochement) allows us to examine in a new light various clinical observations regarding borderline personality organization. I fully agree with Mahler that a large majority of patients with borderline personality organization present intrapsychic structural organization and conflicts related to those of the rapprochement subphase. A small group of borderline patients however—severely schizoid personalities for the most part— present transference developments and regression that seem more related to the differentiation subphase. In this connection, placing the degree of self-object differentiation within a developmental continuum, I have described (1978a) the following spectrum of psychopathology stemming from before object constancy is achieved.

First, we have the fixation at or regression to psychotic identifications in Jacobson's (1954a, b) terms, or the symbiotic stage of development in Mahler's (Mahler and Furer, 1968) terms, in which the differentiation of self from nonself is abolished and self- and object representations re-fuse: here we find only idealized, ecstatic merged states, and terrifying, aggressive merged stages. The chief emphasis in such cases has to be on gradually helping the patient to differentiate his internal life from the therapist's psychological reality, on stressing the reality of the immediate therapeutic interaction, and on being alert to the dangers in the patient's life derived from the breakdown of ego boundaries outside the therapeutic situation. It seems to me that Searles's work with schizophrenic patients (1965) speaks to this point.

Second, there are patients in whom the regression and/or fixation is primarily to a stage of differentiation preceding the typical borderline pathology (reflected in the splitting of "good" and "bad" self- and object representations) but more advanced than that of psychotic refusion. Usually, these are patients in whom schizoid characteristics predominate, but most patients with schizoid personalities present typical borderline pathology; in fact, Fairbairn described splitting operations as the key characteristic of schizoid states (see Chapter 4). In a minority of schizoid patients, however, the prevailing level of regression relates to the early differentiation subphase of separation-individuation, and these patients require, as part of the treatment approach, "holding" (Winnicott, 1965) — being empathized with and yet permitted to maintain their autonomy vis-à-vis the therapist — at least as an important aspect of the treatment technique in certain stages of therapeutic regression. A temporary regression to this early developmental subphase may signify a potential for new ego growth, as both Balint (1968) and Winnicott (1953, 1960) have suggested.

Third, the next level of regression and/or fixation is precisely the one typical of the large majority of patients with borderline personality organization. Here, the problem is no longer the need to protect the gradually emerging autonomous self of the differentiation subphase, but rather to focus on the integration of split-off aspects of self- and object representations, which reflect pathology linked largely — as Mahler (1971, 1972a, b) found — with the rapprochement subphase. In other words, in these patients, the issue is not between autonomy or merger, or between true and false self, but between nonintegrated and integrated self, nonintegrated and integrated object relations. The treatment approach I have outlined for borderline patients is consistent with this conception.

I have suggested (1975, 1976a, b) that the principal therapeutic tasks with borderline patients are to transform primitive into advanced transferences (manifest by the transformation of primitive, dissociated or split object relations into integrated or total object relations) and, related to this, to transform an ego organization characterized by primitive defenses centering around splitting into an integrated ego characterized by defenses centering around repression; this transformation will lead to the differentiation of ego, superego, and id as as integrated structures.

In this process, which is done by means of interpretation, first, the dissociated or generally fragmented aspects of the patient's intra-psychic conflicts are gradually integrated into significant units of primitive internalized object relations; second, each unit (consti-tuted of a particular self-representation, a particular object represen-tation, and a major affect disposition linking these) then needs to be clarified as it becomes activated in the transference, including the alternation of reciprocal self- and object reenactments in the relationship with the therapist; and third, when these units can be interpreted and integrated with other related or contradictory units — particularly when libidinally invested and aggressively invested units can be integrated — the process of working through of the transference and the resolution of primitive constellations of defensive operations characteristic of borderline conditions has begun.

As mentioned before, the principal difference between Mahler's and my approach to the pathology of the rapprochement subphase resides in the major stress, in my work, on the continuity between splitting of "good" and "bad" internalized object relations of the sym-biotic and the separation-individuation stage, in contrast to Mahler's statement referring to the rapprochement crisis (Mahler et al., 1975, p. 99): "Yet splitting the object world has also begun." Again, these are differences in emphasis. The description, in the same book, of splitting operations in a patient during the rapprochement subphase (pp. 82–85) beautifully illustrates the patient's need to defend the good mother against the patient's own destructive rage by splitting the object world into "good" and "bad."

Mahler stresses that in the individual solutions of the rapproche-ment crisis there is a development of patternings and personality characteristics with which the child enters into the consolidation of individuation, an extremely important formulation, which explains the prevalence of preoedipal character constellations in borderline patients and the possibility of directly tracing character structure back to the rapprochement subphase of separation-individuation. Coercion and splitting of the object world, two mechanisms that Mahler has described as particularly characteristic of most cases of adult borderline transference, are typically exaggerated in cases of failure to overcome the rapprochement crisis. In agreeing, I would point to the splitting in borderline patients, which I have stressed, and the relation of coercion to the mechanisms of omnipotence and projective identification (with their implications of efforts to omnipotently control the object onto whom a split-off impulse has been projected).

Regarding the next stage of development, "on the road to object constancy," I would stress my full agreement with Mahler (1975) regarding the intimate relationship between preoedipal and oedipal conflicts, an area where Mahler is still misunderstood. I am referring to the confluence of prevalent conflicts deriving from separation-individuation factors with those deriving from the following oedipal period. This confluence normally evolves in the context of establishing object constancy and the definite integration of the psychic structures. Jacobson, Mahler, and I agree that this stage of development consists in a gradual and more realistic integration of "good" and "bad" self-representations and the parallel integration of "good" and "bad" object representations; in this process, partial aspects of self- and object representations become integrated or, respectively, total self- and object representations. The completion of the stage of separation-individuation and the establishment of object constancy permit the development of differentiated oedipal relations.

Differentiated oedipal relations presuppose the capacity for a differentiated concept of the parental couple, including their sexual characteristics, and differentiated relations to them which take into consideration their sexual identity. Absence of these preconditions are typical for patients with borderline personality organization, whose preoedipal conflicts, particularly around aggression, infiltrate all object relations. In addition to reinforcing and fixating primitive defensive operations centering around splitting, excessive aggression also contaminates the later object relations characteristics of the Oedipus complex. This creates characteristic distortions in the oedipal constellation, reflected in features I have described elsewhere (1977b; see also Chapter 9). Here, in agreement with Mahler (1975), I am stressing that consequences of severe preoedipal conflicts derived from the pathology of development that precedes object constancy include the pathological development of oedipal conflicts, but not an absence of them. Masterson (1972, 1976) applies a theoretical frame of reference derived from Mahler's work to the psychotherapeutic treatment of adolescent and adult borderline patients, which in my opinion treats these patients as if they were fixated at the conflicts of separation-individuation to the exclusion of the developments and transformations that these conflicts undergo under the influence of oedipal developments. The application of Mahler's thinking to psychoanalysis and the psychotherapeutic treatment of children as carried out by herself and her close co-workers take transformations and condensations of preoedipal and oedipal issues fully into consideration.

TECHNICAL ISSUES

Although Mahler has not so far presented a systematic approach to the treatment of borderline conditions based on her developmental and psychopathological findings, it is my impression that she is in general agreement with the approach that I have recommended for the treatment of adolescent and adult borderline patients, namely, a modified psychoanalytic approach or psychoanalytic psychotherapy. Based on her views, Rinsley (1977), Masterson (1972, 1976, 1978), and Furer (1977) have proposed psychotherapeutic approaches to the treatment of borderline patients that are, essentially, in harmony with the psychoanalytic psychotherapy I have suggested for these conditions (1975, 1976a, b, 1978a).

Rinsley's conclusions stem from a combination of Mahler's, Masterson's, and my views. He states (1977, p. 67): "Psychoanalytic therapy of borderline personalities requires confrontative and interpretive exposure of the split object-relations unit within the therapeutic transference, which, if successful, catalyzes the development of the therapeutic alliance with ensuing restructuring of the patient's endopsychic representations ('healthy object-relations unit'). The resultant depressive working through enables the patient to achieve developmental stage 4, typified by a sense of personal separateness and wholeness." His succinct statement, however, does not make clear to what extent he is also in full agreement with Masterson and, therefore, in potential disagreement with some aspects of my approach.

Masterson (1972, 1976, 1978) proposes a psychotherapeutic approach specifically geared to the resolution of the "abandonment depression," and the correction and repair of the ego defects that accompany the narcissistic oral fixation of these patients by encouraging growth through the stages of separation-individuation to autonomy. He recommends that psychotherapy with borderline patients start out as supportive and suggests that intensive reconstructive, psychoanalytically oriented psychotherapy is usually an expansion and outgrowth of supportive psychotherapy. He stresses the importance of the analysis of primitive transferences, and has expanded on the description of two mutually split-off part-object-relations units (the rewarding or libidinal part-object-relations unit and the withdrawing or aggressive part-object-relations unit), thus combining an object relations viewpoint of intrapsychic structure, following my findings, with a developmental model based upon Mahler's work.

In that Masterson stresses the importance of analyzing primitive transference and the need to interpretively resolve the split-off internalized object relations of borderline patients, his approach is quite close to mine. However, what Masterson describes as the early supportive stage of the treatment seems to imply a combination of supportive and interpretive techniques that I have found questionable in the treatment of borderline patients. Supportive and interpretive techniques tend to cancel each other out, and, in contrast to the possibility of combining them in patients with less severe illness, I think that the cleavage between the two approaches should be sharp and definite in the treatment of patients with borderline conditions. (I deal with the reasons for this conclusion in Chapter 10.)

In addition, I disagree with what I consider the relative simplification of primitive transferences in Masterson's two-part object relations units. I think one sees a wider range—both more fragmented and more integrated—of self- and object representations in borderline patients, and that primitive transferences have a more complicated nature than is implied in his clinical analyses. Also, in Masterson's almost exclusive emphasis, from the beginning of treatment, on interpreting primitive transferences in light of the vicissitudes of the developmental stage of separation-individuation, he conveys the impression that he neglects oedipal implications of the material, particularly the typical condensation of preoedipal and oedipal conflicts that one finds in borderline conditions—and that one could also assume to be present from his published clinical material. In short, I think Masterson may not be doing full justice to the complexity and subtlety of Mahler's theoretical and clinical approach.

Regarding similarities and differences in the application of Mahler's and my conceptions to standard psychoanalytic technique, the only person I am aware of, so far, who has systematically applied Mahler's approach to the standard psychoanalytic technique is Kramer (1979). Richards (1978), examining Kramer's (1979) and my presentations (see Chapter 9) in a panel discussion, succinctly commented on both theoretical and technical agreements and disagreements of our views, and, given my basic agreement with his analysis, I can do no better than quote the pertinent passages.

> I think what both Mahler and Kernberg are implying is that their theoretical conceptions represent a special point of view which is readily integrated within the psychoanalytic theoretical framework that includes the tripartite model; that it is an extension and an elaboration from the angle of dyadic relationships rather than a new clinical theory or a new metapsychological point of view. I think both Drs. Kramer and Kernberg would disagree with the theoretical pluralists who talk about different psychoanalytic models, viewed either hierarchically or in parallel, which are suitable for different kinds of psychopathology and have consequence for and result in sharply distinctive psychoanalytic and psychotherapeutic techniques.
>
> Given, then, their basic agreement about theory, it is not surprising that Drs. Kramer and Kernberg agree on technique. They hold similiar views about the relationship between preoedipal and oedipal conflicts and about the importance of preverbal communication.
>
> Finally, they agree that ego defect or ego deficiency does not preclude conflict or require us to abandon an analytic stance.

Richards correctly stresses these areas of major agreement. He also points to a possible area of disagreement between Kramer and myself, namely, the relationship in the analytic situation between transference, genetic history, and early development. As I shall be elaborating on later (in Chapter 9), I believe that in cases of severe psychopathology or when severe regression occurs in the transference, the road from current transference developments to the genetic or intrapsychic history of organization of the material is more indirect than in better-functioning patients; and the earlier the points of fixation or regression of the psychopathology, the greater is the gap between actual childhood experiences, the intrapsychic elaboration and structuring of such experiences, and the nature of transference developments. Under these conditions, paradoxically, early childhood experiences can be reconstructed only in advanced stages of the treatment; hence, the danger of equating primitive transferences with "early" object relations in a mechanical, direct way, and the misleading temptation to "reconstruct" the earliest intrapsychic development on the basis of primitive transference manifestations.

I would therefore probably be much more cautious than Kramer in attempting to reconstruct psychopathology derived from separation-individuation phases, and in subphase reconstruction. Kramer conveys the impression that she thinks our knowledge about early phases of separation-individuation can be directly applied from the early stages of analysis on, in contrast to my emphasis on the gradual activation and clarification of these early phases in the context of transference regression. With this proviso, I would agree fully with Kramer in that the nonverbal communication of the patient (including changes of affect and mood, bodily states, anal or genital sensations, flushing, headaches, transient pain, dizziness, desires to urinate or defecate, to suck, to smoke, to keep the eyes open or closed, to struggle against remaining on the couch or in the office or against leaving the analytic session) may reflect preoedipal material expressed in the personal interaction with rather than in the verbal communication to the analyst.

Kramer, quoting Mahler, points out that the residues of preverbal and preoedipal conflicts may emerge in the nonverbal communicative processes of patient and analyst and that they can be diagnosed by the analyst's empathic understanding of the total interactional process at that point. My observations on regression in the communicative process in the analytic situation (see Chapter 9) underline the importance of differentiating true regression to stages of development that predate object constancy from fantasies about such regressive states or experiences. True regression to such early stages is usually accompanied by formal regression in the transference, which permits the analyst to differentiate these two kinds of situations.

In conclusion, I consider my theoretical formulations stemming from the application of an object relations framework to the structural analysis of patients with borderline personality organization, and the implications of this framework for psychoanalytic and psychotherapeutic technique, to be basically in harmony with Mahler's object relations approach, her developmental formulations, and their potential applications to the diagnostic evaluation and technical approach to regressive transferences. Mahler's fundamental contributions to the understanding of infantile and early childhood development and their relationship to structure formation and psychopathology have probably helped more than any other psychoanalyst's work in closing the gap between the formulation of theories of normal and pathological early development derived from adult psychopathology and psychoanalytic exploration, and actual psychoanalytically derived observation and exploration of the child's early development of intrapsychic experience and structure formation.

Part Two

APPLICATIONS TO PATHOLOGY AND TREATMENT

Chapter Seven

Normal Narcissism in Middle Age

Because psychoanalytic studies of normal tasks and crises of adulthood are surprisingly scarce, it seems advisable to preface a discussion of pathological narcissism in middle age with a description of
normal narcissism in that age group.

A few studies on the vicissitudes of internalized object relations in
mid-life and with aging have opened the field for further exploration. In this connection, the work of Erikson (1959), Melanie Klein
(1963), and Jaques (1970) are particularly relevant. Erikson (1959,
p. 98) describes the issue of "integrity versus despair and disgust" as
a basic life task in mature age. He refers to integrity as ". . . the
acceptance of one's own . . . life cycle and of the people who have
become significant to it as something that had to be and that, by
necessity, permitted of no substitutions. It thus means a new . . .
love of one's parents, free of the wish that they should have been different, and an acceptance of the fact that one's life is one's own
responsibility. . . ."

Clinically, Erikson goes on,

the lack or loss of this accrued ego integration is signified by
despair and an often unconscious fear of death: the one and only

121

life cycle is not accepted as the ultimate of life. Despair expresses the feeling that the time is short, too short for the attempt to start another life and to try out alternate roads to integrity. Such a despair is often hidden behind a show of disgust, a misanthropy, or a chronic contemptuous displeasure with particular institutions and particular people—a disgust and a displeasure which . . . only signify the individual's contempt of himself.

Melanie Klein (1963, pp. 16–17) stresses the successful resolution of excessive envy and rivalry as a precondition for normal adjustment to adulthood and old age: "When envy and rivalry are not too great, it becomes possible to enjoy vicariously the pleasures of others. In childhood the hostility and rivalry of the Oedipus complex are counteracted by the capacity to enjoy vicariously the happiness of the parents. In adult life, parents can share the pleasure of childhood and avoid interfering with them because they are capable of identifying with their children. They become able to watch without envy their children growing up."

And she adds (p. 113), "A child, who, in spite of some envy and jealousy, can identify himself with the pleasure of gratifications of members of his family circle, will be able to do so in relation to other people in late life. In old age he will then be able to reverse the early situation and identify himself with satisfactions of youth. This is only possible if there is gratitude for past pleasures without too much resentment because they are no longer available."

She concludes this chapter and the book—one of her final contributions—with a pessimistic statement: "In conclusion I wish to restate my hypothesis that although loneliness can be diminished or increased by external influences, it can never be completely eliminated, because the urge towards integration, as well as the pain experienced in the process of integration, spring from internal sources which remain powerful throughout life."

Jaques (1970), in a paper strongly influenced by Melanie Klein's theories, suggests that the recognition in mid-life—which he places approximately in the middle and late thirties—of eventual death, of the existence within oneself of hate and destructive impulses is inevitable. He suggests that the recognition of death and human destructiveness brings about a depressive reaction in the course of which the "depressive position" must be worked through once again, with an increasing consolidation of the capacity for love while accepting the unavoidable fusion of love and aggression as part of human nature. ". . . The misery and despair of suffering and chaos unconsciously brought about by oneself are encountered and must be surmounted for life to be endured and for creativity to continue. . . . The successful outcome of mature creative work lies thus in constructive resignation both to the imperfections of men and to shortcomings in one's own work. It is this constructive resignation that then imparts security to life and work" (p. 45).

Jaques focuses on the unconscious meaning of death—death as persecution by dead objects and as the loss of good internal and external objects and concludes that in mid-life, the establishment of a satisfactory adjustment to the conscious contemplation of one's own death depends upon the capacity to integrate love and hate, to mitigate destruction by tenderness, and to resolve the reactivation of the depressive position by reparation and sublimation. What is now needed, Jaques suggests, is to "begin to mourn our own eventual death. . . . Such a working-through is possible if the primal object is sufficiently well established in its own right and neither excessively idealized nor devalued" (p. 61).

Others who have described developmental tasks for the middle years include Cath (1962), Levin (1965), Lidz (1968), Vaillant (1977), and Levinson (1978). K. R. Eissler (1975b) has focused on shifting cathexes of narcissistic investment, and on their effects on the structural conflicts and equilibrium between ego, superego, and external reality. He describes how an increased narcissistic cathexis of the superego and the ego ideal may develop, with the consequent dangers of rigidity, compulsiveness, intolerance, and involutional depression; or a narcissistic overcathexis of the ego may lead to an increased expectation of admiration and self-affirmation. In other instances, the accretion of narcissistic cathexis may be distributed over the entire personality. Eissler suggests that aging decreases the demands of passionate drives so that it may result in a lessening of the tendency toward conflict. Under these circumstances, superego and ego are also less separated and there is less tension between these two agencies.

In attempting to spell out, in the light of what others have found and my own clinical experience, some key life tasks in middle age, I have found Erikson's perspective on the life cycle particularly helpful. While I think Erikson underestimates the importance of infancy and early childhood in identity formation and overemphasizes the importance of adolescence, his efforts to integrate a psychoanalytic and psychosocial perspective provide a useful frame, which I will attempt to develop further. I think one cannot be too rigid in defining "middle age." I am focusing on the years from the late thirties to the early sixties. Perhaps "middle adulthood" would be a more appropriate term; but it would also be less familiar.

LIFE TASKS IN MIDDLE AGE

Shift in Time Perspective

Normally, in early introjections and identifications, there is an internalization of reciprocal roles of self- and object representations. Many of the identifications the child makes remain relatively dormant or inactive until a future time when objective reality reactivates them; only then can some past identifications be fully experienced. Young adulthood and middle age normally create many opportunities for relationships in reality that replicate past relationships with inverted roles, typically that of middle-aged parents with their young and adolescent children. When repressive barriers are not excessive, the affect-laden memories of the relations with one's own parents become part of the relations with one's children, and past and present begin to merge more strongly than was previously possible. The middle-aged person not only remembers clearly, but also begins to understand more about his past as the present replays it with roles inverted. The increasing understanding of the past also increases the understanding of one's own, now aging, parents and reinforces the awareness of the future — and the passage of time. The growing insight about what one's parents were in the past facilitates a stronger identification with them, including their present roles as persons experiencing and coming to terms with old age. This process, naturally, extends to other young and old people who represent, respectively, one's past self- and parental images, and provides new role models for coming to terms with the difficult integration of past and future. Thus, the activation of reciprocal roles stemming from internalized object relations of the past brings about an increasing awareness of and coming to terms with identifications reflecting the entire life span.

The new perspective implied in exploring the past interactions with — and the internal life of — an older generation on the part of the middle-aged person extends to past relations with grandparents. It has been said that grandchildren and grandparents get along well with each other because they have a common enemy. The usually limited contact between grandparents and grandchildren fosters their idealizing of one another, simultaneously with the displacement — or splitting — of hostility toward the generation separating them. A child's oedipal ambivalence may be defended against by fear and hatred of the father coupled with idealization and longing for the grandfather. Such normal or neurotic idealization of the grandparents — and of aging parents — fosters normal adaptation to the aging process. A child's loving relations toward his grandparents and his identification with the giving grandparents may constitute a basis for the later capacity to accept his own parents' aging without excessive guilt, and for an easier transition toward the normal reversal of roles in old age when parents may have to depend at least to some extent on their children. Normal overcoming of oedipal guilt is, of course, an extremely important factor in accepting the role reversal with one's own aging parents without excessive anxiety over what unconsciously may also represent the triumph over the oedipal rival.

Normally, a renewed preoccupation with one's past childhood and adolescence and with one's future adaptation to old age expresses the growing awareness of the total life cycle, and also prepares the middle-aged person for dealing with old age.

Reversal in External and Internal Rates of Change

Under ordinary circumstances, throughout childhood and adolescence, the rate of subjective intrapsychic change and of bodily changes reflecting growth and maturation by far exceeds that of the interpersonal environment and the inanimate world. It is as if the child's parents and relatives, his home and neighborhood remain relatively stable, while he himself experiences a sequence of seemingly unending metamorphoses. Particularly in the shift from childhood to adolescence and from adolescence to adulthood, the impressive difference between massive changes within the youngster and the relative stability of his parents' generation is in sharp contrast to the reversal of this situation when the middle-aged see their children grow rapidly and leave home and their parents' generation age rapidly and disappear. Even the stability of the inanimate world now seems threatened: the cities one knows from the past change, neighborhoods change, and these external changes may symbolize and reinforce all mourning processes regarding loss and separation.

The awareness of the ephemerality of human life becomes a very concrete and powerful force which increases mourning processes — and growth connected with them — and fosters an orientation to both the past that is gone and the future that now seems nearer.

The Limits of Creativity

Each of us has our own timetable for establishing a home, for being ready to marry and have children, for learning and carrying on a profession. A mathematician's most creative contribution may come when he is in his twenties, a surgeon's in his forties, and a good many artists' and philosophers' when they are in their sixties or even later. For most people, however, a time comes sooner or later, and usually during middle life, when they perceive with clarity the limits of their past and especially of what they can accomplish in the future, and they have to learn to accept themselves within such limits. Here again, one must come to accept that other people's achievements will at some point surpass one's own.

The acceptance of these limitations implies the mastering of oedipal tasks—overcoming oedipal rivalries—and preoedipal tasks—overcoming preoedipal envy. And, as Jaques has pointed out, the tolerance of the limits of one's creativity also tests the sense of inner conviction that love is stronger than hate in one's relations with oneself and with significant others. Normal resolution of this painful learning process increases the capacity to identify with what others create, to experience enjoyment and gratitude rather than jealousy, shame, and envy.

Ego Identity in the Perspective of Time

Middle age adds a new dimension to the consolidation of ego identity, which starts in infancy and childhood and normally is reconfirmed in the identity crises of adolescence. In middle age, one should be able to come to terms with the limits to change derived from one's character, one's personality structure, and with the related repetitive cycles of activation of one's internalized object relations, which are enacted, again and again, as a limited repertoire of "personal myths."

The resolution of pathological oedipal fixations does not eliminate the oedipal organization of life experience. The personal unconscious myth concerning the oedipal situation and the still earlier vicissitudes of dyadic object relations continue to contribute to the habitual behavior patterns that express in action what ordinary daydreams express in fantasy, namely, the particular way to recreate, again and again, a cycle of personal experiences that provides meaning and continuity, but also reactivates old conflicts and a renewed search for their resolution. To accept oneself within such limits is an important aspect of emotional maturity that is in contrast to narcissistic rationalization, to denial, to resignation and cynicism, and to masochistic self-blame.

The new knowledge about the limitations in one's personality functioning derives from the experience throughout time of repetitive cycles of significant reactivated object relations. It represents a consolidation of ego identity beyond that of adolescence, which still suffered from serious restrictions of time boundaries. Ego identity now not only delimits one's own personality from all others and integrates further self-perceptions with social confirmation, it also integrates the knowledge of what one will not be able to do or to be; and it also includes a painful and yet illuminating awareness of where one's creativity should or could lead next — and yet will not. Paradoxically though, self-acceptance now also means to accept the adventurous part of living, knowing that the road one takes has its dangers and limits, and yet accepting that this is one's destiny. The task of middle age is to reconcile one's knowledge of one's future derived from knowledge about one's past, with the acceptance of risk.

Knowledge about the limits — as well as the temptations to break beyond those limits — stemming from one's personality have particular relevance to the middle-age task of consolidating a stable sexual relation, whether in marriage or not, and such stability implies the capacity for intimacy, the tolerance of conflict, and maintained mystery in the love relation. To accept the inherent conflicts in love and marriage and to contain them in a stable object relation is perhaps the major task of middle life.

Coming to Terms with External Aggression

The "average expectable environment" includes aggression, sadism, corruption, and envy, especially as part of the group processes in organizational and institutional life in which most adult work functions are carried out. Apart from those few who manage to live in ivory towers, we are constantly confronted with the full impact of narrow-mindedness, prejudice, envy, bias, and other forms of more or less rationalized aggression that we have to deny within ourselves.

The task is to face these attacks realistically, and rather than exploit them sadistically, to stand up to them without denial, masochistic submission, or blind rebelliousness, or, indeed, to be corrupted by them. Ego identity in middle age includes abiding by the ideals first consolidated in adolescence and now put to a definite test. To accept the fact that an individual's final responsibility is to himself is one more task of middle age.

Loss, Mourning, and Death

The increasing awareness of passing time in middle age is accentuated by the accumulation of losses of parents, siblings, relatives, and friends from childhood. The manifestations of aging that affect physical effectiveness, well-being, and appearance reinforce the awareness and acceptance of the possibility of physical illness and death at any time as a real personal fate. The capacity to realistically face these issues in middle age without denial or pathological anxiety is strengthened by normal narcissistic development. Gradually throughout adult life, the pleasure in self-fulfillment and creativity becomes fused with the pleasure of giving and dedicating oneself to those one loves and to the ideals for which one stands. Normal narcissism and normal object relations tend to go hand in hand (Kernberg, 1975, Chapters 8 and 9), and, although self-interests may sometimes clash with one's relations to significant others, normally, life goals integrate these two polarities of existence, so that the mourning processes over personal loss and failure include sadness over the loss, distancing from, or letting down those one loved, together with the sense of loneliness stemming from objective impoverishment and from deeper sources of guilt connected with all loss. In contrast, the unconscious sense that one's creativity has contributed to the strength and permanence of the "good" internalized object relations and that one has fulfilled one's duties toward those one loves, permits a diminution in the anxiety over one's own death and the related unconscious concern and guilt about the survival of the inner world and external loved objects. The sense of accepting what one has accomplished, with all its limitations, helps in accepting death as a final statement of "mission accomplished."

Intimately connected with this issue is the realistic capacity "to start all over again." The potential for accepting real shattering loss and failure with a sense of sufficient inner resources to be able to continue accepting oneself and trusting one's capacity to reconstitute a meaningful life is a key test of the normal accomplishment of the tasks of middle age. Many individuals are fortunate in not having to pass this test, but serious failure in work or social life, in marriage, or in relation to close friends or one's own children, are examples of real challenges and the consequent question to oneself whether, indeed, starting from rock bottom is possible. The rehabilitation of patients with severe, crippling physical illness or severe emotional illness hinges on this question; first, there is the issue of facing reality without denial, and then, whether coming to terms with this reality can be done without despair: here, we come back to Erikson's definition of the basic life task in maturity as the issue of integrity versus despair and disgust.

Oedipal Conflicts

By now, it is a common observation that the Oedipus complex, after its repression in the context of the integration and consolidation of the superego, reemerges again in puberty and adolescence together with the powerful reactivation of sexual and aggressive drives and a partial redissolution and reorganization of the superego. Clinical experience also points to the reactivation of the oedipal complex at later stages of life. Apart from the consistent reactivation of oedipal currents in social and group life, the concrete experiences of adults, when their own children are at the height of their infantile oedipal strivings, and again when their children are adolescents, activate unconscious oedipal conflicts and defensive constellations.

When children in late adolescence consolidate their autonomy and leave home, new facets of the oedipal constellation are activated for both parents and children. The new generation, with new social structures, values, and power, challenges the fantasies and reality of the previous generation's social values, structures, and power. Yesterday's "revolutionary" parent discovers himself, by an unanticipated shift in his immediate family constellation, today's defender of authority and potentially "reactionary." The creation of new meanings to life, in the context of the discovery of the roads that link eroticism, tenderness, sexual excitement, and rebellion has passed on to a new generation.

When, in addition, the young adult son can carry out the same functions as his father but with more vigor and persistence, external reality seems to have recreated even further the intrapsychic reality of the struggle between the generations. Oedipal wishes reemerge as impulses toward incest and filicide. As Devereux (1953) has pointed out, we strangely tend to neglect that the Oedipus legend starts out with Laius' efforts to kill Oedipus, a theme that, as Abadi (1960) suggested, is a universal myth, which perhaps most strikingly confronts us in God's order to Abraham to kill his son Isaac. In fact, Rascovsky (1973) argues that it is easy to find evidence for culturally sanctioned filicidal impulses and behavior. The tyranny of the old over the young in organizational life is well known, and the initiation rites of adolescence speak to the oedipal conflicts and fantasies of the older generation as well. As Herodotus said, in peace time sons bury their fathers, while in war fathers bury their sons. The hatred against the new naturally coincides with the hatred against the young.

The normal resolution of both aggressive and sexual strivings of the older generation vis-à-vis their children derives from the normal integration of love and hate under the dominance of love. A normal task of adulthood is the achievement of the function of the "generous parent" (Braunschweig and Fain, 1971), the mature parents whose love for their children and respect for their autonomy blend with the mourning process for the loss of their own parental functions of power and control and with accepting the transfer of authority and of centrality, in social and cultural terms, of sex and power to a younger generation.

The normal reactivation and renewed resolution of oedipal conflicts in middle age involves numerous psychological tasks. To begin, there is a blending of normal self-assertion, competitiveness, and independence in creative work, with the acceptance of the limitations of one's influence on the triumph and persistence of values and ideas. The physical and spiritual products of work eventually transcend and outlast their individual creators, and to accept one's contribution to a shared generational goal with a willingness to concede one's control or power over it is another way of stating this task. In contrast, the desperate need to cling to power and control reflects the pathological ascendence of unresolved oedipal (in addition to narcissistic) conflicts.

In addition, the consolidation of personal autonomy and independence from group pressures, and the increasing reliance of the middle-aged parental couple on their newly emerging, separation from the extended family reflect the achievement of the task of stabilizing their own love relation and protecting it from the invasive challenge of group processes around them. The middle-aged couple may become freer than ever before from their previous dependence on social structures and conventional values. At the same time, the parental couple, freed from the entanglements in reality of inter-generational conflicts, may recreate in their own dyadic structure the world of their own parents, whose death in reality is a universal challenge of middle age.

In *Mourning and Melancholia* (1917), Freud pointed to the resolution of the process of mourning by means of identification with the lost object; the gradual, painful working through of this loss in all areas culminates in such an identification. The analysis of middle-aged patients often reveals that even under normal circumstances the process of mourning for their parents is not a self-limited period, and that the extension over years of pathological mourning has its counterpart in the extension, as a life task, of normal mourning processes. Such subtle but extended periods of mourning for the real loss of the parents may represent a final, normal integration of oedipal conflicts into the personality.

I am referring here particularly to the mourning for the world of the parents which constitutes the background, in the child's memories, of his specific interactions with them: the parents' habits, memories, and traditions, the fantasies that their daily life and inter-actions evoked in the child. As long as parents are alive, they are still the depositories of that personal history, those fantasies and memories. It seems to me that it is only the death of both parents (partic-ularly in the absence of an extended family of their generation) that transforms radically an external reality into an internal one.

I am using the term *internal* in the sense of the intrapsychic relation with the object world, an inner life of fantasied relations with one's parents that persist hand in hand with identifications with them. This is a special instance of our present understanding that identificatory processes do not replace object relations, but, nor-mally, consolidate them both internally and in external reality.

Goethe (1807) implied that we all die twice: first with our own death, and second with the death of all those who loved us and remembered us. Keeping alive the world of our parents is a deep and gratifying personal need and sensed responsibility, an intrapsychic task that can only be shared in limited ways outside the intimacy of the marital couple, one's children, very close friends — and psychoanalysis. This awareness of and sense of responsibility for the past is also painful, a pain that does not decrease with the passage of time, but rather increases with the growing awareness of the limited nature of one's own life span and the receding nature of the past — the aging of photographs and gravestones.

This mourning, like mourning processes in general, requires an unconscious working through of the ambivalence toward the parents, a renewed overcoming of the Oedipus complex. This mourning process typically contains elements of guilt on a preconscious level (frequently, not having appreciated enough, or not having responded enough to the love of the parents) and, at a deeper level, guilt over aggression toward them mixed with sexual strivings and ambivalence toward both parents; it blends incestual and aggressive strivings with sublimated love and longing.

The repeated work of recreating and consolidating the world of one's parents also increases the tolerance for the ambivalence of and toward one's children, and the freedom for maintaining, increasing, and deepening the interest in their now independently growing world. The sense of security derived from the strong internal reality of a world of the past diminishes envy of the young and the fear of direct or projected aggression in competitiveness with them.

Here, object relatedness and normal narcissism blend in ways which make it difficult to separate the one from the other and to separate oedipal from preoedipal constellations. This growing internal world is a new source of creativity. The wish and capacity to share one's own past with a younger generation stems, not from unconscious envy of what is new, but from a sense of responsibility and love for what has been valuable before; it is presented to the young as a gift, not an imposition. By the same token, this internal world of the past linked with mourning for the parents diminishes the envy of the young, the envy of horizons that the now older generations may envision but will not be able to reach.

The reinstatement of the parents as object representations, and of their world as an internal object world reflects the love toward them and a persistent object investment in them and what they stand for. This process has to be differentiated from and is parallel to the internalization of the demanding and prohibitive aspect of the parental images into the superego. Parricide and filicide are the constant temptations and dangers of unresolved oedipal conflicts, but not their destiny: awareness of these temptations and dangers, and their resolution as part of the normal process of mourning throughout adulthood (or in the course of psychoanalysis) seem to me to reflect more broadly the range of alternatives open in the working through of the Oedipus complex.

Patients with pathological narcissism have enormous difficulties in achieving this normal task. Frequently, the death of their parents when the patients are in middle age leaves a void, a further dimming of their own past, an increased sense of internal abandonment, and an intensification of narcissistic defenses.

Chapter Eight

Pathological Narcissism in Middle Age

Let us now examine the nature of the processes operating in narcissistic personalities that worsen narcissistic pathology in middle age. In summary of my previous work in this area (1975), normal narcissistic gratification not only increases self-regard or self-esteem, but—because it is intimately linked to satisfactory relations with others—also strengthens the investments of others with love, appreciation, and gratitude. These investments, in turn, strengthen the representations of these objects, and a good and strong world of internalized object representations offers enrichment and support to the self. Thus, narcissistic gratification from external sources is augmented by secondary narcissistic gratification from internal sources. In addition, insofar as normal narcissistic gratification goes hand in hand with satisfactory, pleasurable, and successful investments in work and daily activities, in creativity and value systems, there is also an internal build-up of a nonpersonal world of nature and things, of internal values and communications with them reflected both in the ego's—or rather the self's—harmonious relation with the ego-ideal aspects of the superego, and with conscious ideals and goals. The enjoyment of and gratitude for "things in themselves" as they are—because they exist rather than belong to one—contributes to self-enjoyment.

All these processes fail to a major extent in the case of pathological narcissism. Here, the identity diffusion characteristic of borderline personality organization has been compensated for by the crystallization of a pathological grandiose self at the cost of further deterioration of internalized object relations by massive processes of devaluation of objects and object representations, and by projective mechanisms that displace devalued part self- and object representations upon the external world (Kernberg, 1975). The pathological grandiose self does not charge the battery, so to speak, of internal object representations and internalized value systems. What is received from the outside, particularly admiration, reconfirms the narcissistic gratification of the grandiose self. Admiration is "extracted" with an unconscious greed that empties the source of pleasure and gratification, which, once emptied, is left valueless. This extraction also fuels the tendency to depreciate and devalue others, particularly those who have been emptied, who now seem mediocre, inferior, or useless — basically, external objects onto whom dissociated or repressed devalued object representations and devalued self-representations are now projected. The devaluation protects the patient against envy, but at the price of a pervasive subjective sense of emptiness. And so the grandiose self, lacking internalized object representations and value systems, feeds on itself within a vacuum. The result is that there is no protective reserve available of libidinal investment in others and in their object representations for times of loss, failure, or crisis: the enjoyment of daily life, of what is constantly or repeatedly available, suffers.

Success, applause, and admiration, once received, are absorbed and yet, strangely enough, soon become "spoiled." The patient's relentless greed, his avid and yet destructive incorporation of what he envies, the consequent deterioration of his object representations, his wanting things because they are not his rather than because of their intrinsic value, all increase endless greed while impoverishing and destroying what he receives. This affects the narcissistic patient's relationship to his past and to the future. He longs for a new narcissistic "refueling," but discovers that lasting satisfaction is never to be found; consequently, he restlessly hopes for and yet fears the future. Also, paradoxically, past success or satisfactions are a double threat: insofar as they raised expectations, they create the potential threat that the future will not live up to the past and that narcissistic aspirations, therefore, will be shattered. And, insofar as the patient has experienced past satisfactions as centering around the self (to the exclusion of satisfactory investment of others and of values), he has available no past experiences with others and of the external world as something meaningful which has been lived and enjoyed, which he can carry within himself and reinvest in present and future relations with others and in values. Typically, patients may remember themselves in past interactions, but only vaguely the other people involved, their struggles and their feelings. The narcissistic patient has no gratitude for what he has received in the past, experiences the past as lost, wishes he had it now, and is painfully resentful that it is no longer available to him. At bottom, the narcissistic middle-aged patient is painfully envious of himself in the past, having had what he no longer has.

Another complicating factor that reduces the capacity to enjoy what has been received in the past is the lessening of the temporary idealization of what is greedily wanted and not yet available, the acquisition of wealth and expensive objects, for example, or the avid exploration of new places to visit, and, above all, the excitement of new sexual conquests and affairs. Insofar as temporary idealizations of all these previously unavailable and wanted objects made their acquisition a feast of narcissistic gratification, they provided a source of renewable pleasure. But, insofar as the narcissistic components of those gratifications rapidly wore off (as the devaluation and spoiling of "conquered" sexual objects, for example, brought about disappointment, boredom, and the need to escape into new relations) such temporary idealizations eventually languish. The narcissistic person learns from experience that the "exciting new" is one more edition of the "disappointing old"; and he misses what is really new in any relationship because of his serious limitations in grasping the depth and uniqueness of human beings.

Unconscious aggression and rage over past frustrations, linked to greediness and envy, is the source of the destruction of what was first desperately needed, later greedily incorporated, and finally devalued. The patient may end up disgusted with his own past hopes and expectations. Misanthropic generalizations of such dashed hopes may be rationalized as a pessimistic philosophy of the "vanity" of all pursuits for gratification.

Viewed in terms of a broad period of time, then, the grandiose self always has been, and remains, alone and in a strangely atemporal world of repeating cycles of wants, temporary idealizations, greedy incorporation, and disappearance of supplies by spoiling, disappointing, and devaluation.

The overall effect of these mechanisms on the aging process is a gradual deterioration of the narcissistic patient's internal past. It is as if he lived in an eternal present; the passage of time and aging represent an external situation that overcomes him in a bewildering way, without the normal sensitive awareness and preparation for the changes that occur with time. This may quite often be reflected in a particular "youthfulness" in middle-aged narcissistic patients, as if literally, time had not touched them. The normal idealization of the future, characteristic of youth, is exaggerated in the narcissistic personality, for whom the future represents exalted narcissistic gratifications in the area of physical attractiveness, power, wealth, prestige, success, and admiration. When external reality gradually demonstrates to him that these fantasies are no longer viable, when aging reduces the function of idealization of the future, a vicious circle is established.

The narcissistic devaluation of the past is compounded by the painful awareness that the narcissistic gratifications of youth and past triumphs are no longer available, and, in order to avoid painful envy of his own past, the narcissistic patient is forced to devalue even his own past achievements and accomplishments. The narcissistic patient is "eternally young" not only in the sense of not being psychologically prepared to acknowledge the passage of time but also in his lack of accumulation of an internal life that provides sustenance and compensation for later loss and failure. This lack of emotional wealth is compounded by the need to escape from feelings of regret and guilt over lost opportunities in the realm of interpersonal relations, particularly over lost opportunities to accept, enjoy, and reciprocate love and gratitude. The question "where has life gone?" is common even in normal people, but the feelings that prompt it are painfully maximized in narcissistic patients.

The middle-aged patient with narcissistic pathology has particular difficulties in facing the growing independence of his adolescent children. To empathize with this growing world of adolescence while feeling subtly and increasingly excluded from it requires maturity and empathy with others, which compensate for the natural sense of loss and mourning, overcoming or neutralizing the universal feelings of envy. The longing for the past, the regret over the passage of time, and the subtle feelings of guilt for what was missed in the past, all normal accompaniments of the separation from adolescent children, are particularly difficult for narcissistic patients, given the limitations in what they were able to give to and receive from their children. Realistic appraisal of failure in their past relations with their adolescent children combines with guilt over their present envious attitude toward them; or the incapacity to tolerate guilt feelings activates devaluation processes and hatred of their growing children — defenses against and expressions of such envy. Above all, these parents miss the sheer enjoyment of their children's growth and independent development.

One patient in analysis, a businessman in his early fifties with two adolescent daughters, saw his older daughter as arrogant, selfish, and ruthless, and he loathed these qualities in her. He idealized his younger daughter who in many ways represented his own idealized version of himself. During the treatment it became evident that the distrust of his older daughter was related to his projection onto her of the envious and exploitative aspects of himself he could not tolerate and which resulted from his identification with the horrible image he had of his mother. His younger daughter represented a split-off image of an idealized, perfect, mother. As the treatment progressed and he gradually became aware of his internal conflicts about his older daughter and began to appreciate and to love her, he grew increasingly anxious at the prospect of losing the relation with her now that she was about to leave home and go to college. He felt she was abandoning him, but on a deeper level he was struggling with the anxiety produced by strong feelings of guilt and regret for having missed opportunities in the past for developing a good relation with her. The old temptation to devalue her, to withdraw from her, and "forget her altogether" tempted him, but at the same time now seemed an impoverishment to him. To attempt to "start all over again," at the last moment seemed a more human and hopeful situation in spite of the pain involved; but it meant facing his guilt and the incapacity to fully repair whatever damage he felt had been done to their past relationship.

DEFENSIVE DEVELOPMENTS

Denial

One type of reinforcement of pathological narcissistic character traits in response to aging centers around the mechanism of denial: Typically, patients employing this defense show an increase or reinforcement of behavior patterns that provided narcissistic gratifications in the past but no longer do so. The exaggerated, artificial, and sometimes almost grotesque pseudo youthfulness of aging narcissistic personalities, some love affairs middle-aged men and women have with adolescent partners, a hypomanic undertaking of activities that would ordinarily diminish or be restricted by the aging process are other examples of such denial.

These patients attempt to deny the process and consequences of aging and to escape from the necessary normal mourning and sublimatory processes connected with it. The most dramatic effect of the denial of aging in narcissistic personalities can be seen in their artificial maintenance of a façade of "adolescent beauty." They may inappropriately persist in doing what brought success and applause in the past and stubbornly refuse to accept the naturally occurring diminution of appreciation by others of their past performances; they repeatedly dwell on what they achieved, who they were, and the like. The gratification derived from financial wealth may now turn into a tendency to hoard and a desperate clinging to possessions and financial power, so they can no longer even enjoy what they have. The clinging to power by old men who are envious of the young is proverbial in institutional psychology, and has narcissistic as well as oedipal implications.

A woman in her middle fifties who dressed and acted as if she were a late adolescent became aware during treatment of how afraid she was that younger women would depreciate her for being old and spent, as she had depreciated older women when she was young and beautiful. But she was even more concerned at losing the sense of triumph over her contemporaries — she had the illusion that she was still the youngest among them and the most attractive — and if she dressed appropriately for her age, other women would triumphantly enjoy the breakdown of her superiority. She could not go back to visit her home town, her family and friends of the distant past, because they all would notice how much she had aged, while they, living together, would be oblivious to their own aging.

The normal acceptance of shortcomings related to aging is reflected in the need to maintain autonomy and independence and yet to accept dependence and external support under conditions of stress or when objectively needed. Above all, to be able to continue one's interest and investment in an area that is no longer under one's control is a crucial consequence of normal — in contrast to pathological — narcissism. The aging person who can still love being in the mountains when he can no longer climb them illustrates this point.

Under optimal circumstances, support from others reinforces self-esteem and fosters further autonomy. In the case of pathological narcissism, however, realistically needed support or dependence induces shame, a sense of failure and humiliation (because of the projection of the superior and depreciatory attitude of the grandiose self onto those on whom the patient needs to depend).

The narcissist's distorted perceptions of the past, the failure in his capacity for empathy with his own parents, and his — projected — fear of depreciation by the young now interfere with growth and maturation, with learning about himself from the young, particularly his children, and with coming to terms with the cyclical nature of human life. The normally growing capacity to project oneself into the future and the related capacity to come to terms with it suffer in consequence.

Under conditions of pathological narcissism, the early idealization of grandparents is frail and unrealistic and can easily break down (as all idealizations do, typically, in the case of narcissistic personalities). Depreciation of the old may become the prevailing feature in the relation, first to grandparents and later to parents and other aging people. The reversal of the situations of infantile dependency—that is, the fact that aging parents increasingly depend on their narcissistic (and now adult) child—may become a triumph for the latter, with narcissistic as well as oedipal features, particularly in a sense of narcissistic triumph and superiority over the now dependent parent. By the same token, however, confrontation on the part of the middle-aged narcissistic patient with his own aging process and his acquisition of the grandparent's role are fraught with dangers: to contemplate having to depend is to be shamefully inferior, to be exploited and depreciated; no gratitude or love, only pity or depreciation can be expected from grandchildren or the young. This increases the dread of aging and of old age and reinforces denial.

In addition, narcissistic pathology, with its general limitations in fully experiencing guilt feelings, reinforces the difficulties of overcoming and working through oedipal guilt. Therefore, aging parents are frightening to these patients; to perceive themselves in the role of such aging, helpless, and dependent parents is in turn a frightening, even uncanny experience that has to be denied and fought against. The fear of loss of bodily functions, unconsciously perceived as an attack from envious, resentful enemies, is an important factor in the development of hypochondriacal concerns in narcissistic patients.

Devaluation of External and Internal Reality

Some patients, confronted with a loss of physical attractiveness, with limitations in their social or political power, with limits in their work, in the advancement in their professional or artistic skills or career—now devalue what no longer offers them new fantasied and real narcissistic gratifications. They defend themselves against intense envy of others who still possess these hopes, capacities, or potential for further advancement (particularly those who are younger) by devaluing them and their work. They also devaluate interests or investments that formerly seemed of great importance to them — because they promised narcissistic gratifications — resulting in a sense of emptiness and loss of meaning in their daily life. Such devaluation may sometimes be rationalized in terms of a pessimistic or misanthropic life philosophy, a pseudo conservatism that is really destructiveness directed at what is new, full of enthusiasm, and hopeful.

A more subtle form of devaluation is a certain sterile eclecticism, wherein all new ideas or findings, new forms of artistic expression or creativity, are devalued by focusing on their limitations with a skepticism that implicitly makes the patient the superior arbiter of the new and questionable.

While these patients may appear less inappropriate than the group who used denial, they are likely to offer more intense and at times even insurmountable resistance to treatment. The devaluation may also be directed against the efforts of those who attempt to help them — who presumably have something new and good to offer and who are therefore envied: Distrust, bitterness, or cynicism regarding any professional help are frequent rationalizations of their devaluation of the therapist.

Devaluation is a significant narcissistic defense reflecting the reaction to the passage of time and to aging, and it may be observed in patients from their middle thirties on. All of what I said earlier about the defensive devaluation of the past and the present applies here. In order to avoid the dreaded fantasied situation of being the devalued object of a projected grandiose self attributed to others, present object relations, particularly dependent ones, have to be denied and devaluated in turn.

A patient with narcissistic personality, an intelligent professional woman in her late forties, presented a combination of denial and devaluation. She worked in the personnel office of a large business firm in charge of evaluating job applications. She had gone through two marriages in which her relentlessly domineering, queenly attitude toward the husbands had led to their leaving her; she could not tolerate the better marriages of her friends, and gradually devaluated them as conventional and empty (in fact, projecting her own sense of emptiness onto them as a defense against envy), and she withdrew into a pseudo counterculture style while feeling lonelier and lonelier. Denial was evident in her convictions that her counter-cultural style reflected an unchanging youthfulness, and her deval-uation of "bourgeois" values gradually extended to most of her former friends and relatives. The patient found herself more and more bored, incapable of empathizing with others, particularly with younger people whom she had to evaluate, and she relied increas-ingly on various drugs to induce an artificial state of emotional awareness to be able to empathize, even if at a rather primitive level, with her friends. She felt her children from both marriages to be a burden, but gradually began to cling to outings with them because she did not know what to do with her time; and she began to fear aging and old age with an almost panicky quality, all of which led to her treatment. Consciously, she experienced emptiness and dread of the future; unconsciously, her distrust, hatred, and depreciation of all those whom she needed — particularly her therapist, had induced a shopping spree from analyst to analyst, premature treatment disruptions, and a maligning of all the therapists she had seen.

The effect of pathological narcissism on the equilibrium of a couple is an important issue in marital conflicts and divorce at middle age. The normal maturation of sexual interests linked to an interest in a total person is in sharp contrast to the gradual divergence of sexual excitement from investment in the person that occurs when there is severe narcissistic pathology. Here, eternally youthful bodies are needed compulsively, regardless of the face, the person, the attitudes with which such bodies relate to the patient. Normally, men and women should be able to fall in love, remain in love, and be sexually excited with persons of the other sex of their own age group; and if anything, a capacity for a lasting sexual relation with a person from a broadening age group of the other sex should develop.

The disillusionment with sexual "freedom," with repeated affairs and various kinds of sexual experimentation, may bring about, in some narcissistic patients, what seems to be an improvement in their sexual life: greater stability of the marriage in some cases, and a questioning of the "swinging" style of life in others. However, an increased marital stability is often accompanied by an obvious or subtle depreciation of the marital partner, a willingness to settle for a "stable" relationship in which the partner is really a servant or a convenient fixture, and where depreciation and resentment are institutionalized in chronic aggressive behavior. Where the partner is willing and able to tolerate such a state of affairs, a relatively comfortable equilibrium may be reached at the cost of mutual distancing, or with the patient's sense of freedom "from having to pretend" or for abusing the other person with impunity. The marital partner's strong masochistic needs, mutual exploitation of narcissistic partners, or other marital psychopathology maintain the stability of the situation.

In other cases, particularly where a conventional marriage was maintained initially, idealized love affairs may disrupt that equilibrium in middle age. Paradoxically, the sexually more inhibited narcissistic character of early adulthood may now initiate the road to sexual promiscuity and various sexual deviations which other narcissistic patients are already abandoning in middle age because of their accumulated experience of dissatisfaction with the search for narcissistic gratification in sexual encounters. Thus, middle-aged narcissistic personalities with a long history of chaotic sexual encounters may be less prone to this kind of acting out during analytic treatment when it is initiated when they are in their late forties or fifties. Their experience of long-standing sexual disappointment and a sobering awareness of their cycles of idealization and devaluation may actually foster emotional introspection and motivation for change.

The dread and hatred of dependency of narcissistic personalities may bring unavoidable conflicts at a time when objective failure forces them to such a dependency on external sources. The envy and hatred of those they have to depend on and whose importance they can no longer deny may bring about a staggering combination of demandingness, suspicion of how what is received from others has been given, devaluation of what they have received, and sadistic attacks on or exploitation of those they need. The incapacity to experience gratitude, the sense of humiliation at needing the other person, and the deeper difficulty of facing the intense guilt over having destroyed potentially good relations with others make for very pathological, even dramatic complications in the narcissistic patient's objective dependency upon his spouse, relatives, or caretaking personnel.

This becomes particularly evident in these patients' inability to really depend on the analyst. Their almost hypomanic denial of any need to depend is replaced by a frightening sense of emptiness and loneliness together with a subtle depreciation and devaluation of what the analyst might give. Because of the conflicts over dreaded dependency, many patients have to first go through a string of relationships with many therapists before coming to terms with the fact that, after all, they need one human being in spite of his "imperfections." While contemptuous behavior, narcissistic rage, and rapid devaluation of whatever is received is characteristic of narcissistic personalities in intensive treatment at all stages of life, these features become particularly dramatic when it becomes obvious to the patient himself that only the therapist stands between him and a life in which narcissistic gratifications are no longer forthcoming.

Depression and Pathological Mourning

The sources of depression in narcissistic personalities faced with the conflicts of aging are several; first, there is the direct manifestation of mourning over loss of narcissistically invested functions, often with a sense of impotent rage, shame, and humiliation — and fantasied triumph, contempt, and depreciation on the part of others. This is a manifestation of failure of denial. Depression may also reflect the painful awareness of aloneness, of lack of human warmth and relatedness when devaluating processes have emptied the world of people and of values. In addition, depression may be caused by the regret and guilt over what the patient gradually recognizes as his own participation in the problems he experiences as a consequence of pathological narcissism. The patient may regret among opportunities lost that of giving to and receiving from others, and his neglect of his healthier and more valuable potentialities in the pursuit of narcissistic gratification.

A patient in his late forties divorced his wife because he could no longer sustain the image of a triumphant hero admired by a frail woman, which had constituted the main compensating mechanism against intense unconscious envy and feelings of inferiority toward his wife. He divorced her and established relationships with other women with whom he felt he could reestablish the lost narcissistic gratifications. The patient finally became aware of how much he had really come to appreciate and love his wife's qualities, and the sense-lessness, the self-destructive nature of his separation from a woman who had been essentially loyal, dedicated, and in love with him. He now developed a severe depression which initiated a lengthy treat-ment in which the initial goal of recovering his lost wife — which was no longer possible — could be replaced by an effort to make the best of his life as it was and to consolidate his relation with another woman whom he could accept in her own right.

Depression in narcissistic personalities tends to appear with grow-ing frequency and intensity in middle age. Although these patients give evidence of much more suffering and often a greater loss of social functioning, than either of the two groups mentioned before (patients presenting denial and/or devaluation), they are also more accessible to treatment. Depressed narcissistic patients may be more able to accept psychoanalytic treatment that acknowledges their realistic motives for depression and loss of self-esteem, but also holds out the hope for opening up new emotional resources as part and consequence of the reexamination of their narcissistic personality structure. One complicated issue in advanced stages of psycho-analytic treatment of these patients is their potential for suicidal thoughts and behavior. Mourning and guilt may prove intolerable, and suicide a solution that condenses, in an illusory way, the expia-tion of guilt and the protection of the sense of a core goodness by kill-ing what is "bad" inside. The therapist needs to explore with the patient the two directions into which depression may evolve: self-awareness and growth, or despair and suicide.

Other Symptoms, Defenses, and Developments

While denial, devaluation, and depression might be described as a continuum of defensive operations increasingly important in narcis-sistic personalities in middle age, other types of compromise forma-tions can also be seen, usually reflecting more complex secondary developments in these patients. First, hypochondriacal reactions and compensatory health fads and rituals may be expressing fear related to the breakdown of the denial of the aging process, a projection of dissociated aggressively invested object representations onto the body and body functioning, and a defensive withdrawal from external reality. Efforts to omnipotently control the body functions, and a regressive replacement of control over external objects by such control and fears connected with it are other frequent mechanisms involved.

Second, some narcissistic personalities find a protective idealization of a value system — a religious belief or cult — compensation for the frightening devaluation of their previous interests and for narcissistic failure and loss in middle age. One patient became interested in the occult and combined a sense of mystical oneness with the universe with an elitist ideology regarding the few selected ones able to grasp the occult. Some narcissistic personalities may actually find a new sense of humility and selflessness in their identification with an ideal embracing all of humanity; one sometimes finds a love for all human beings curiously combined with a depreciation of the patient's immediate social environment. Rarely, cases where severe aggression infiltrates the pathological grandiose self may gravitate toward a more malignant idealization of a sadistic and paranoid belief, ideology, or cult, and develop rationalized antisocial behavior precisely at a time when other patients with antisocial personality features seem to "burn out" their antisocial behavior.

Third, some patients may find a niche for themselves in some subordinate function or capacity, surrounding themselves with people they — consciously or unconsciously — consider inferior, and thus maintain the fiction (or the reality) of the great man wandering unknown among the ordinary people. A broad variety of situations may evolve, from very adaptive dedication to a group or ideal to a devastating waste of the patient's potential in a self-defeating life situation. One patient, for example, a brilliant specialist, worked in a poverty-stricken area where his leadership was of great human value (although his special skills went unused). Another patient never managed to get his degree as a lawyer, unconsciously rebelling against the "insult" of having to submit himself to tests and examinations. He worked in a subordinate capacity in a business firm, acting like an impoverished but proud, mysteriously suffering aristocrat. With regard to treatment, the extent to which a patient has actually ruined important opportunities in his life may become crucial in evaluating whether his denial should be challenged.

Fourth, some patients with polymorphous perverse sexual traits may elect, at least for a short time, a homosexual relation — in contrast to previously maintained highly turbulent heterosexual ones; unconsciously, the homosexual relationship may protect them against loneliness and a dreaded emptiness; because in their fantasy the relation is unreal, it does not threaten their self-esteem. More generally, "deviant" lifestyles as camouflage or an escape against self-awareness may have parallels in chronic alcoholism or drug addiction as "self-erasing" mechanisms.

Finally, some middle-aged narcissistic personalities may "settle down" in a relatively routine, strangely flat, and nondescript social life; a "burning out" seems to have occurred, a self-effacing and anesthetizing abandonment of their previous aspirations and grandiosity. This comes more easily to patients without significant intellectual, artistic, or cultural backgrounds, whereas patients having a rich intellectual and cultural background may suffer from severe depressions when treatment confronts them with their neglect or abandonment of their lost self-interests. To eliminate self-awareness is one way out of the consequences of narcissistic frustration or failure. All the developments mentioned here illustrate how poorly narcissistic personalities really love themselves (Van der Waals, 1965).

TREATMENT CONSIDERATIONS

It is my growing conviction that the prognosis for psychoanalytic treatment of some narcissistic patients may be better when they are in their late forties or fifties than when they are younger. Their gradual learning from experience, the decrease of narcissistic gratifications, and, above all, the impact of the deteriorating quality of narcissistic defenses may increase both self-awareness and motivation for treatment.

The chief question we have to ask ourselves, and eventually discuss with our patients, is to what extent it is possible to clarify and confront a patient with severe narcissistic character pathology which has remained untouched for so many years. To what extent can a narcissistic lifestyle be changed in middle age? The problem is sometimes made easier by the obviously inappropriate, self-defeating, and potentially dangerous manifestations of severe denial or devaluation or chronic depression.

Patients suffering from depression with elements of regret, concern, and guilt, with remorse for time and opportunities wasted, have a much better prognosis than those who react with the more primitive feeling of empty rage and a sense of defeat mixed with attributing blame to others. The former, despite their serious character pathology, have been able to learn from experience, and their depression reflects authentic concern for themselves and for those they have been able to love notwithstanding their own limitations. In other words, some patients are able to "jump over their shadow," to become aware over the years how they spoil or destroy their own enjoyment of life and their relations with those who are most important to them. I am stressing here the significant qualitative differences in the experience of depression in middle-aged narcissistic patients.

In all cases, a key question is also whether the middle-aged narcissistic patient really has something better to look forward to than his present psychological equilibrium and life situation. Certain criteria favor the indication of psychoanalysis or psychoanalytic psychotherapy: (1) the possibility of clarifying and confronting the patient with the specific manifestations of denial of narcissistic failure or loss without development of paranoid reactions toward the diagnostician, and a clinical predominance of depressive over paranoid reactions in the early transference; (2) the patient's capacity to understand how his tendency to devalue what he does not have and envies (on a conscious level) contributes to the impoverishment of his present life (patients who are spontaneously concerned over the consequences of their loss of interest in, of enthusiasm or respect for others may hereby reflect an important capacity for introspection); (3) the patient's capacity for advanced or higher level depressive reactions, with elements of concern, guilt, and wishes to repair damage done, in contrast to primitive depression characterized by paranoid, blame-distributing features; in more general terms, whether aggression is more externalized (paranoid trends) than internalized (depression) is prognostically relevant; (4) the prognostic criteria I have stressed in previous work (1975, Chapter 4): the patient's capacity to invest in people and value systems beyond his own narcissistic needs, which includes the quality of object relations, the degree of superego integration, and the patient's capacity for sublimation.

One crucial underlying feature of these prognostic criteria is the patient's propensity for paranoid reactions when the narcissistic equilibrium is disturbed. It is impressive how frequently minor paranoid distortions may never be resolved fully in the analytic process, but silently accumulate over a period of months or years and finally emerge as what amounts to an almost delusional massive projection onto the analyst of a primitive persecutory maternal image. In addition to its intrinsic dynamic meanings, such a projection may serve multiple functions: to protect the idealized quality of the pathological grandiose self; to rationalize disappointment reactions, devaluation of the analyst, and acting out in general; to prepare the road, so to speak, for a premature abandonment of the treatment (as an expression of the need to "expropriate" the therapist's knowledge, to frustrate his satisfaction over the patient's improvement, and to reassert the patient's self-sufficiency). I would say that an early evaluation of this paranoid potential is supraordinate to the other criteria I have described.

In contrast to this paranoid potential, the patient's genuine capacity for mourning, his genuine regret for the consequences of his narcissistic illness are prognostically favorable. In older patients, those in their late forties or early fifties, a "healing process" may set in, in which depression and mourning combine with developing gratitude for what they are receiving from life in spite of their "badness." For example, the love from a marital partner previously depreciated and now acknowledged may evoke gratitude and relief. The permanence of beauty in nature, of values in religion, ideas, science, or art (for those patients with the capacity to appreciate them) may also initiate a reassurance against the fantasied devastating effects of their aggression.

Narcissistic patients who consult in their late forties or fifties often have already undergone various psychotherapeutic experiences, and the careful and detailed evaluation of such past experiences may clarify their distortions — above all, devaluations in their perceptions of their previous therapist. Of course the analyst has to reserve his judgment regarding what happened objectively in the past, but the rapid oscillations of idealization and devaluation, or typical splitting operations involving previous therapists are often striking. The advantage in treating such patients is that past treatment failures may facilitate the initial evaluation and permit "preventive interpretation" of acting-out potential which may disrupt the treatment; but these patients' "sophistication" regarding psychoanalysis may obscure subtle resistances, including the acting out of envious "stealing" of the analyst's knowledge. The patient may unconsciously want treatment to learn about one more approach, one more "gimmick" he has not yet tried, patiently waiting to incorporate it and then drop the therapist (for one more try — or many others — with someone else).

A particular difficulty is presented by patients who report having benefited from other treatment before, but then of interrupting treatment, having "reached a limit of how far one can go" with the previous analyst. These patients often present a specific difficulty in acknowledging gratitude and in depending on the analyst as a real good object. They have to extract, unconsciously, what he has to give, and to escape before what they receive from him is "contaminated" by dissociated and projected rage; at other times, the experience of having "emptied out" the previous therapist expresses their unconscious convictions that the therapeutic relationship, as all others in their life, is between an exploiter and an exploited.

The patient's lack of emotional relatedness to the analyst may be masked by an eager alertness to any of the analyst's comments, which gives the impression that the patient is dependently seeking nurturing in each session. It is only when this eagerness is interpreted and the patient expresses his frustration at having to associate "without getting anything in return" that the devaluation of the analytic process and the fantasies of being exploited by the analyst unless the patient "extracts" something from him — a typical underlying narcissistic resistance — may become apparent.

The analyst's honest tolerance of the possibility of failure and his communication to the patient from very early on that the treatment may indeed fail and that it is hard to predict how this particular association of patient and analyst will turn out may be very important in protecting the analyst from developing excessive paranoid or guilt-ridden feelings when treating patients with narcissistic pathology.

The analyst's conviction that the middle-aged patient still has the time, the opportunity, the potential for substantially changing his life by resolving his pathological character structure will help him to help the patient in the difficult process of coming to terms with his present and past life. I suspect that the analyst's attitude to his own conflicts about aging, his trust in the possibility of facing and resolving such conflicts in himself, has something to do with how far he will dare to go with his patient.

Chapter Nine

Object Relations Theory
and Psychoanalytic Technique

Object relations theory has added enormously to the understanding and treatment of patients with severe regression in the transference; it also has other applications for psychoanalytic technique, many of which have long been integrated with that technique.

Within an object relations framework, unconscious intrapsychic conflicts always involve self- and object representations, or rather, conflicts between certain units of self- and object representations under the impact of a determined drive derivative (clinically, a certain affect disposition) and other, contradictory or opposing, units of self- and object representations and their respective affect dispositions reflecting the defensive structure. Unconscious intrapsychic conflicts are never simple conflicts between impulse and defense; rather, the drive derivative finds expression through a certain primitive object relation (a certain unit of self- and object representation); and the defense, too, is reflected by a certain internalized object relation. The conflict is between these intrapsychic structures. Thus, all character defenses really reflect the activation of a defensive constellation of self- and object representations directed against an opposite and dreaded, repressed self- and object constellation. For example, a man who is excessively submissive may be operating under the influence of a unit

consisting of a self-image submitting happily to a powerful and protective parental (object) image. But this set of representations is
defending him against a repressed self-image rebelling angrily
against a sadistic and castrating parental image.

While, therefore, the consolidation of the ego, superego, and id
results in an integration of internalized object relations which
obscures the constituent units within these structures, in the course
of psychoanalysis one observes in the transference the gradual
redissolution of pathogenic superego and ego structures, and the
activation of the constituent internalized object relations in the
transference. In this regard, Glover's (1955) classical formulation of
the transference as reflecting an impulse and an identification may
easily be translated into the transference as always reflecting an
object relation under the impact of a certain drive derivative.

In other words, the unconscious intrapsychic conflicts that are
producing neurotic symptoms and pathological character traits are
always dynamically structured, that is, they are rooted in a relatively permanent intrapsychic organization consisting of contradictory or conflicting internalized object relations. At severe levels of
psychopathology, where psychoanalysis is usually contraindicated
(certain types of severe character pathology and borderline conditions), dissociative mechanisms stabilize such dynamic structures
within an ego-id matrix and permit the contradictory aspects of these
conflicts to remain — at least partially — in consciousness.

On the other hand, with patients presenting less severe character
pathology and psychoneurosis, the dynamically structured intrapsychic conflicts are repressed and truly unconscious. They are
intersystemic conflicts between ego, superego, and id and their
advanced, high-level or "neurotic" defense mechanisms. Here, in the
course of the psychoanalytic process, the development of a regressive
transference neurosis will gradually activate in the transference the
constituent units of internalized object relations that form part of ego
and superego structures, and of the repressed units of internalized
object relations that have become part of the id. At first, rather
global expressions of ego and superego functions make their appearance, such as guilt feelings about unacceptable impulses, or broadly
rationalized ego-syntonic character traits. Eventually, however, the

transference is expressed more and more directly by means of a certain object relation which is used defensively against an opposing one reflecting the repressed drive derivatives. In the case of both defense- and impulse-determined object relations, the patient may reenact the self-representation of the unit while projecting the object representation onto the analyst, or, at other times, he may project his self-representation onto the analyst while identifying with the object representation of the unit. (These shifts are illustrated in the clinical example below.)

Because in the ordinary psychoanalytic case these transitory identifications emerge in the context of a well-integrated tripartite structure and a consolidated ego identity so that the patient has a clear concept of himself and significant others—including the psychoanalyst—the patient is able to maintain a certain distance from, or perspective on, this momentary activation of a certain distortion of self- and object representation without necessarily losing the capacity for reality testing in the transference. This capacity permits the analyst to deal with the regressive transference neurosis from a position of technical neutrality, by interpretive means; and it permits the patient to deal with interpretations introspectively, searching for further self-understanding in the light of the analyst's interpretive comments. In spite of temporary weakening of reality testing during affect storms and transference acting out, this interpretive quality of the psychoanalytic process is one of its outstanding specific features.

The analyst, while empathizing by means of a transitory or trial identification with the patient's experience of himself and his object representations, also explores empathically the object relation that is currently dominant in the interactional or nonverbal aspects of the transference, and, in this context, the nature of the self- or object representation that the patient is projecting onto him. The analyst's subjective experience at that point may include either a transitory identification with the patient's self-experience—as is the case in concordant identification—or with the patient's currently dissociated or projected self- or object representation—as is the case in complementary identification (where the analyst, rather than identifying with the patient's self or ego, identifies with his object representation, dissociated self-representation, or superego [Racker, 1968]).

Throughout this process, the analyst first transforms his empathic understanding into intuitive formulations; he later ventures into a more restrictive formulation that incorporates a general understanding in the light of all available information (Beres and Arlow, 1974). The empathy with, the intuitive understanding, and the integrative formulation of the patient's affect states during this process clarify the nature of the drive derivative activated and defended against in the object relation predominating in the transference.

The theory of technique just described takes into consideration the structural characteristics, defensive operations, object relations, and transference developments of patients who are fixated at or have regressed to a structural organization that antedates the integration of the intrapsychic structures, as well as of patients whose tripartite structure has been consolidated. I am suggesting that this theory of psychoanalytic technique facilitates the application of a nonmodified psychoanalytic technique to some patients with severe psychopathology, clarifies certain modifications of the standard psychoanalytic technique for cases where psychoanalysis is contraindicated for individual reasons, and, most importantly, implies a reconfirmation of standard psychoanalytic technique for the patient with solid integration of the tripartite structure. I shall now attempt to illustrate this approach by means of a clinical vignette from a standard psychoanalytic treatment.

CLINICAL EXAMPLE

The patient, a mid-western professional in a field of the behavioral sciences, came for treatment in his middle forties because of chronic marital conflicts, severe work inhibition — particularly in the creative aspect of his research functions — and occasional sexual impotence with his wife. He was potent with prostitutes, and at the time of the episode to be described, in the second year of his psychoanalysis, sadistic sexual behavior with prostitutes had become a major form of acting out. The patient's father had been a prominent politician whom the patient both feared and depreciated. His mother was a rather submissive, but complaining and guilt-evoking woman who seemed totally controlled by a powerful husband and escaped from his demands and dissatisfactions by means of chronic hypochondriacal complaints.

We had already explored the patient's submissive behavior toward his wife, his chronic fear of displeasing her, and we understood the revengeful enactment of sadistic behavior against other women as a displaced expression of his hatred toward her. Only beginning to emerge was that, on a deeper level, his sexual relations with prostitutes represented a dissociated identification with his sadistic father with whom he did not dare identify out of profound oedipal guilt.

For several months it had become apparent that the patient was presenting me with his "shameful" and self-defeating submission to his wife. For example, because of the strict regulations he felt she imposed upon him (regarding her hours of going to bed, feeding their animals, and her requests for silence in the home which interfered with his research work), his work inhibitions were allegedly further increased, for which he implicitly blamed me. He also contrasted my efforts to help him gain understanding without giving him advice with the more active encouragement and sympathy he had obtained, he said, from his previous therapist. In fact, I gradually learned that he had seduced his previous therapist into giving him advice on how to handle his wife, and eventually "proved" that therapist to be totally impotent in really influencing his marital difficulties.

The patient was also constantly examining my interpretations in the light of what he had learned in his professional training about psychoanalysis. He often reacted to my interpretations with an amused, ironical expression, implying that I could do better than that, or that I was not in my best form in giving that interpretation, or that I should pay more attention to him than to my theories. The "spoiling" and devaluation of my interpretations, his efforts to "learn" what I had to teach him and to use it in his work without really absorbing my comments, gave the sessions a strong quality of narcissistic resistance. However, he showed a capacity for differentiating in depth his concepts both of himself and of the significant people in his life, which reconfirmed for me that he was not a narcissistic personality proper. (This case illustrates the presence of narcissistic resistances in an essentially neurotic character structure.) My overall hypothesis at the time was that the patient was attempting to maintain me at a devalued, impotent level in order to avoid developing a frightening image of me as a brutal, overpowering father.

For several sessions preceding the one to be described, I had experienced a sense of impotence, an incapacity to know how I could convey to him an understanding that would be useful to him. This insecurity on my part was matched by the patient's shift from his previous attitude of ironic superiority (which he had in the past attributed to other men he experienced as rivals in his work) to a complaining, nagging protest over not getting any better, the uselessness of this treatment, the enormous sacrifices he had to make, and my failure to offer any "original contributions" to what he knew about himself.

When, one day, I felt myself in a role similar to the role he described himself in vis-à-vis his nagging wife, I verbalized my sense that he was repeating in this session his relation with his wife with inverted roles. The patient now became tense and remembered that I had pointed out to him in the past that he had been attracted by masculine features in his wife. He said he felt I was accusing him of identifying with his wife and implicitly telling him that he was a homosexual.

His associations then shifted to his wife's rage with him because once, when he attempted to penetrate her orally, she had felt brutally attacked and now, years later, still accused him of having behaved sadistically toward her. He then thought of prostitutes he had engaged to participate masochistically in sexual games in which he "playfully" acted like a sadist and had fantasies about giving such prostitutes enemas. He next remembered his mother and father jointly holding him while giving him enemas in his childhood.

Throughout these associations, I sensed an increasing fearfulness in him, and when I pointed this out to him, he remembered that I had blown my nose forcefully in the previous session, and that this seemed something "brutally uninhibited" to him. He then thought that I wouldn't take all that abuse from his wife if I were married to her, and also imagined me standing up to his boss very effectively, in fact, intimidating him, in contrast to the patient's always trying to play the nice boy. At this moment, I also experienced a sudden sense of intellectual clarity and power, quite in contrast to the helpless insecurity that I had experienced earlier. I felt that I now represented his powerful and brutal father forcing him into homosexual submission, and that he was engaged in a pathetic effort to identify with me in his sadistic role with prostitutes, while leaving—in his fantasy—his wife and his work to me.

I proceeded to interpret the patient's image of me as a powerful man, strong, ruthless, and brutal with women—as he had perceived his father—and I raised the question whether his fear of my branding him as a homosexual might reflect his fear of his masculinity's being destroyed if he dared to compete with me, as father, in his behavior toward his wife and toward his boss. I later added that his intense search for sadomasochistic relations with prostitutes in recent weeks might serve the purpose of reassuring him against his fear of me and his temptation to submit to me (father). After some silence, the patient said that it was very painful to think that because of his neurotic behavior he had lost valuable opportunities for advancement in his research work. He added, with a kind of shudder, that he had never before thought that the reason he had no child with his wife was because he had never dared to stand up to her unrealistic excuses for not wanting to have a child, and now it was probably too late.

It was now my turn to be shocked; although I had all along had the evidence that his not having had a child reflected the neurotic character of his marriage, I had never before been able to formulate this hypothesis—his not daring to have a child out of oedipal guilt and fear—precisely in my mind: presumably, I think, because of the intensity of his denial, and his secondary rationalizations of this problem in earlier stages of his analysis. My emotional reaction now became one of concern and strong positive feeling for the patient: I felt that, almost unwittingly, I had helped him to gain an understanding of a painful reality which indeed—given his present circumstances—probably reflected a missed opportunity. I said it must be very painful for him to review the past joint decision with his wife not to have a child in light of this new understanding, and the patient acknowledged his sense of my having understood him. There followed a long silence, in which I experienced a strong current of empathy for him.

I have tried through this case to illustrate the rapid shifts in my empathy and transitory identification from, first, with a projected self-representation of the patient (the helpless little boy masochistically submitting to a nagging mother) while the patient identified with the object representations of mother-wife; then my empathy with his powerful and "brutal" father while the patient became his fearful and insecure self; and finally, my empathy with the patient's central self-experience. The first two identifications enacted in the transference were clearly of the complementary type, the last one concordant.

From a broader perspective, the patient was expressing in the transference his characterological defenses of superiority and irony against directly experiencing fear of and submission to a powerful, castrating father image. He then experienced this fear more directly, and also became more aware of the related masochistic submission to his wife, of his not daring to compete with father.

I have elsewhere (1976a) spelled out modifications of psycho-analytic technique for patients with borderline personality organization; I shall now spell out some applications of this reformulation from the standpoint of object relations theory for the standard psycho-analytic technique. It must be stressed that, with this reformulation of aspects of the theory of psychoanalytic technique, the basic technique itself does not change, but, by an expansion of its application, is enriched in daily practice. What follows is not an exhaustive list of applications, but rather refers to frequent clinical situations for which the aforementioned ego psychological theory of object relations and the related theory of technique seem to me particularly useful.

APPLICATIONS TO CLINICAL INTERVENTIONS

The Nature of the Conflicts to Be Interpreted

The earlier the development of psychopathology, the more seriously it affects, not only the development of ego and superego structures (which in the treatment is reflected in a premature activation of the constituent internalized object relations that ordinarily are integrated within more global ego and superego functions in early stages of a psychoanalysis), but also the capacity for entering a normal oedipal situation. Under these conditions, preoedipal conflicts, particularly conflicts around preoedipal aggression, infiltrate all object relations. In addition to reinforcing and fixating primitive defensive operations centering around splitting, excessive aggression also contaminates the later object relations characteristic of the Oedipus complex.

This creates characteristic distortions in the oedipal constellation, reflected in the following frequent findings: Excessive splitting of the preoedipal maternal image may be complicated later on by a defensive devaluation, fear, and hatred of the oedipal mother and an unstable idealization of the oedipal father which easily breaks down and is replaced by further splitting of father's image. This reinforces oedipal rivalry in men and penis envy in women, excessive fear and guilt over sexuality in both sexes, and the search for desexualized and idealized relationships, which influence the development of homosexuality having its roots in a preoedipally distorted oedipal phase in both sexes. A predominance of sadistic and masochistic components in genital strivings are other consequences of this situation. Under these circumstances, the differentiation of parental images along sexual lines, typical for triadic oedipal relationships, may be complicated by splitting mechanisms which make one sex good and the other bad, or by pathological fusion of the respectively idealized or threatening aspects of both sexes, so that unrealistic combined father/mother images develop: the "phallic mother" is only one example of these developments.

I am stressing that consequences of severe preoedipal conflicts include pathological development of oedipal conflicts but not an absence of them. I believe that the controversy regarding the predominance of oedipal versus preoedipal conflicts in regressive conditions, or when early ego distortion or lack of development of the definite tripartite structure exists, really obscures some of the significant issues. Not even in nonanalyzable borderline conditions or in cases with severe pathology of object relations, such as the narcissistic personality, have I ever been able to find a patient without evidence of crucial oedipal pathology: the question is not presence or absence of oedipal conflicts, but the degree to which preoedipal features have distorted the oedipal constellation and have left important imprints on character formation (Blum, 1977). It is only at advanced stages of resolution of severe psychopathologies stemming from the preoedipal period when one may indeed find a "clearing up" of the condensed oedipal-preoedipal transference. In this clearing up, the early dyadic relationships with the preoedipal mother are reactivated in relatively undistorted ways, and conflicts between search for closeness and even merger and the need for autonomy (or differentiation) appear relatively directly in the transference. In contrast, in the advanced stages of psychoanalytic treatment of narcissistic personalities, when the pathological grandiose self has been systematically analyzed, the full-fledged oedipal conflicts typically predominate—with varying degrees of preoedipal condensation—as the core underlying conflicts.

Transference, Genetic History, and Early Development

Oedipal conflicts condensed with pathological preoedipal object relations contribute to creating highly unrealistic transference developments. The prevalence of partial, nonintegrated self- and object representations when early ego defenses predominate also contributes to creating unrealistic transference developments. Therefore, the earlier the points of fixation or regression of the psychopathology, the greater is the gap between actual childhood experiences, the intrapsychic elaboration of such experiences, the structuring of these intrapsychic elaborations, and the nature of transference developments.

Although in all patients the predominant transference paradigm may be conceived as a "personal myth" which condenses conflicts from various stages of development, when total object relations and intersystemic conflicts in the transference prevail, the genetic link between the nature of the transference and the antecedent childhood experiences is more direct, more readily available, and makes it possible to offer reconstructions earlier than in cases of severe psychopathology or when severe regression occurs in the transference. In these latter cases, the road from current transference developments to the genetic or intrapsychic history of organization of the material is more indirect, and, paradoxically, early childhood experiences can be reconstructed only in advanced stages of the treatment. Hence, the dangers of mechanically equating primitive transferences with "early" object-relations, and "reconstructing" the earliest intrapsychic development on the basis of primitive transference manifestations.

It is important to differentiate patients who have not reached object constancy, where the syndrome of identity diffusion and the preponderance of primitive defense mechanisms indicate the presence of borderline personality organization, from patients with stable ego identity and, therefore, the prerequisites for object constancy, total object relations, and the capacity for maintaining reality testing in the transference even under conditions of severe regression. In these latter cases, when primitive transferences are activated in advanced stages of the treatment, an interpretive stance and technical neutrality can be maintained while utilizing the understanding that object relations theory provides as one way to resolve these primitive transferences by means of interpretation.

In many neurotic patients and in patients with nonborderline character pathology, regressions to primitive transferences do occur in the analysis. Because of the intense affective developments, the temporary weakening of reality testing, the projective tendencies, and the chaotic interactions that develop at such times, the analyst is sometimes tempted to move away from a technically neutral and strictly interpretive attitude. Such moves are often rationalized by the assumption that the patient has reached a stage of "ego deficit" or "fragility of the self" or "maturational arrest." In fact, what occurs at such points of regression is that the patient has regressed from some stage of his infantile (yet integrated) self relating to an infantile (yet integrated) parental object to a stage that predates object constancy. Now, both the self- and object representations activated in the transference are partial and represent dissociated or split-off aspects of an integrated object relation which the patient experiences as intolerable because of the intense ambivalence or contradiction between love and hate involved. Hence, the analysis of intrapsychic conflict in terms of defense and impulse is no longer facilitated by the organizing features of intersystemic conflict. Rather, it is that contradictory ego states — or ego-id states — constitute the polarities of the conflict: both sides include primitive impulse derivatives imbedded in a primitive unit of internalized object relation. Under these circumstances, defense and content can rapidly be interchanged in shifting equilibria of such activated part-object relations, and contradictory impulses are conscious and mutually dissociated or split off rather than unconscious — that is, repressed. Here, the nature of consciousness and unconsciousness no longer coincides with what is on the surface and what is deep, what is defense and what is content. The extensive clinical example at the end of this chapter illustrates these developments.

The analysis, at such stages, of the nature of the immediate object relation in the transference and the defensive operations connected with its dissociation from other, contradictory, object relations helps the analyst to clarify the meaning of the transference, the defensive aspects of the object relation activated, its motivation in protecting the patient against a contradictory or opposite object relation, and the implicit conflict between primitive ego structures. In metapsychological terms, while the topographic approach to interpretation (the ordering of the material from surface to depth) no longer holds, the economic, dynamic, and structural aspects of interpretation as spelled out by Fenichel (1941) are still fully relevant. If, at this point, the analyst first interprets the part-object relation activated and its affect state, and later, its defensive function against other, contradictory, parallel or previously conscious affect states linked to other part-object relations, dramatic change and new understanding may be gained while the patient's reality testing returns to normal. This interpretative approach, however, requires that the analyst first ascertain whether the patient is still able to maintain some degree of self-observation and reality testing in the transference. Otherwise, it is crucially important to start out by clarifying the reality aspects of the psychoanalytic situation, then to focus upon the patient's "interpretation" of the analyst's interpretative comments, and, if this is not sufficient to restore the patient's analytic work, the analyst may have to apply the general approach recommended for cases in which there is a regression in the communicative function (see below).

The more the transference developments present the characteristics of activation of part-object relations, predominance of primitive defensive operations, and condensation of preoedipal and oedipal conflicts, the more it is indicated to interpret the transference in an "as if" that is, nongenetic mode. For example, I interpreted a patient's chronic frustrations with me at a certain advanced stage of her treatment as a search for a warm and giving, endlessly patient, and understanding father with strong maternal features, "as if" she were reliving a time in which she would have wished to have a father with breasts and a penis from which milk would flow endlessly. This interpretation stemmed from many dreams, masturbatory fantasies, and complex interactions in the transference, and I did not "place it historically" because of the reasons mentioned before. Such an "as if" qualification to genetic reconstructions permits the analyst to sort out the initially condensed, mixed, compressed material stemming from various stages of development, and to gradually crystallize, on the basis of this primitive transference pattern, a sequence of early and later stages of development as issues within the same transference constellation.

For example, a patient's urgent demands that I listen to her with unwavering attention, accept her ongoing sharp criticism of me without arguing with her, and not say anything unless specifically asked seemed to reflect at one point an effort to control me sadistically and yet to feel reassured that I continued to love her, to be close to me and yet avoid my overwhelming her with my thoughts — all of which seemed to relate to a derivative constellation of the rapprochement crisis. However, this same transference disposition seemed to reflect, at a later stage of her treatment, a suspicion that all that was coming from me was bad, like poisoned food she should not ingest, while she still felt that I was the only source of potential satisfaction, of any kind of good; so she pleaded with me to give her good and not poisoned food. I interpreted all this as relating to a still earlier period of oral dependence, projection of aggression, and consequent fears of being poisoned by a malevolent, though desperately needed, feeding mother. I must point out that the actual reconstruction of developments from the patient's second to fifth year of life followed much later, so that the sequence of my interpretive comments reflected a layering — or the internal structure — of her "personal myth" and not yet a hypothesis regarding the actual sequence of developments that had taken place in her past.

It is important to differentiate actual regression to modes of functioning that predate object constancy from patients' fantasies about such regression. Patients might, for example, have fantasies about "merger" with the analyst. These fantasies may have many meanings and do not by themselves indicate that regression to a symbiotic or early stage of differentiation of self has taken place. Such merger fantasies may express regressively wishes for total dependence; or efforts to escape from guilt feelings by blurring the responsibility of, respectively, patient and analyst; or, quite frequently, regressive forms of expression of sexual impulses. Actual regression to subphases of separation-individuation or even symbiosis occurs rarely in the analyses of well-selected (in the sense of their suitability for analysis) patients, requires a long time to develop, and, above all, is reflected in significant regressive changes in the total therapeutic interaction, in the patient's nonverbal as well as verbal behavior, and in a regressive increase in his responses to the total psychoanalytic setting — more of this later. Psychoanalytic fashions may artificially increase a "language of regression," partially induced by inappropriate introduction of the analyst's theories into the interpretive comments.

Regression in the Communicative Process

Patients with well-integrated tripartite structures are usually able to communicate verbally to the analyst their internal world, their subjective experience in the broadest sense. Naturally, under the effect of repression and other defense mechanisms, such communication is restricted in certain areas. However, by means of ordinary empathic listening and transitory identification with the patient, the analyst is able to construct in his own mind a picture of the patient's experience, his personality, and his interactions with significant others. In addition, of course, the analyst utilizes his direct observations of the patient's nonverbal communications, his attitudes and attire, all the behavioral elements that provide a key counterpart to the verbal communication and the subjective world it opens. It might seem trivial to repeat this well-known aspect of the psychoanalytic process were it not that the patient's very awareness and communication of his subjective world may become blurred, distorted, and mostly inoperative at points of severe regression when part-object relations predominate in the transference.

Under these conditions, the normally subdued influence of the psychoanalytic setting comes into the foreground of the analytic process, and the patient's communication of his subjectivity is replaced by severe distortions in the interactions with the psychoanalyst. I am not referring here to the ordinary acting out of a specific, clearly circumscribed transference reaction in the psychoanalytic situation, but to the more subtle, often uncanny combination of strange or unusual modes of behavior and relationships to the analyst that impress themselves strongly though confusingly upon the analyst's mind, and make it very difficult for him to maintain empathy with the content of the patient's verbal communications. Here, in short, communication occurs by means of the transformation of the patient's relation to the psychoanalytic setting and his expression of the uncanny in the interpersonal field, rather than by the ordinary predominance of shared subjectivity, that is, the patient's communicating his subjective world to the analyst by verbal means.

True regression to stages of development that predate object constancy — in contrast to fantasies about such regressive states or experiences — are usually accompanied by this formal regression in the transference, which permits the analyst to differentiate these two kinds of situations. The analyst will recognize this state of affairs by noting that his interpretations are ineffective, his words no longer seem to count; the patient begins to use language that seems aimed more to provoke or block the analyst's actions than to provide him with information. Also, at this point, dramatic acting out and the communication to the analyst of a general sense of urgency may occur. In addition, the patient may appear more and more oriented to the immediate environment of the analytic situation, the analyst's room and its furniture, the duration of the hour, the analyst's availability and absences, the tone of the analyst's communication, rather than the content of what he is saying. Long periods of silence from the patient that evoke unusual fantasy formations in the analyst, or a sense of paralysis of understanding in the analyst may also develop. The patient's incapacity to listen or interact by means of verbal communication may coincide with a total loss of what appeared previously as a good capacity for introspection or insight. The patient may experience no emotions (thus reflecting, for example, severe splitting or fragmentation of affect, or a subjective sense of total artificiality or emptiness), or intense, overwhelming affects, or a chronic sense of confusion. In some cases somatization or hypochondriacal tendencies come to the fore at this point.

Under these circumstances, the analyst's sense of confusion or paralysis may appear to be a severe countertransference development, but if he explores it over a period of time by means of introspection, it may emerge as a condensation of the analyst's countertransference potential with a stimulation in him of affects reflecting the patient's primitive object relations. The analyst's efforts to maintain emotional contact with his patient at times of regression fosters a special receptivity in the analyst, which lends itself to or fosters the development in him or her of such an emotional response (Kernberg, 1975). Of particular importance here is the projection onto the analyst of split-off aspects of the patient's self, so that, in rapidly alternating reversals of the reciprocal enactment of self- and object representations in the transference, the analyst represents the patient's part-self-representation interacting with the part-object representation enacted by the patient himself, and vice versa in cyclical fashion. In short, the rapid "cycling" of self- and object representations and the unrealistic qualities of these representations and the respective interactions activated in the transference reveal the primitive nature of these part-object relations. Here, the analyst's effort to empathize with the patient's central subjective experience needs to be broadened to include empathy with the aspect of the currently dominant object relation the patient is projecting onto the analyst. In other words, the analyst's empathy has to incorporate the partial aspect of the self as well as the partial aspect of the object representation involved in this interaction, and empathy with mutually contradictory aspects of the patient's intra-psychic life that he himself cannot tolerate or, therefore, integrate.

This is a stressful situation for the psychoanalyst. He may be tempted to respond to the patient's incapacity to verbally communicate his subjectivity by a redoubled effort to interpret the material verbally, thus unwillingly shifting into what might be called an authoritarian use of interpretation as a defense against the difficulty in tolerating such vaguely experienced contradictory material in himself. Or else he may be tempted to abandon the patient emotionally by the thought mentioned before that the patient presents ego defects that no longer have conflictual implications and require modifications of technique.

But if the analyst fully explores his own emotional reactions, sorting out objective reactions to the patient's reality and transference from what might be his countertransference dispositions, he may be able to formulate, to himself first and to the patient later, how the patient is perceiving him and/or attempting to "redesign" him. The immediate meaning of the patient's relation to the analyst under such conditions has to be constructed out of the total emotional situation that now exists in the analysis. At such points, past and present are condensed so fully into one transference situation that it can be temporarily analyzed only in terms of the immediate relation, the "here and now." There are extreme circumstances in which even the stress on reality may have to be temporarily suspended, or at least left open. If the patient, for example, seems too involved in a severe paranoid distortion, perceiving the analyst as a dangerous, hostile, sadistic enemy whom, however, he desperately needs, the analyst needs to acknowledge that this is the current unshakeable vision that the patient has of him, that this conflict between need and suspicion is what the patient is struggling with, and that both patient and analyst have to tolerate the coincidence of very different ways of looking at the reality of this interaction.

Here, two major technical tools may prove very helpful. One is the analyst's effort to integrate cognitively the confusing and contradictory manifestations of the patient's immediate behavior, including his use of language, the nature of the acting out, the contradictory behavioral manifestations in the hours, and the emotional reactions induced in the analyst. This cognitive function temporarily makes the analyst an auxiliary ego to the patient within the preservation of a technically neutral position.

A second helpful attitude is what Winnicott (1958, 1965) has called the "holding" function of the analyst, namely, his ongoing emotional availability to the patient at points of severe regression, which includes at least three aspects: (1) the analyst's respecting the patient's autonomy, his not "impinging" on the patient at such points of vulnerability where the patient's "true self" may emerge; (2) the analyst's "survival" in the face of the patient's aggression, his "ruthlessness" before integration of good and bad self- and object representations has been achieved; and (3) the analyst's empathic availability for the provision of an emotionally supportive environment at points of significant regression.

The analysis of regressive transference developments, particularly when severely paranoid transferences emerge, is always difficult and its outcome uncertain. Although I am suggesting that the application of an object relations focus as described improves the prognosis for a psychoanalytic approach and facilitates the maintenance of a technically neutral attitude, this cautious optimism should not be interpreted as an assurance of success in all cases.

There is a tendency among some analysts working with severely regressed patients to adopt an exclusively intellectual or cognitive stance. Others tend to abandon their efforts at intellectual understanding and stress the purely affective "holding." I think the analyst needs to maintain a balance between the two. He must maintain authentic concern and persisting efforts to cognitively understand the patient, even if verbal communication has to be temporarily adjusted to the limited degree to which the patient can understand and incorporate the analyst's contributions. As mentioned before, the analyst's attitude also needs to incorporate empathy with what the patient cannot tolerate in himself—with the dissociated aspects of self- and object representations. This transcends ordinary empathy with the central subjective experience of another person, and brings us to our next point, the role of empathy.

Empathy and Regression in the Transference

My emphasis on the need for empathy for patients with severe regression or severe psychopathology (including the narcissistic personalities and the borderline conditions) might lead to a misunderstanding. I do not mean that the more severe the patient's ego distortion, the more it becomes necessary to replace a position of technical neutrality (which would permit interpretation of the transference) with the analyst's availability as an empathic, friendly person who permits the patient to internalize him and thus to compensate for an arrested or incomplete early mother/infant dyad.

It seems to me that this quite prevalent misconception stems from a misunderstanding of Loewald's (1960) and Winnicott's (1958, 1965) contributions. Loewald has focused on the therapeutic effects of the patient's internalizing a benign or positive dyadic interaction in the psychoanalytic situation, an interaction that reflects the relation between a mature, understanding, integrating person and an immature, uncertain, dependent one. This internalization strengthens the primal basis for all transferences stemming from a good mother/infant relation, consolidates the self, and permits identification processes to develop which strengthen ego functions.

It needs to be stressed, however, that such interaction and internalization processes imply a relatively normal early development — the achievement of object constancy — and should be considered an important yet unobtrusive mechanism of action of psychoanalysis which constitutes a nonspecific effect of psychoanalytic technique in contrast to the specific effects of interpretations. In a different context, Winnicott's description of the analyst's "holding" function under certain conditions of severe regression in the transference referred to patients in whom, presumably, severely regressive conflicts expressed in intensely ambivalent transferences had been analyzed extensively before this particular regression occurred.

In other words, the analyst's empathy and intuition permit growth to occur in patients with good ego strength (or well-integrated tripartite structure) in the course of a standard psychoanalytic situation, and are also helpful at certain points of severe regression with

patients in whom sufficient working through of regressive transferences has occurred.

To infer that, for patients in regression, it is the therapist's
empathic presence — rather than his interpretation — that is really
helpful, that it is the patient's identification with this mothering
function — rather than his coming to terms with his intrapsychic
conflicts — that is important would be to misunderstand the function
of empathy. An empathic and concerned attitude on the part of the
analyst is a necessary precondition in all cases of psychoanalysis.
And, as mentioned before, at levels of severe regression, the analyst
has to be empathic not only with the patient's central subjective
experience at any particular point, but also with what the patient
cannot tolerate in himself and has to dissociate or project. Empathy
is a prerequisite for interpretive work, not its replacement.

In this connection, the dissociated or repressed material that
patients defend themselves against may be clinically expressed in
any of several ways: (1) it may be repressed and only indirect
manifestations of it are present in the content of the patient's free
associations or in the transference; (2) it may be dissociated in mutually contradictory ego states that are alternatively conscious; (3) it
may be expressed in acting out; and (4) it may be reflected solely in
the nature of the interactional processes in the analysis, in the creation
of an "uncanny" emotional atmosphere which does not, in a strict
sense, belong to the patient's subjective experience and has to be
diagnosed by the analyst's empathic awareness of the total emotional
situation in the analytic hours. This requires a special "analytic
empathy" that transcends ordinary mothering functions and has to be
part of the analyst's capacity to diagnose all these various manifestations of unconscious intrapsychic conflicts in the analytic situation.

CLINICAL EXAMPLE

A history professor in his late thirties had consulted because of
sexual inhibition, lack of interest in sexual relations with his wife,
passivity, and procrastination in his work. He was diagnosed as an
obsessive personality with some infantile features and referred to

psychoanalysis. In the first year of treatment, submission to, fear of, and unconscious rebellion against authority by means of passive resistance were predominant features; in the transference was a fear that the analyst would criticize the patient for sexual fantasies and wishes toward women other than his wife and a pseudo compliance together with a deeper rejection of the analyst's comments as an imposition from what appeared to be an oedipal authority. I must stress that at no time did the patient appear to have borderline features or a narcissistic character structure; to the contrary, he impressed me in the analysis as presenting a rather well-consolidated tripartite structure and ego functioning.

In the second year of analysis it became clearer that severe repressive barriers interfered with his memories of any aspect of his childhood — a bare few were available from before age eight. He had a sense of chronic, almost total distance from both parents. He stressed that he had hardly mourned his mother's death, which had occurred several months before he started analysis, and experienced his father as cold, critical, and nagging.

The repeated interpretation of the patient's surface submission to me and his deeper underlying rejections of my interpretations did not lead to further awareness, but to the emergence of a new symptom: he fell asleep in the session every time I tried to focus on the transference. This symptom expanded to such an extent that even my indirect comments that the patient suspected might relate to the transference immediately elicited sleep, first for a few seconds, then, gradually, over longer stretches of time until he was sleeping during some one-fourth to one-third of his sessions. At the same time, it gradually became clearer that he now experienced me as cold, distant, and nagging, but also shy and withdrawn: all characteristics he had experienced in his father.

It then became possible to distinguish between two very different kinds of sessions. There were sessions in which the patient paid lip service to free association and self-observation but fell asleep easily and repeatedly without any apparent feelings of anxiety or guilt. And there were other sessions during which he seemed very anxious, guilt-ridden because of his sleeping and yet extremely limited in his capacity to free associate. He seemed unable to tolerate in himself the expression of any thought or feeling he considered inappropriate, such as sexual impulses toward women other than his wife or angry thoughts about me. In this seemingly neurotic man, the relatively extreme loss of the ordinary capacity for reasoning and self-observation in both these mental states was startling.

At the same time, while complaining that analysis was not helping him, he not only came punctually, but also checked on whether I was giving him his allotted time. This was a permanent feature of both the sleepy and the guilt-ridden sessions, so that he might be fast asleep toward the end of the session, wake up following a comment of mine indicating that time was up, and, still half asleep, look at his watch as he rose from the couch before leaving. It also became clearer that in both his mental states there was a subtle but permanent opposition to me, a hidden rejection of everything I was saying, linked to chronic suspiciousness of me.

Toward the end of the third year, the patient began to develop rage attacks in his home, treating his children tyrannically, feeling very regretful afterward, and eventually linking these attacks of rage with the sessions in which he slept. My interpretations, which had centered around oedipal conflicts in the first year of his analysis and had focused on the analysis of his behavior in the sessions in terms of the same, primarily oedipal, conflicts during the second year, now shifted to the analysis of the common features of the two apparently contradictory mental states: his desperate need to receive something from me without ever being able to achieve it, his fear and suspicion of me as cold and indifferent but also exploitative and dishonest (my intention to rob him of his time, and the displacement of rage against me onto his own children because of this perception of me).

I interpreted this total situation "as if" he saw me as a cold, indifferent person from whom he wanted very much to receive love and support, but whom, at the same time, he had to control and suspect because I wanted only to extract money and time from him. I left it open what transference object that might be, and the patient spontaneously said that all this had nothing to do with either of his parents because he had never expected anything from his father and his mother was always very giving (although she also required that everybody behave very properly, was disgusted by messiness and disorder, and was afraid that the neighbors spied on them in order to have something to talk about!). I then told the patient that, in the sessions he slept in, he was treating me as if I were his father, and in the sessions he tried desperately to be a good boy, as if I were a harsh mother demanding perfection; I added that he felt there was nothing to hope for from me just as he had felt disappointment from both his parents. I also said that the rage attacks toward his children — he consistently had denied any emotion of anger toward me — was a displacement of rage against me representing both his parents.

The patient then experienced me more clearly as an authority who was trying to trick him: I was pretending to be warm and interested so that he would be forced to talk about his unacceptable sexual impulses and his rage, that is, all his badness, only so I could despise and punish him further by rejecting him, and he was not letting himself be tricked. These understandings were gained in brief intervals of communications during sessions in which he felt very guilty about his sleeping, at not giving thought to what I was saying, at forgetting me completely between the hours, and at depreciating me and my treatment. Now his sleeping during the hours increased even further, and so did his monotonous statements that the treatment was getting nowhere and that all this made no sense at all.

Simultaneously, however, the patient began to talk about his older and younger brother — how much he hated and depreciated the former, who was violent, derogatory, and totally insensitive psychologically. In contrast, his younger brother was friendly, patient, obedient, had always been loving and respectful toward their parents — strikingly different from the patient's own indifferent abandonment of them. I now interpreted the patient's alternate ego states in the hours as his identification with now his older and now his younger brother. I said he was trying to avoid the terrible conflict between feeling that if he were spontaneous and open he would be like his horrible older brother, and I would therefore hate and depreciate him; or, if he were like his younger brother, he would have to renounce any change toward independence and would have to be a good boy who experienced no sexual urges or rage. I also added that he must have experienced a lack of emotional support from his mother to feel that his impulses were so unacceptable. I later connected this with his submission and rebellion toward his father: he did not dare express rebellion toward his father because all emotional expression was forbidden by the combined action of both parents. The fear of father's punishment had combined with mother's rejection of his sexual curiosity to induce total repression of his oedipal urges, and his solution was to remain withdrawn and passively resistant at home. I also reminded him that at age seventeen he had rather abruptly left home and all memories of his past, just as he was leaving me every session without giving me any further thought, or abandoning me in the sessions themselves by means of sleep.

The patient now began to experience me as a very patient, tolerant, understanding mother, and at the same time developed feelings of guilt because of his lack of feelings around the death of his own mother. For the first time, he cried in the session, and expressed gratitude because of what he experienced as my patience with him. He began to understand that the incapacity to integrate his identifications with both his brothers was reflected in a combination of his sense of badness and the fear of rejection and attack from both parents. His emotional attitude toward himself in the hours changed, and he became able again to meaningfully observe and communicate what was going on in him, for the first time developing curiosity about himself and his internal life. I later interpreted his caring for himself as an identification with his caring mother and with me representing her, an identification he had earlier been unable to achieve because of his unconscious guilt toward her.

Gradually, his transference shifted again into a predominantly oedipal level, and toward examining the sexual inhibition with his wife. It turned out that, at one level, his wife was like a superficially good mother who really replaced his own internal, bad, and guilt-provoking mother, toward whom he had to be a well-behaved little boy lest she severely attack and depreciate him (if, for example, he was sexually freer with her). At a different level, he felt that his marriage, with all its problems, was such an improvement over the marriage of his parents that he could not tolerate this triumph over his own father.

I have tried to illustrate how, in an ordinary neurotic transference, primitive dissociation or splitting in the transference (the contradictory ego states), regressive shifts from verbal to nonverbal communication, and temporary weakening of reality testing in connection with the activation of primitive defensive operations (splitting, projection, denial) were resolved analytically in a case that, at a certain point, might have been considered nonanalyzable.

To conclude: Object relations theory permits us to sharpen our understanding and technical handling of the various types of psychopathology and degrees of regression in the transference. A cohesive, holistic theory of technique, it seems to me, is far preferable to attempting to develop *ad hoc* theories of technique for various psychopathological conditions. Such *ad hoc* formulations contain within them the potential for disregarding contradictory implications in terms of psychoanalytic theory and technique and our understanding of normal and pathological development.

Chapter Ten

A Theory of
Psychoanalytic Psychotherapy

Having described how object relations theory can be fruitfully applied to both the theoretical and technical aspects of psychoanalysis, I turn now to its application to and relevance for psychotherapy.

HISTORICAL ROOTS OF
PSYCHOANALYTIC PSYCHOTHERAPY

Psychoanalytic exploration of the defenses and resistances, the transferences and drive derivatives of patients with severe character pathology and borderline personality organization has shown that the intrapsychic structural organization of these patients seems very different from that in better-functioning patients. This finding has imposed serious constraints upon the traditional theory of psychoanalytic psychotherapy. Of particular concern is that the structural characteristics of borderline patients defy applying the model of psychoanalysis to psychoanalytic psychotherapy unless the model is modified. At the same time, many studies of pathological early development and object relations theory aimed at understanding severe psychopathologies implicitly or explicitly recommend only standard psychoanalytic techniques. We seem to have, on the one hand, a theory of psychotherapy that is not applicable to many patients in psychotherapy and, on the other hand, theories of pathological development and severe psychopathologies that might relate to new models of psychotherapy, but are presented in terms geared mostly to psychoanalytic technique proper. One purpose of this chapter is to try to resolve this paradox.

Gill's (1954) definition of psychoanalysis as the establishment of a therapeutic setting that permits the development of a regressive transference neurosis and the resolution of this transference neurosis by means of interpretation carried out by the analyst from a position of technical neutrality contains two important implications for the theory of psychoanalytic psychotherapy. First, if the analyst's position of technical neutrality, the use of interpretation as a major psychotherapeutic tool, and the systematic analysis of the transference define psychoanalysis, then psychoanalytic psychotherapies may be defined in terms of modifications in any or all of these three technical essentials. In fact, I think the definition of a spectrum of psychoanalytic psychotherapies ranging from psychoanalysis to supportive psychotherapies is possible in terms of these three basic features.

Second, it needs to be stressed that the analysis of the transference is simultaneously the analysis of instinctual urges and defenses against them, and of a particular object relation within which these instinctual urges and defenses are played out. As Glover (1955) pointed out, all transference phenomena must be analyzed in terms of the principal stage of libidinal investment activated and the principal identification involved. Both contemporary ego psychology and object relations theory take their departure from this dual nature of the transference.

It seems to me that the major contributions to the theory of technique — in contrast to theories of development and psychopathology — of modern ego psychology stem from Wilhelm Reich's *Character Analysis* (1933–1934) and Fenichel's *Problems of Psychoanalytic Technique* (1941). With these works, the analysis of resistances — including the transference as a principal resistance and source of information in the psychoanalytic situation — expanded into the detailed analysis of the resistance function of pathological character traits. These contributions also pointed to the intimate connection between the predominance of character defenses in cases of character pathology and the activation of these defenses as part of the prevailing transference resistances in all analytic treatments.

The analysis of character may well be the most dramatic practical application of psychoanalytic technique to the treatment of the neuroses. Psychoanalytic character analysis is a fundamental challenge to the traditionally pessimistic attitude of psychology and psychiatry toward the possibility of changing personality structure. From the early focus on reaction formations and inhibitory character traits to the later focus on impulsive character traits and impulse-ridden characters in general, there remained only a small step to the psychoanalytic focus on the nature of global ego defects — and on the puzzling relationships between ego "defects" and pathological character traits (in the sense of the question whether a character "defect" is a resistance, or whether a character resistance is a reflection of an ego defect).

The ego psychology theory of psychoanalytic psychotherapy as proposed by Gill (1951, 1954), Stone (1951, 1954), Eissler (1953), Bibring (1954), and others may be defined as a psychoanalytically based or oriented treatment that does not attempt to systematically resolve unconscious conflicts, and therefore, resistances, but rather to partially resolve some and reinforce other resistances, with a subsequent partial integration of previously repressed impulses into the adult ego. As a result, a partial increase of ego strength and flexibility may take place, which then permits a more effective repression of residual, dynamically unconscious, impulses and a modified impulse-defense configuration which increases the adaptive — in contrast to maladaptive — aspects of character formation. This definition differentiates psychoanalysis from psychoanalytic psychotherapy in terms of both goals and the underlying theory of change reflected in these different goals.

Wallerstein formulated this difference when he proposed (1965) that the procedural stance of psychoanalysis is characterized by goallessness (in terms of the open-ended nature of analytic work), but the goal of psychoanalysis is that of fundamental character realignment. In contrast, psychoanalytic psychotherapy focuses on certain individual circumscribed goals in that it aims for desirable modifications of behavior and character structure without the broad goal of resolving character pathology.

The techniques employed in psychoanalytic psychotherapy were all devised to facilitate these goals and to bring about a partial shift of the dynamic equilibrium among the tripartite structures. I would modify Bibring's (1954) description of psychotherapeutic techniques to include, first of all, partial interpretation, meaning both (a) preliminary interpretations which would remain limited to conscious and preconscious areas or clarification and (b) full interpretations of some limited intrapsychic segments (while others would be left untouched). The effect of these techniques would still be "analytic" in a strict sense, that is, uncovering, at least partially, unconscious motives and conflicts. Direct efforts to facilitate abreaction would permit the expression in the therapeutic situation of suppressed or repressed emotions, thereby presumably reducing intrapsychic pressures, owing to the sense of being accepted by the therapist as a tolerant and empathic parental figure and, in this connection, also by means of other transference gratifications. Suggestion, a broad spectrum of psychotherapeutic techniques, comprising rational counseling and giving advice and emotional suggestions (including hypnosis), would be effective due to the transference implications of direct support and command from an important parental figure, the reinforcement of adaptive characterological solutions to intrapsychic conflicts, the (at least temporary) decrease of superego pressures (by their externalization and, in this process, modification), and the facilitation of identificatory processes with the therapist's active and supportive stances toward the patient. Manipulation would affect the intrapsychic balance of forces by indirect means, such as by fostering a more favorable social environment for the patient, eliminating or controlling regressive and conflict-inducing situations in the environment, and favoring derivative expressions of the patient's unconscious needs by providing specific social outlets or situations.

Some common mechanisms by which all of these psychotherapeutic techniques may affect the patient in psychoanalytic psychotherapy have been described in the literature, such as the "corrective emotional experience" implied in the positive relationship developed in the course of psychoanalytic psychotherapy; the particular transference gratifications symbolically achieved in the course of the therapist's suggestive, manipulative, abreactive, and even clarifying and interpreting interventions; and, most importantly, the activation of identification processes in the patient by means of all of these interventions: adaptive ego identifications with the therapist would increase ego strength directly.

Combining the techniques employed in psychoanalytic psychotherapy, the ego psychology approach defined two major modalities of treatment (Gill, 1951, 1954). First, exploratory, insight, uncovering, or simply, expressive psychoanalytic psychotherapy; and second, suppressive, or supportive psychotherapy.

Expressive psychotherapy is characterized by the utilization of clarification and interpretation as major tools. Partial aspects of the transference are interpreted, and the therapist actively selects such transferences to be interpreted in the light of the particular goals of treatment, the predominant transference resistances, and the patient's external reality. Technical neutrality is mostly maintained, but a systematic analysis of all transference paradigms, or a systematic resolution of the transference neurosis by interpretation alone is definitely not attempted.

Supportive psychotherapy is characterized by partial utilization of clarification and abreaction, but chiefly by the use of suggestion and manipulation. Insofar as supportive psychotherapy still implies that the psychotherapist is acutely aware of and monitoring the transference and is carefully considering transference resistances as part of his technique in dealing with character problems and their connection to the patient's life difficulties, this is still a psychoanalytic psychotherapy in a broad sense. By definition, however, transference is not interpreted in purely supportive psychotherapy, and the use of suggestion and manipulation implicitly eliminates technical neutrality. A comprehensive overview of the ego psychology theory of psychoanalytic psychotherapy can be found in Dewald's (1969) textbook.

All the ego psychology theoreticians I mentioned earlier have stressed the difference between structural change achieved in psychoanalysis and the more limited changes achieved in psycho-therapy. Structural change as obtained in psychoanalysis implies a radical change in the equilibrium of conflicting forces involving the tripartite structural system, that is, reduction in superego pathology and pressures on the ego, reduction in the rigidity of the ego's defensive structures, sublimatory integration of previously repressed unconscious impulses, and significant increase in the scope and flexibility of adaptation to internal and external reality derived from such changes in intersystemic equilibrium.

In contrast, the changes obtained in psychotherapies would be largely behavioral. Increase in the adaptive functions of certain impulse-defense configurations would predominate in the outcome of these psychotherapies. Instead of obtaining mostly structural intrapsychic change on the basis of an interpretive approach, the therapeutic changes would be in large part adaptive, obtained by at least partially "structuring" approaches (in the sense of environmental manipulation) which would help the patient deal with an environment that has become more manageable for him, or by educational influences on his behavior by means of consistently guiding him toward better ways of adjusting to the environment.

As suggested earlier, the major problem with this technical theory of psychoanalytic psychotherapy has been the contradiction between the theoretical model from which it stems and the structural intra-psychic organization of many patients with whom it has chiefly been used. Thus, the ideal indications for expressive psychoanalytic psychotherapy (from here on, I will use the term psychoanalytic psychotherapy as equivalent to expressive psychotherapy) would be for mild cases where the "major surgery" of psychoanalysis is not warranted, and for serious psychological illness (severe character pathologies, etc.) where psychoanalysis seems contraindicated (Wallerstein and Robbins, 1956). In effect, psychoanalytic psycho-therapy with patients having relatively mild psychological illness is highly effective, and even brief psychoanalytically oriented psycho-therapy or "focal" psychotherapy (Balint et al., 1972) with patients who have good ego strength and motivation can be effective. More-over, the theoretical model underlying this approach holds remark-ably well for patients with good ego strength.

The application of this psychoanalytic psychotherapy model to patients with severe psychopathologies, however, led to the findings I described in Chapter 1. In short, the cases for which the ego psychology approach had transformed classical psychoanalytic theory into a theory of change by less than strictly psychoanalytic means did not seem to fit the theoretical model on the basis of which these cases were approached therapeutically.

This leads us to the third psychoanalytic approach (in addition to the classical and contemporary ego psychology one) which attempts to deal with the phenomena just described — namely, psychoanalytic object relations theory. As I said before, there is a paradox in the fact that object relations theories offer answers to problems that originally developed within ego psychological psychoanalytic psychotherapy, while many object relations theoreticians, particularly those of the British Schools, steadfastly refuse to consider any theory of technique and any technical approach to patients with severe character pathologies and ego weakness other than psychoanalysis. What follows is an application to a theory of technique of psychoanalytic psychotherapy of my model of psychoanalytic object relations theory integrated with ego psychology.

In the severe psychopathologies, early, primitive units of internalized object relations are directly manifest in the transference as conflicting drive derivatives reflected in contradictory ego states. In these cases, the predominance of a constellation of early defense mechanisms centering around primitive dissociation or splitting immediately activates in the transference mutually contradictory, primitive but conscious intrapsychic conflicts. What appear to be inappropriate, primitive, chaotic character traits and interpersonal interactions, impulsive behavior, and affect storms are actually reflections of the fantastic early object-relations-derived structures that are the building blocks of the later tripartite system. These object relations determine the characteristics of primitive transference, that is, of highly fantastic, unrealistic precipitates of early object relations which do not reflect directly the real object relations of infancy and childhood, and must be interpreted until the more realistic aspects of the developmental history emerge. In the treatment, structural integration through interpretation, as I stressed in the preceding chapter, precedes genetic reconstructions.

The interpretation of primitive transferences—which includes the systematic interpretation of splitting mechanisms and other primitive defenses—requires special psychoanalytic methods. First of all, the danger of severe acting out and of blurring the boundaries of the psychoanalytic situation requires considering the need for establishing parameters of technique and/or structuring the patient's external life in order to protect the psychoanalytic situation. Second, insofar as, at primitive levels of fixation or regression, language as a communicative function may itself be disturbed, and severe psychopathology is typically expressed nonverbally (the same applies generally to character pathology), the analyst's focus may have to shift from the content of free association to the total material expressed in the patient/therapist interaction, and to the patient's experience of and reaction to the psychoanalytic setting, which frequently becomes a major channel of expressing the transference. Third, under these conditions, the immediate meaning of the present interpersonal relation in the transference—in terms of the activation of primitive transference dispositions—has to be interpreted with a special consideration of the patient's predominant unit of self- and object representations reflected in such interaction. Some authors have used the notion of psychoanalytic "space" (Winnicott, 1958, 1965, 1971; Bion, 1967, 1970) to refer to this type of translation of nonverbal interaction into a primitive object-relations structure. They have stressed the integrating function of the analyst's cognitive and emotional absorption and tolerance of the chaotic material and his utilization of his integration of that material in interpretive comments (the affectively "holding" and cognitively "containing" functions of Winnicott and Bion). Fourth, countertransference dispositions are particularly activated in these cases and require particular methods so that the analyst's emotional reactions can be controlled and therapeutically utilized.

In contrast to the facilitation of integrated ego functioning by means of the ego's overall defensive structure in the case of patients with good ego strength, primitive defensive operations in patients with severe psychopathology have a serious ego-weakening effect.

Therefore, interpretation of such primitive defensive constellations (of splitting, projection, projective identification, denial, omnipotence, idealization, devaluation, etc.) improves ego strength and permits the gradual development of an observing and integrated ego function (Kernberg, 1976a). Thus, within an object relations framework, interpretation of defenses as clinical resistances, and of the transferences as internalized object relations may — and actually should — be applied throughout the entire spectrum of psychopathology. Jacobson (1971), for example, has applied her findings regarding the psychopathology of depression and depressed borderline patients to the psychoanalytic treatment of these conditions.

However, while Jacobson and Mahler and theoreticians oriented to ego psychology object relations viewpoints have generally been careful in selecting cases for psychoanalysis and question the indiscriminate application of the same psychoanalytic technique to all patients, the British object relations group, particularly the Kleinians, have, as I said earlier, applied the same unmodified technical approach to all patients. In the light of much accumulated clinical experience, I consider this erroneous and think that it can lead to disastrous results.

In contrast, some British "Middle Group" clinicians have generally tended to blur the distinctions between psychoanalysis and psychoanalytic psychotherapy, which can lead to considerable confusion. The approach of the British School represents, precisely, the other side of the paradox mentioned earlier, namely, that the theoretical and technical contributions of most interest for the psychoanalytic psychotherapy of patients with severe psychopathologies have been developed without regard for the theoretical and technical differences between psychoanalysis and psychotherapy.

I think it is possible to formulate a theory of psychoanalytic psychotherapy that utilizes the concepts derived from ego psychology and object relations theory.

A THEORY OF PSYCHOANALYTIC PSYCHOTHERAPY

At all levels of psychopathology where psychoanalysis or psychoanalytic psychotherapy are clinically indicated, symptoms and pathological character traits reflect intrapsychic conflicts. These conflicts are always dynamically structured, that is, they reflect a relatively permanent intrapsychic organization of contradictory or conflicting internalized object relations. At severe levels of psychopathology, such dynamic structures are dissociated, thus permitting the contradictory aspects of the conflicts to remain in consciousness. Here, interpretation of defenses and of primitive transferences permits ego integration to occur and fosters the consolidation of the tripartite structure and the simultaneous transformation of primitive into advanced or typically neurotic transferences. Under these conditions, interpretation of the transference may bring about an alteration of the equilibrium of the forces in conflict, as well as structural intrapsychic change in the sense of integrating part- into total object relations, consolidating ego identity, and reinforcing the boundaries of ego, id, and superego. The analysis of the transference is carried out by a direct analysis of the total analytic situation, with particular emphasis on the psychoanalytic setting and its relation to reality.

At less severe levels of psychopathology or in the standard psychoanalytic case, the dynamically structured intrapsychic conflicts are unconscious, and are manifest largely in intersystemic conflicts between ego, superego, and id and their typical defense mechanisms. Here, the interpretation of defense mechanisms induces a partial redissolution — or rather, a loosening and shifting of the boundaries — of the tripartite structure, facilitates the establishment of a regressive transference neurosis, and gradually, by means of the systematic analysis of ego and superego defenses, the unfolding of a regressive transference that has more integrated characteristics than the initial transferences of patients with severe psychopathologies. The analysis of the transference in patients with well-integrated tripartite structure is facilitated by the patient's observing ego and the related therapeutic alliance. It requires that the focus be chiefly on free association and its distortions by the manifestation of various defense mechanisms; the focus on the analytic setting itself recedes into the background. The integration of complex repressed impulses reflecting entire constellations of repressed object relations (most importantly, the oedipal constellation) permits an enrichment of ego functions and experiences and a reduction in the rigidity and constraining nature of ego defenses and superego pressures.

Although individual considerations always have priority in determining the type of treatment, generally speaking, patients with milder forms of psychopathology have a preferential indication for psychoanalysis, except when special circumstances warrant brief psychotherapy or psychoanalytic psychotherapy. For patients with good ego strength, the definition of psychoanalytic psychotherapy as originally proposed by the ego psychologists I referred to earlier still stands, and so does the possibility of using various expressive and supportive techniques. (Gill [1978], however, has questioned the advisability of combining expressive and supportive techniques for patients with good ego strength, and has presented strong arguments for maintaining a strictly expressive approach with these patients.) In any case, the three paradigms of (1) the principal technical tools (clarification and interpretation versus suggestion and manipulation), (2) the extent to which the transference is interpreted, and (3) the degree to which technical neutrality is maintained jointly define the nature of psychotherapy within the expressive-supportive range of treatment.

In cases of severe psychopathology—with a few exceptions where for well-documented, individual reasons psychoanalysis is indicated or feasible—the treatment indication is for psychoanalytic psychotherapy. Here, however, the characteristics of psychoanalytic psychotherapy can no longer be described in ways similar to those for patients with well-integrated tripartite structure. Maintaining the three basic paradigms upon which differentiation of psychoanalysis proper from psychoanalytic psychotherapy can be established, psychoanalytic psychotherapy for severe psychopathology might be described as follows.

Because primitive transferences are immediately available, predominate as resistances, and, in fact, determine the severity of intrapsychic and interpersonal disturbances, they can and need to be focused upon immediately, starting with their interpretation in the "here and now," and leading into genetic reconstruction only at late stages of the treatment (when primitive transferences determined by part-object relations have been transformed into advanced transferences or total object relations, thus approaching the more realistic experiences of childhood that lend themselves to genetic reconstructions). Interpretation of the transference requires maintaining a position of technical neutrality. For there can be no interpretation of primitive transferences without a firm, consistent, stable maintenance of reality boundaries in the therapeutic situation, and without an active caution on the part of the therapist not to be sucked into the reactivation of pathological primitive object relations by the patient. Insofar as both transference interpretation and a position of technical neutrality require the use of clarification and interpretation and contraindicate the use of suggestive and manipulative techniques, clarification and interpretation are maintained as principal techniques.

However, in contrast to psychoanalysis proper, transference analysis is not systematic. Because of the need to focus on the severity of acting out and on the disturbances in the patient's external reality (which may threaten the continuity of the treatment as well as the patient's psychosocial survival), and also because the treatment, as part of acting out of primitive transferences, easily comes to replace life, transference interpretation now has to be codetermined by (1) the predominant conflicts in immediate reality, (2) the overall specific goals of treatment—and the consistent differentiation of life goals from treatment goals (Ticho, 1972)—and (3) by what is immediately prevailing in the transference.

In addition, technical neutrality is limited by the need to establish parameters of technique, including, in certain cases, the structuring of the patient's external life and establishing a teamwork approach with patients who cannot function autonomously during long stretches of their psychotherapy. Technical neutrality is therefore a theoretical base line from which deviations occur again and again, to be reduced by interpretation. The therapist's interpretation of the patient's understanding (or misunderstanding) of the therapist's comments is an important aspect of this effort to reduce the deviations from technical neutrality. Further exploration of the differences between psychoanalytic psychotherapy with patients presenting ego weakness and with patients having good ego strength requires a sharper focus on the mechanism of action — and the effects — of psychotherapeutic techniques, our next issue.

The Therapeutic Action of Psychoanalytic Psychotherapy

Interestingly, little concern was expressed in the nineteen-fifties regarding the potentially contradictory effects of combining various interpretive and supportive technical interventions in terms of their effects. Although psychoanalytic psychotherapies were classified along a spectrum ranging from the purely expressive to the purely suppressive, it was assumed that a mixture of supportive and interpretive techniques and effects was perfectly harmonious.

In retrospect, such a mixture of supportive and exploratory techniques seems feasible for patients with good ego strength. For example, a therapist's suggestive and manipulative interventions in the course of an exploratory psychotherapy that mostly focuses on transference developments and their relation to the patient's immediate reality may not distort such transference developments excessively, except, naturally, in reducing the intensity of transference regression (particularly in driving underground the severer aspects of the negative transference dispositions or displacing them toward other objects). Or else, the therapist's empathic attitude in helping the patient to deal with an immediate problem in his external life may indeed lead to a favorable ego identification, without activating a primitive, pathological idealization of the "good" therapist as a defense against the activation of paranoid fears of the "bad" therapist (the potential receptacle for projected early sadistic superego forerunners).

In other words, ego identification with the therapist and transference gratification may indeed take place in the context of a mixture of supportive and expressive technical approaches with patients who have sufficiently good ego strength to be able to perceive, understand, and integrate the more positive aspects of the therapeutic relationship in spite of the underlying ambivalences in the transferences. However, this combination of expressive and supportive techniques and the respective mechanisms of their action may become inoperative in the case of patients with severe psychopathologies. In patients with predominantly primitive transference dispositions reflecting part-object relations, all these psychotherapeutic techniques (except interpretation per se) and the mechanisms by which they are supposed to bring about therapeutic change raise new questions.

First, the selective interpretation of some resistances while leaving others untouched in order to protect ego integration runs counter the clinical observation that the predominant constellation of primitive defensive mechanisms in these cases has ego-weakening effects, and that the systematic interpretation of such defenses — largely manifest as transference resistances — has an ego-strengthening effect.

Second, the very fact that the conflicting impulses — the pathologically condensed sexual and aggressive drive derivatives expressed in dissociated or split-off part-object relations — are conscious makes it imperative to deal with them: ignoring such exigent needs and impulse expressions in these patients only increases their fear of their own impulses and displaces the most significant instinctual conflicts from the transference situation onto other relationships, thus increasing acting out.

 Third, the therapist's effort to provide a stable, reliable, and empathic parental figure, which may permit the patient's emotional growth by processes of ego identification and transference gratification, is often made impossible by the development of severely negative transferences reflected in paranoid dispositions. These paranoid dispositions must be dealt with to prevent the disruption of the psychotherapeutic relationship and to permit some semblance of therapeutic alliance to be established.

Fourth, and most important, the gratification of certain transference demands (in practice, the patient's most strongly pressed-for transference gratification usually stems from the need to protect the good, idealized relationship in the face of a threatening breakthrough of conflicts around aggression) significantly distorts the patient's perception of the therapist and of the therapeutic situation.

In short, the flexible capacity to take the best from the therapist, which patients with good ego strength have and which, I think, has much to do with the fact that these patients are able to respond favorably to a broad range of exploratory-supportive psychotherapeutic techniques, is missing in cases with severe psychopathology.

Identification in the latter cases, instead of being with the benign aspects of the psychotherapist, are rather reconfirmations of highly idealized projected forerunners of the ego ideal, idealizations which potentially weaken the patient's capacity to feel that he will ever be able to live up to them and which undermine his autonomous growth. A related problem derives from the misunderstanding of the importance of empathy on the part of the therapist for patients with severe psychopathology, which I have already discussed at some length in the previous chapter.

For all these reasons, a supportive technique runs counter to the therapeutic needs of patients with severe psychopathology, particularly borderline conditions, where a modified psychoanalytic procedure or psychoanalytic psychotherapy is attempted. These patients require a purely expressive approach. I shall now proceed to spell out the three technical paradigms that jointly define psychoanalytic psychotherapy with borderline personality organization, and the specific effects of these techniques.

(1) *Interpretation.* Interpretation is a fundamental technical tool in psychoanalytic psychotherapy with borderline patients; in fact, in order to protect—as much as possible—technical neutrality, suggestion and manipulation are practically contraindicated here, except when the potential for severe acting out requires structuring the patient's external life and, with it, a team approach, which implies limit-setting and other interventions in the social field. Such socially structuring or manipulative efforts should be considered parameters of technique, to be interpreted as much and as comprehensively as possible in working toward their gradual dissolution.

The question has been raised how it is possible that patients with severe psychological illness and ego weakness are able to respond to interpretation. Do these patients really accept interpretations because of their actual meaning or as manifestations of the therapist's interest, that is, because of their magical, transference meanings? Empirical evidence indicates that patients with severe psychological illness are indeed able to understand and integrate interpretive comments, particularly if the patient's interpretations of the therapist's interpretations are examined and interpreted in turn. In other words, the patient's difficulty in integrating verbal

communication is in itself a product of primitive defensive operations, which can be interpreted, particularly as they are activated in
the patient's reactions to the therapist's interpretations.

However, the very facts that the patient's interpretations of the
therapist's interpretations must be explored so fully and that clarification of the immediate reality of the therapeutic situation—the
meaning of what the therapist has been saying in contrast to the
patient's interpretation of what that meaning was—requires such
consistent attention result in clarification taking precedence over
interpretation. This technical demand creates quantitative differences
between this kind of psychotherapy and psychoanalysis.

(2) *Maintenance of Technical Neutrality*. This is an essential technical
tool, indispensable for the possibility of interpretive work to occur.
Once more, technical neutrality is in no contradiction to an
empathic, authentic, warm attitude on the part of the therapist, and,
to the contrary, may best reflect such warmth and empathy under
conditions in which emergence of the patient's regressive aggression
in the transference would naturally bring about counteraggressive
reactions in the therapist. The therapist's capacity to emotionally
maintain his empathic attitude under such circumstances (the therapist's "holding" action) and his capacity to cognitively integrate
("contain") the fragmentarily expressed transferences are important
components of such technical neutrality.

However, because the potential for severe acting out, and the
development of life—and/or treatment-threatening—situations on
the patient's part may require structuring, not only of the patient's
life but of the psychotherapy sessions themselves, technical neutrality is constantly interfered with, threatened, or limited, and a good
part of the therapist's efforts will have to concentrate on returning,
again and again, to the point of technical neutrality. To put it differ-
ently, in patients with severe ego weakness or ego distortions where
the nondefensive or observing part of the ego (which would ordinarily contribute to the therapeutic alliance or working relationship
with the therapist) is not available, the provision of such auxiliary
ego functions in terms of clarifying the immediate reality simultaneously shifts the interpretations into clarifications and may bring
about deviations from technical neutrality, requiring later reductions

of such deviations by interpretive means. Again, this quantitative reduction in technical neutrality implies a difference from psychoanalysis proper.

(3) *Transference Analysis*. I mentioned earlier that transference interpretation is limited in these cases, that it is codetermined by a constant focus on the immediate reality of the patient's life and the ultimate treatment goals. Also, because the interpretation of primitive transferences reflected by part-object relationships gradually leads to the integration of such part-object relations into total object relations, and, by the same token, a transformation of the transference from primitive into advanced or neurotic, there are relatively sudden shifts in the transference of borderline patients. More neurotic or advanced transferences reflecting more realistic childhood developments first appear infrequently and then with increasing frequency throughout the treatment. As a result, the processes of transforming primitive transference structures into their integrated counterparts evolve in discontinuous, qualitatively shifting phases throughout the treatment, which gives an overall timelessness to the genetic reconstruction and interferes with its historical placement (see Chapter 9). These developments require the interpretation of the transference in an atemporal, "as if" mode over extended periods of time, an additional reason for considering transference interpretation in these cases less than systematic, and therefore different from, the standard psychoanalytic situation.

Nevertheless, while transference analysis is less than systematic under these conditions, the interpretation of defensive constellations is quite systematic: In contrast to exploratory psychotherapy with better-functioning patients—where certain defenses may be selectively interpreted while others are not touched—the systematic interpretation of defenses in severe psychopathology is crucial to improve ego functioning and to permit the transformation and resolution of primitive transferences. The interpretation of the constellation of primitive defensive operations centering around splitting, therefore, should be as consistent as their detection in the patient's transferences and his extratherapeutic relationships permits.

The basic mechanisms of change implied in this psychoanalytic psychotherapy have already been alluded to, and I will briefly summarize them at this point. The most important mechanisms of change implied in this approach, that is, the effects specifically attempted by means of interpretation of primitive transferences, are the resolution of primitive defense mechanisms in the therapeutic situation, the integration of part-object relations into total-object relations, and the related integration and development of ego functions, particularly of ego identity, with the corresponding integration of the self concept and object constancy.

Elsewhere (1976a, Chapter 6) I have described the interpretive steps that gradually transform primitive into advanced transferences, steps that consist, first, in defining the predominant human interaction activated at any particular time in the transference; second, in defining the self- and object components and the affect disposition (reflecting libidinal or aggressive drive derivatives) linking them in this interaction; and third, in integrating the mutually dissociated or split-off self- and object representations under the impact of libidinal and aggressive drive derivatives.

This specific effect of interpretation, that is, transformation by integration, is supported by the relatively nonspecific effect derived from the auxiliary ego functions carried out by the psychotherapist, particularly his emotionally and cognitive integrating function reflected in his capacity to tolerate what the patient originally could not tolerate in himself. This permits the patient to accept what was previously too painful to be integrated in his own subjective experience and, in the process, provides an implicit and silent assurance that, in contrast to the patient's fantasies, aggression does not necessarily destroy love and the possibility of having a sustained and meaningful relation with another. These nonspecific effects may be considered "supportive," but then, all interventions are potentially supportive in their effects, in contrast to being supportive techniques. It has been rightly stated that psychoanalysis is the "most supportive" form of therapy.

In summary of these considerations, psychoanalytic psychotherapy with borderline patients is characterized by technical tools similar to those of psychoanalysis and by mechanisms of action of these technical tools which differentiate this treatment from the effects of the same technical tools when they are utilized in exploratory psychotherapy with patients presenting ego strength (see Table 1).

TABLE I
PSYCHOANALYTIC PSYCHOTHERAPY

Technical Tools	Mechanisms of Action	
	With good ego strength	*With ego weakness*
Interpretation	by reducing defenses permits emergence of repressed material	increases ego strength by resolving primitive defenses
Transference analysis	of selected transferences permits their gradual resolution	of primitive into advanced transferences permits their eventual resolution
Technical neutrality	fosters transference regression; permits interpretation by not gratifying transferences	protects reality in the therapeutic situation; permits interpretation of primitive trans- ferences

There is one more dimension along which psychoanalytic psycho-therapy for patients with severe character pathology and borderline conditions may bring about significant transformations in the direc-tion of therapeutic change. This dimension has to do with the patient's increased capacity to experience what was previously disso-ciated and expressed in the distortions of his interpersonal realm and behavior. One mechanism of change in the psychoanalytic psycho-therapy of severely regressed patients is the transformation of the patient's relations to the psychotherapeutic setting, and of his expres-sion of the uncanny in the interpersonal field, into the patient's subjective awareness. This effect is similar, at this level of pathology, to the incorporation into consciousness of what was repressed in patients with well-integrated tripartite structure. Again, this is a particular effect of an analytic approach that quantitatively sepa-rates psychoanalytic psychotherapy with regressed patients from the standard psychoanalytic situation, as well as from psychoanalytic psychotherapy with patients presenting good ego strength.

The differences between them notwithstanding, the similarity between psychoanalytic psychotherapy and psychoanalysis is much greater in cases of severe psychopathology than in cases of milder psychological illness. One might say that, with the former, the tactical psychotherapeutic approach to each session is almost indistinguishable from psychoanalysis proper, and only from a long-term, strategic standpoint do the differences emerge. However, although the technical approach to borderline patients resembles that of psychoanalysis, the therapeutic atmosphere is quite different: the way in which nonverbal communication and the examination of the total interaction predominates over the patient's communication of subjective experiences and his intrapsychic life creates a special therapeutic climate.

By the same token, the cleavage between psychoanalytic psychotherapy and supportive psychotherapy is sharp and definite in patients with severe pathology, whereas it may be more gradual and blurred with those less severely ill. In other words, it is not possible to bring about significant personality modifications by means of psychotherapy in patients with severe psychopathology without exploring and resolving primitive transferences, and this requires an analytic approach, although it is not psychoanalysis proper. In my view, it is very helpful to maintain a clear distinction between psychoanalytic psychotherapy and psychoanalysis in all cases.

There are patients for whom psychoanalytic psychotherapy is contraindicated (psychoanalysis, of course, would be even more contraindicated in such cases), and if a patient with severe character pathology, narcissistic personality, or borderline personality organization has such a contraindication, I think that a strictly supportive approach is best. Such supportive psychotherapy requires, in turn, a very sophisticated way of utilizing suggestive and manipulative techniques and of dealing with primitive transferences noninterpretively: All our understanding regarding supportive psychotherapy may have to be reexamined and reformulated in the light of what we now know about severe psychopathology.

CLINICAL ILLUSTRATION

The following segment from the psychoanalytic psychotherapy of a 34-year-old single woman, a mathematician who had been unable to work for over six years and whose personality structure combined intense schizoid and masochistic features, occurred toward the end of the fourth year of treatment when, after significant improvement, a severe negative therapeutic reaction developed over a period of five months. During this time, the patient responded with subtle mockery and provocations to any of my efforts to clarify the meaning of her frequent silences, her emotional withdrawal from me, and her keeping me ignorant of important occurrences in her daily life. Over a period of months, she gradually became aware that the severe blockings and long silences in the hours reflected an internal prohibition against further improvement because of intense guilt, a sense that change could occur only at the cost of her mother's suffering in reality and of the destruction and loss of her attachment to mother inside of her.

On the surface, the patient's attacks on me were an attempt to make me withdraw emotionally and counterattack, which would then have permitted her to externalize her cruel maternal image on me. In fact, there were times when a partial compromise solution took the form of her attacking me as a representation of her mother — thus partially rebelling against her — while maintaining a good surface relation with her mother in reality — thereby apparently submitting to her and keeping the treatment situation stable. She attacked her mother by bitterly complaining because her mother was cold, dominating, and yet rejecting of her. Some of the patient's descriptions of her clinging to an overpowering and aggressive mother corresponded to actual aspects of her infantile past. But all opportunities present in the therapeutic situation that would have permitted a true dependency on me were internally forbidden and unavailable to the patient, for which she blamed me.

Within this context, the following episode took place. Following a stormy session, the patient sent me a letter. What follows is a summary of that letter and of the two sessions following my reception of it. Both because the treatment was conducted in a bilingual mode, and the letter was in a foreign language, the salient features of it will be paraphrased in translation. The patient had left for approximately a week to visit her mother, who lived in a different state. She wrote the letter soon after her arrival there, and the letter reached me the day before our next session.

The patient wrote that she was furious at me because she felt I was just "tolerating" her, she hated my sitting "patiently" through her angry outbursts or nagging demands. She was not denying her anger or demands, but all of this was made worse by what she experienced as my detached "professional" tolerance which aggravated her even more. She had fantasies of making me suffer terribly, of hurting my feelings very deeply. Without any transition, she went on to tell me how much she hated me because I never gave her any credit for anything good that she did and never made her feel good about herself in any way. She also felt that I never acted as if we were working together and I never showed any sense of accomplishment or pride in the progress she had made. She felt that my emotional detachment was unfair because the progress in her treatment was not only her own work. She found my attitude one of artificial concern for her, as if I were giving her lessons in "positive feelings," and then added that one thing she hated about the treatment was that I never erred, that I never forgot I was the therapist or slipped from that role.

The letter then went on to say that she was perfectly aware what "transference" meant, that she would have to be mentally retarded not to understand this after years of treatment. But this did not take away her sense of loneliness, her sadness about not being involved in a satisfying and fulfilling relationship. And further, she added, when she did talk about this in the sessions, I twisted it around so that the problem always involved me, resulting in her feeling that I did not care at all. She really wanted to feel loved and appreciated, and instead of examining what she expected of the relationship, I only suggested endlessly that she did not appreciate what I had to give to her.

She then wrote, in an abrupt shift, that instead of being angry at her parents directly she felt angry at me for not fulfilling her parental ideals. She wanted to be loved and felt nobody loved her. In conclusion, she added that she also sometimes hated me for not being compassionate with her; she felt reduced to self-pity. She really hated me, she wrote, for the pain I had caused her over the past years—without thinking twice about it. Finally, she didn't think that I deserved any good feelings from her because I never gave anything back, and she didn't need lessons in expressing "positive feelings."

In spite of the intensity of the anger expressed in its contents, the letter also conveyed feelings of warmth and gratitude; I experienced the letter as a clear indication of the patient's increased tolerance of ambivalence, her awareness of the complexity of her emotional relation with me. In short, I was very touched by it.

In the session following my receiving the letter, the patient complained bitterly that I did not love her, that I was "professionally" objective and cool and had no real feelings for her. As these complaints were repeated insistently, I was struck by several things: by the patient's sadistic tone of voice and triumphant smile; by my perception of a "frozen" quality inside myself, as if indeed I had no feelings for her, and a sense of guilt—as if I owed her some real feelings. This was in striking contrast to the strong positive feelings I had experienced for her at the beginning of the session. I was also struck by the contrast between her almost unusually clear, coherent, and modulated way of expressing herself, and the contents of the accusations which expressed how I was frustrating her. In the past, great anger had had a disorganizing effect on her communications. Finally, I noticed her references to how angry she had been with me since the last session, and how this anger had only decreased temporarily during the visit to her mother, after which she felt much better. She remarked, however, that her mother had told her she now looked "dangerously healthy." (!)

After attempting to stimulate the patient to explore how all the features I was observing might fit together, I realized that she was cutting me off every time I tried to speak, almost triumphantly making me shut up, and only remaining silent when I in turn remained silent. I told her I felt she was putting many of her internal conflicts into me because she could not tolerate them, and that she wanted to shut me up in order to avoid that I return to her what she was putting into me because she couldn't tolerate it. I said that behind her "simple" feeling that I had no feelings for her was a condensation of many conflicts and a fear on her part that I would undo that condensation and face her with the conflicts that were buried in her assertion that I did not care for her.

The patient said she did feel afraid; I said she felt afraid I would try to help her understand what was going on, which was indeed very frightening. At the same time, I continued, one part of her also wanted to know what was going on, so that her fear expressed the struggle between the part of her that wanted to know and the part that simply wanted to get rid of her internal problems and of me.

Now the patient said she wanted me to tell her how I understood what was going on (she was no longer interrupting me). I said I felt there were several layers of problems expressed in her feeling that I did not care for her. First, she felt that I was like a cold and rejecting mother with whom she was enraged for not giving any love; second, she was taking revenge against this mother by herself becoming an aggressive, sadistic, and triumphant mother who was accusing me (representing the frightened little daughter) of not having good feelings toward her mother to whom I (she) owed everything; third, in reenacting her relation with her mother with interchanged roles, she was also attempting to spoil the good aspects of her relation with me because she felt guilty about her improvement in psychotherapy: to attack me by accusing me of not loving her permitted her to protest against her mother while at the same time maintaining her submission to mother.

The patient's expression changed markedly at this point; she became sad and thoughtful. She said she was aware that her mother wanted her to stop her psychotherapy, that her mother had accused her of having a much easier life than the rest of the family, and what right did she have to continue spending so much money and time on herself when other members of the family had far greater problems? And she added that I must know that her mother was also friendly and loving, and at times warm and enthusiastic. I said that it was not I she was trying to reassure that her mother could have good as well as bad sides, but herself; and that it was because she was so afraid that her hatred of her mother would also destroy everything good she felt she had received from her and thus leave her completely alone that she could not acknowledge that hatred more directly, or accept the simultaneous existence of loving and hating feelings for me (mother).

For the first time in several months, the patient was now able to explore further aspects of her relationship with mother, her perception of the mother's personality, and her fear of becoming independent and grown-up.

In the following session, the patient began by saying she had left the last session very sad, that she had cried when returning home, and had gradually begun to feel that I had accused her of being cold and unfeeling. She said she thought that she was not cold and unfeeling and that I was accusing her of problems she had resolved long ago. She complained that I only saw her difficulties, that I could not acknowledge her improvement, and that in the middle of all of this I always maintained a self-satisfied and contented attitude stemming from my "happy satisfaction" with my own family at home. She also added that she knew that she exaggerated, but this was still the way she felt.

I told her that I understood this reaction to be a reversal of the earlier session, in which she had accused me of being cold and unfeeling and in which I had interpreted her identifying herself with her mother in a self-satisfied, aggressive, and superior way, accusing me of being cold and ungrateful in the same way her mother had accused her. I pointed out that, in accepting my interpretation, she had felt guilty for attacking me when she realized that I was really concerned and interested in her. I added that this feeling of guilt had then changed into her sense of being the impotent victim of a sadistic mother who accused her of being cold and unloving, a reversal to the childhood experience we had discussed earlier in that session (a change reflecting the reprojection of her sadistic superego). I added that while this was going on she was aware that there was something unrealistic about her reaction, that her perception of my comments as an attack reflected her own exaggerated, self-critical oversimplification of my comments, and that I felt that she was still capable of maintaining, in one part of her, a good image of me in spite of her anger and suspicion about me (implying that she was now better able to tolerate her ambivalence toward me).

The patient, much relieved, then said she felt it would be much more important to discuss her sexual difficulties rather than to focus so much on her difficulties with her mother; there had been such emotional storms in recent hours with me that she had not been able for several sessions to discuss her relations with her boyfriend. She also said that I was unaware of how intensely sexual her feelings about me sometimes were.

I remained silent, with an attitude of expectation of further communication on her part; but she also became silent, and I finally interpreted her silence, saying that her conflicts with her mother were forcing themselves all over her mind to such an extent that she did not have internal freedom to explore her sexual difficulties. I also said that she might be attributing this interference to me, and that, in the last resort, it was her sadistic mother inside who was attempting to prevent her from describing her sexual feelings to me and from resolving her sexual inhibitions in the process. The patient replied that she understood better how several contradictory things were occurring in her mind, and how she had difficulties in keeping them together, so that it was as if different people were experiencing different problems inside of her. I sensed considerable emotional warmth at the end of that session, that the patient felt reassured by my interest and dedication without having to explore this issue verbally at the moment.

This session illustrates the persistence of the subject matters of the earlier one, the faster "replay" of the earlier resistances as part of working through, and the patient's growing awareness of the relationship between dissociative or splitting mechanisms, on the one hand, and the conflict with a sadistic primitive superego represented by her maternal image, on the other.

Both sessions illustrate some technical characteristics of the process of structural intrapsychic change in the context of the working through of primitive transference paradigms. First, the initial manifestation of part-object relations in the early part of the first session (rapid alternation between patient and therapist of the enactment of self- and object representations reflecting the conflicts with mother in an overall confused or chaotic transference situation) changed rapidly in the second half of the first session and throughout most of the second one into the more organized transference disposition of a higher or "neurotic" level.

Second, the material illustrates how the painful experience of not being loved could be analyzed in its genetic components consisting of conflicts over both love and aggression. In other words, although the transference repeated an earlier experience of not being loved by mother, that earlier experience (as well as its repetition in the transference) reflected a more complicated set of conditions. The experience of not being loved was the final outcome of the combination of the expression of need for love, envy, and jealousy of mother; frustration and aggression stemming from mother; counteraggression and its projection onto her; and the spiraling effect of the projection of aggression onto the image of a frightfully sadistic and destructive mother. The therapist's availability as a real object permitted a diagnosis, as part of the total perception of the transference/countertransference situation, of these various components and their analytic resolution.

A contrasting approach would have been to gratify the patient's transference demands by indicating that she was indeed "special" to the therapist by shifting from a position of technical neutrality into that of an orally giving parent. There are therapists, for example, who at such points might offer extra time, express directly their positive feelings for the patient, or even hold the patient's hand. I think such an approach ill-advised and harmful in the long run; one pays a high price for the temporary relief that the patient experiences when transference demands for love are met.

Third, the sequence illustrates the shift from a predominantly dyadic, pregenital transference into the beginning of a triadic and oedipal one as the pregenital components are elaborated in the transference. The patient's envy and jealousy of the therapist's family contained elements of oral envy (the therapist prefers his children over the patient and feeds them with all his love) and also oedipal elements (jealousy of the relation between the therapist and his wife and/or his adolescent daughter). In the second session the patient also directly referred to sexual fantasies and desires for the therapist, as well as concern for her remaining sexual difficulties with her boyfriend.

Fourth, the overall sequence illustrates that the primitive transferences cannot be explored separately from the working through of ordinary neurotic transferences, and that there are repetitive cycles in which primitive transference dominates, is understood and worked through, then shifts into a neurotic transference with which it is genetically connected, illustrating in the process the intimate relation between pregenital and genital conflicts in cases with severe character pathology.

Perhaps I should repeat that the sequence I have described occurred after approximately four years of treatment, that the patient had been quite obviously on the road to improvement, in terms of symptoms, social functioning, and the development of the transference. In summary, the stalemate reflecting the patient's submission to and identification with a sadistic primitive maternal image could be resolved analytically by working through the primitive transference reflecting this internalized object relationship.

Part Three

THE INDIVIDUAL
IN GROUPS

Chapter Eleven

Regression in Groups

My initial interest in group processes stemmed from my explorations of the subject of love (on which, more in Part Four). I have found a psychoanalytic study of large-group processes of particular importance on several counts. First, it permits us to apply psychoanalytic understanding to organizational and administrative functioning and thus to gain an additional dimension to the problem of "morale" (the direct manifestation of group processes within organizational structures). Then too, applying object relations theory to large-group functioning increases our understanding of the regressive temptations and dangers to the individual in such groups. Finally, the study of large groups helps to explain processes that take place in small groups, which, in turn, illuminate the intricate interplay between groups and individuals.

My starting point is Freud's pioneering work *Group Psychology and the Analysis of the Ego* (1921). The translation of the title of that work requires a short digression. The most accurate English word for the German *Masse* is a crowd or, even better, horde or mob. A crowd is a large human conglomerate without any formal organization; a horde or mob is a crowd that has a certain rudimentary but clearly visible organization in terms of direction, purpose, or motivation, usually characterized by its high emotional quality. One might say that mobs are temporary hordes and that certain social and political conditions may transform a crowd into a mob.

Insofar as Freud was referring to the psychology of large human groups characterized by some organized but highly affective and irrational behavior, he was describing hordes or mobs. The term mob, however, has depreciatory connotations that are absent in the German *Masse*: it should be stressed that this connotation is inappropriate and irrelevant in the discussion that follows.

Freud described the primitive, emotionally driven, unreflective behavior of hordes or mobs, and explained the sense of immediate closeness or intimacy of individuals with each other in mobs as derived from the projection of their ego ideal onto the leader, and the identification of the members of the horde with him as well as with each other. The projection of the ego ideal onto the idealized leader eliminates individual moral constraints as well as the higher functions of self-criticism and responsibility that are so importantly mediated by the superego. The mutual identifications of the members of the mob bring about a sense of unity and belonging that protects them from losing their sense of identity but is accompanied by severe reduction in ego functioning. As a result, primitive, ordinarily unconscious needs take over, and the mob functions under the sway of drives and affects, excitement and rage stimulated and directed by the leader.

Freud linked these concepts with the ideas contained in "Totem and Taboo" (1913), suggesting that the leader of the primal horde was the original father, killed by the alliance of the sons and replaced by the totemic law that regulates the life of the horde and protects it from self-destructive rivalry among the sons and from incestuous endogamy. In his postscript to *Group Psychology and the Analysis of the Ego,* Freud refers to the myth of the hero as a reflection of the ritualization of the fantasy that the youngest son was able to kill his father, thus becoming the idealized hero of the other sons and permitting them, through unconscious identification with him, to participate in the success of parricide without acknowledging their guilt. The leader of the horde represents the idealized, mythical hero; but, by the same token, the idealization of the leader also includes the original idealization of the oedipal father.

Bion (1961) described regressive processes that occur in small groups. His observations were based on the fantasies, fears, and behavior in unstructured groups of eight to twelve members whose leader consistently refused to participate in any decision or structuring of the group other than to observe its behavior. Bion's theory of small-group processes probably constitutes the most important psychoanalytic contribution to understanding group behavior since Freud. My observations of large groups, both structured and unstructured, confirm Bion's findings, and because his ideas are so relevant to my thesis, I shall recapitulate them here (see also Kernberg, 1976a, Chapter 9).

Bion described the regressive processes he observed in small groups in terms of basic emotional assumptions ("basic assumptions group"): the "fight-flight" assumption, the "dependency" assumption, and the "pairing" assumption. These assumptions constitute the basis for group reactions that potentially exist at all times, but are particularly activated when the task structure ("work group") breaks down.

The "dependency" group perceives the leader as omnipotent and omniscient and themselves inadequate, immature, and incompetent. Their idealization of the leader is matched by desperate efforts to extract knowledge, power, and goodness from him in a greedy and forever-dissatisfied way. When the leader fails to live up to such an ideal of perfection, the members react first with denial and then with a rapid, complete devaluation of him and a search for substitute leadership. Thus, primitive idealization, projected omnipotence, denial, envy, and greed, together with defenses against these, characterize the dependency group. Its members feel united by a common sense of needfulness, helplessness, and a fear of an outside world vaguely experienced as empty or frustrating.

The "fight-flight" group is united against what it vaguely perceives as external enemies. This group expects the leader to direct the fight against such enemies and to protect the group from in-fighting. The group, however, cannot tolerate any opposition to the "ideology" shared by the majority of its members and easily splits into subgroups which fight each other. Frequently, one subgroup becomes subservient to the idealized leader, while another attacks the first subgroup or is in flight from it. The group's tendency to control the leader or to experience itself controlled by him, to experience "closeness" in a shared denial of intragroup hostility, and to project aggression onto an out-group, all are prevalent. In short, splitting, projection of aggression, and projective identification prevail, and the search for nurture and dependency characteristic of the dependency group is replaced, in the fight-flight group, by conflicts around aggressive control, with suspiciousness, fighting, and dread of annihilation.

The "pairing" assumption leads the group to focus on two of its members — a couple (usually but not necessarily heterosexual) — to symbolize the pairing group's hopeful expectation that the selected couple will "reproduce itself," thus preserving the group's threatened identity and survival. The fantasies experienced about this selected pair express the group's hope that, by means of a magical "sexual" union, the group will be saved from the conflicts related to both the dependent and fight-flight assumptions. The pairing group, in short, experiences general intimacy and sexual developments as a potential protection against the dangerous conflicts around dependency and aggression that characterize the fight-flight and the dependency groups. The two latter groups have a pregenital character, in contrast to the genital one of the pairing group.

If we compare Bion's findings with Freud's description of the psychology of hordes or mobs, we see that in the small group similar processes of development of irrationality, mutual identification, and idealization of the leader make their appearance, but with the addition of the following features that differentiate small groups from mobs. First, the task-oriented group leader's refusal to assume the roles assigned to him by the group leads to frustration and to the search for alternative ways of dealing with the leadership issue (expressed in the shift among basic-assumption groups), concurrently with the search for alternative leaders within the group who will oblige the group by assuming the role the task leader refused. In this connection, the fact that group members with passive-dependent, hypomanic, or narcissistic features are so easily tempted to take the leadership of the dependent group, and members with severely paranoid features are drawn to the leadership of the fight-flight group, highlights the relationship between individual psychopathology and group processes in the small group.

Second, there is a striking appearance in the small group of defensive mechanisms characteristic of primitive ego organization (splitting, denial, projective identification, idealization, omnipotence) and, in relation to these, of intense aggression with rather primitive features. Le Bon (1895) and Freud (1921) referred to the direct manifestations of violence of mobs; in contrast, the potential for violence is still under control in the small group, not only by the use of the mechanisms mentioned, but also because a certain civilized attitude is maintained in the context of "eye-to-eye contact" and mutual acquaintance, which tone down the aggression. The absence of an "external enemy," however, occasionally raises the group tensions to high pitches. By implication, an external enemy absorbs the aggression generated within groups, but aggression threatens groups that cannot define or locate such external enemies.

Third, the search — in the pairing group — for an idealized couple that will protect the group from the dangers of aggression by means of the couple's sexualized relationship is a counterpart to the animosity and resentment the mob and some social organizations display toward couples, which Freud (1921) described.

Rice (1965) and Turquet (1975) studied the behavior of large unstructured groups, that is, groups of 40 to 120 persons, in ways similar to Bion's study of small-group processes. In such large groups it is impossible for the members to maintain eye-to-eye contact, which differentiates large from small groups; and, in contrast to what happens in mobs, any individual member of the large group can still be heard and responded to by any other member. Turquet stressed the individual member's sense of total loss of identity in large-group situations, and a concomitant, dramatic decrease in the capacity to evaluate realistically the effects of what he or she says and does within such a group setting. The ordinary social feedback to the individual member's verbal communications disappears, there seems to be a general incapacity to listen to anyone, all dialogue is drowned by the discontinuity of communication that evolves, and efforts to establish small, more familiar subgroups typically fail.

The individual is thrown into a void; even projective mechanisms fail because it is impossible to evaluate realistically the behavior of anyone else; therefore, projections become multiple and unstable, and an urgent task for the individual is to find some kind of "skin" by which to differentiate himself from his neighbors.

Turquet described the immediate temptation to withdraw totally from such a social experience, to revert to one's own past as guidance to deal with a large-group situation, and the paradox that such a withdrawal or reversion to the past may control or eliminate the anxiety produced by the loss of a sense of identity, but at the cost of bringing about a total disconnection from the large group, thus further increasing the individual's sense of isolation and impotence. This sense of impotence may motivate him to further withdraw from the group, or else to search for something in common with others in the large group that seems unattainable. For reasons to be mentioned below, only "common-sense" trivialities permit a temporary unification of the large group, and are a further threat to the individual's sense of identity. In essence, severe identity diffusion is both a major aspect of individual members' experience and a general characteristic of unstructured large-group phenomena.

Turquet also described a fear of aggression, of loss of control, and of violent behavior which might emerge at any time in the large group. The fear is the counterpart to provocative behaviors among the individuals of the group, behaviors expressed in part randomly, and mostly directed at the leader. The frequency of mutual attacks, rejections, distortions, and accusations is remarkable, and the intensity of aggression the most remarkable. It gradually emerges that it is those individuals who try to stand up to this atmosphere and maintain some semblance of individuality who are most attacked. It is as if, in the large group, there were a general envy of people who maintain their sanity and individuality. At the same time, efforts at homogenization are prevalent, and any simplistic generalization or ideology that permeates the group may be easily picked up and transformed into an experience of absolute truth. In contrast to the simple rationalization of the violence that permeates the mob, however, in the large group a vulgar or "common-sense" philosophy functions as a calming, reassuring doctrine which reduces all thinking to obvious clichés. One cannot escape the impression that aggression in the large group mainly takes the form of envy of thinking, of individuality, and of rationality.

LARGE-GROUP PROCESSES:
THEORETICAL CONSIDERATIONS

I suggest that some of the strikingly regressive features of small groups, large groups, and mobs may be better understood in the light of our present knowledge of the internalized object relations that predate object constancy and the consolidation of the ego, superego, and id.

Combining the observations made of mobs, large groups, and small groups, I am suggesting that group processes pose a basic threat to personal identity, linked to a proclivity in group situations for the activation of primitive object relations, primitive defensive operations, and primitive aggression with predominantly pregenital features. These processes, particularly the activation of primitive aggression, are dangerous to the survival of the individual in the group as well as to any task the group needs to perform. I think Turquet's description of what happens in large groups constitutes the basic situation against which both the idealization of the leader in the horde described by Freud, and the small-group processes described by Bion, are defending. To blindly follow the idealized leader of the mob reconstitutes a sort of identity by identification with him, as described by Freud, permits protection from intragroup aggression by this common identity and the shared projection of aggression to external enemies, and gratifies dependency needs by submission to the leader. Paradoxically, the essential irrational quality of mobs: that is, crowds temporarily organized into group formation by a shared idealization of a leader and a corresponding ideology—provides better protection against painful awareness of aggression than what obtains in large-group situations with undefined external enemies, and in small groups where it is hard to avoid being aware that the "enemy" is right in the midst of the group itself.

The study of large-group processes highlights the threat to individual identity under social conditions in which ordinary role functions are suspended and various projective mechanisms are no longer effective (because of the loss of face-to-face contact and personal feedback). Obviously, large-group processes can be obscured or controlled by rigid social structuring. Bureaucratization, ritualization, and well-organized task performance are different methods with similar immediate effects.

Large-group processes also highlight the intimate connection between threats to retaining one's identity and fear that primitive aggression and aggressively infiltrated sexuality will emerge. I think that the observations from the study of individual patients, of small groups, and of group processes in organizational and institutional life within which many adult work functions are carried out, confirm the overwhelming nature of human aggression in unstructured group situations.

The point is that an important part of nonintegrated and unsublimated aggression is expressed in vicarious ways throughout group and organizational processes. When relatively well-structured group processes evolve in a task-oriented organization, aggression is channeled toward the decision-making process, particularly by evoking primitive-leadership characteristics in people in positions of authority. Similarly, the exercise of power in organizational and institutional life constitutes an important channel for the expression of aggression in group processes that would ordinarily be under control in dyadic or triadic relations. Aggression emerges more directly and much more intensely when group processes are relatively unstructured.

The multiplicity of primitive self- and object representations that predominate as intrapsychic structures before the consolidation of ego, superego, and id — and, therefore, before the consolidation of ego identity — and the regressive features of part-object relations that evolve when normal ego identity disintegrates are remarkably parallel to the relationships among all individuals within a large-group situation.

The reciprocal reinforcement of a regressive potential in ego structure, on the one hand, and certain social and organizational conditions that promote unstructured large-group processes, on the other, raise two questions. To what extent do normal identity integration and mature ego functioning remain dependent upon the socially determined, that is, the role-aspects of dyadic and triadic internalized object relations? And to what extent are certain types of regressive potentials in individuals much more available than can be ascertained in ordinary social interactions? The chaotic multiple interpersonal struggles that evolve in the large group have their parallel in the ability of borderline patients within a hospital setting to induce conflicts between members of the staff that reflect the enactment of the patients' pathological internalized object relations in the surrounding social field. Within the struggles of small unstructured groups, the fight between factions, particularly in the "fight-flight" group, may be similarly considered an expression, within this social setting, of intrapsychic conflicts that cannot be fully tolerated and integrated by the individual members of the group.

The activation of infantile sexual features in group life is also striking. In the small group, sexuality emerges in the basic assumption of pairing as one defense against primitive aggression; in the large group, sexuality is either denied or expressed in sadistically infiltrated sexual allusions. It usually goes underground, however, and secret formation of couples occurs as a direct reaction to and defense against large-group processes. In the horde, unchallenged idealization of the leader is the counterpart of the group's intolerance of the couple that would attempt to preserve its identity as such (Freud, 1921).

Dissociated and repressed aspects of sexuality, as well as projections of superego-determined prohibitions against infantile sexuality, are easily expressed in all group situations and influence the individual's and the couple's attitudes toward their own sexuality under the impact of the group experience.

There is a striking tendency in large groups to project superego functions on the group as a whole as part of an effort to prevent violence and protect ego identity by means of a shared ideology. The concomitant need of all groups to project and externalize superego functions onto the leader reflects not only sadistic aspects of primitive superego forerunners but also the realistic and protective aspects of more mature superego functioning. The indissoluble union of primitive and advanced aspects of the superego makes this a tragic externalization: the morality of groups and institutions influenced by projection of primitive superego features comes closer to the primitive morality of the unconscious superego than to the conscious morality of the mature individual.

The projection of superego functions and the related submission to authoritarian leadership does protect against violence and against the destruction of couples within the group, but it is condensed with the prohibition against incest and against the most infantile aspects of sexuality. Thus, group morality veers toward a conventional desexualization of heterosexual relations, the suppression of erotic fantasy insofar as it involves infantile polymorphous trends and sensuous eroticism, and toward acknowledging and sanctioning the more "permissible" love relations. The alternative to these defensive efforts — and their miscarriage in repressive ideologies — is the eruption of crude, particularly anally tinged, sexuality in large-group situations, very reminiscent of sexualized group formations of latency and early adolescence.

LARGE-GROUP PROCESSES: CLINICAL OBSERVATIONS

What follows is a review of a three-year experience in conducting a specially designed community meeting at a 50-bed inpatient service geared to the diagnosis and intensive treatment of patients with borderline personality organization and severe character pathology, and a selected group of chronic schizophrenic patients who, after their failure to respond to treatment with ordinary psychopharmacological and rehabilitational methods, were given intensive psychotherapy. As director of that clinical service I had practically full control regarding the admission, treatment, and discharge of the patients, and also appropriate authority for the general educational and research functions on that service. A specially selected and highly qualified nursing staff and social service staff were supplemented by clinical services provided by psychiatric residents assigned full time, for one year to the service and made it possible for two full-time attending psychiatrists and myself to count on adequate resources for a challenging and difficult job.

Every Monday afternoon, a 45-minute community meeting took place, with staff, residents, and patients in attendance. The size of the group fluctuated between 40 and 70 participants, approximately half of whom were staff and half patients. The chief resident conducted the meeting as an unstructured-large-group experience. The primary task of the meeting was to share information regarding issues affecting all members of the therapeutic community and to diagnose themes and conflicts affecting patients and staff. No formal decision-making took place; it was made very explicit that all decision-making occurred in other publicly defined structures. It was also assumed that the knowledge gained from the community meeting would influence all other administrative decision-making, and provide potentially therapeutic functions for patients and educational functions for residents and other trainees.

At the beginning of each meeting, the chief resident reiterated that patients and staff were all expected to discuss freely, without any set agenda, what was concerning them at the time and to observe the nature of the conflicts emerging in the group as the discussion proceeded. I shall mention briefly the findings that seem relevant to the theoretical considerations just discussed.

Condensation of Primitive Aggression and Sexuality

Because late-adolescent and young adult patients of both sexes predominated, intense sexual tensions and conflicts could have been expected. Therefore, neither the extent to which heterosexual and homosexual promiscuity combined with overtly sadistic and masochistic behavior became a major issue in the relations between patients nor the content of dramatic confrontations in group meetings came as any surprise. What was impressive, however, was the group's chronic intolerance of sexual excitement and interests when linked to concern, tenderness, and a sense of mutual responsibility. Clearly, sexuality could only be conceived of as either a primitive form of rebellious, promiscuous, aggressive living-out of polymorphous perverse fantasies or else as a highly conventional, superficial, sentimental portrayal of "pure love," which implied a denial of the relation between love and sexual affirmation. By projection, staff was alternatively experienced as sadistically provocative and gleeful, enjoying the expression of sexual behavior on the part of patients, or else as primitively puritanical, too conventional, and intolerant of any expression of sexuality.

Denial of Projected Aggression

Staff experienced enormous difficulties in overcoming an unconscious collusion with the patients, who sat silently, fell asleep, or appeared to be totally indifferent to what was going on around them. Given the intense affectively charged, often violent nature of interactions on the service throughout the day, this frozen atmosphere took on special significance. Early efforts to interpret it as the patients' defense against very paranoid distortions of staff first met with blatant denial, but consistent interpretation eventually led to the activation in the patients of intense suspicion and hatred of staff, who were perceived as primitive, frustrating, and domineering authorities.

Interpretation along the lines that passivity and indifference were expressing the denial of a dangerous persecutory authority and that that persecutory authority in turn represented the projection onto staff of the patients' own dissociated aggression often permitted dramatic movement from passivity and indifference to more or less open, excited expression of sexualized aggression. Repetitive cycles from passivity to sexualized aggression evolved over a period of months into a greater capacity for integrating within the large-group setting those feelings with loving, dependent, gratifying relationships, which were evolving simultaneously among patients and between patient and staff and which previously had been dissociated in the large-group process.

Depression and Mourning

The integration of the large-group process with the rest of the life on the service, with implications of integrating love and hate, led, particularly in better-functioning patients, to depression and a related integration of ego functioning. This interpretation became a dominant theme when the reasons for the anger at and hatred for staff had been elaborated in detail within a tolerant atmosphere.

For example, when in March of each year, the second-year psychiatric residents in charge of the individual psychotherapy of the patients first mentioned their forthcoming rotation of July and the question of which patient would remain with which therapists arose, important group processes followed. At first, the community meetings expressed a general sense of betrayal, intense envy, and jealousy among the patients as they compared their treatment plans, condensed with strong expressions of pathological mourning. Typically, over several weeks following the announcements about rotation, the patients developed intensely paranoid reactions to staff, together with the denial of all dependency on staff and of any gratitude for what they, the patients, had received. The deadening denial of all emotional reality that temporarily emerged was striking. Under favorable circumstances, this reaction was followed by more direct expressions of rage and the perception of selected staff members as sadistic, ruthless, primitive parental figures. Eventually, patients were able to talk about mourning, longing, guilt feelings, and regrets for the aggressive distortions of all emotional relationships within the service.

The Ascendence of Narcissistic and Antisocial Personalities

One other striking, and at first disconcerting observation was that, under conditions of intense turmoil and stress, the patient group might consolidate in what appeared as a more task-oriented group formation under the leadership of one of the more narcissistic borderline patients, often a patient with clearly antisocial features. It was as if, under conditions of social stress and disorganized large-group functioning, patients with pathological narcissism were better equipped to take on leadership functions than the "ordinary" patient with identity diffusion, or, at times, even "normal" staff members of the large group. There was something frightening about the fact that patients with antisocial features appeared particularly able to relate "realistically" in large-group situations. This finding requires a more general exploration of the reasons for the ascendance of the narcissistic personality in large-group processes.

When large-group processes are operating, two types of individuals are particularly protected from the prevailing identity diffusion. The first is the schizoid personality, for whom total withdrawal from the chaotic conditions of the large group duplicates a well-known path, and who can tolerate the condition of being a "singleton." The second, the person with strong pathological narcissistic tendencies, is particularly well equipped to deal with large-group situations.

The lack of deep conviction regarding his own values makes it easy for the narcissistic personality to swim with the currents of the group. The manipulative, exploitative character of his relations to others, his need to put himself into the foreground of collective attention and admiration, and his immediate realization that the group is searching for a shared reassuring set of ideas that will restore its security may permit him, given he has certain talents for communication, to provide an acceptable ideology and to convey a sense of certainty without triggering the group's envy against individualist thinking, all of which may make him the grand leveler of the group's tensions. Thus, paradoxically, the political opportunist may have important stabilizing functions at times of organizational regression.

The relation between such temporary leadership under large-group conditions and effective political leadership is evident here. I must stress that I am not implying that professional politicians are necessarily narcissistic personalities.

Insofar as small-group processes may also, under conditions of both dependency and pairing, gratify pathological narcissistic needs, the narcissistic personality seems to be particularly well equipped for functioning within both small and large unstructured-group processes, a situation very different from that required for functional leadership over an extended period of time. Groups meeting for a short time may present the danger of facilitating adaptive processes of some narcissistic participants who will utilize—rather than learn from—the group experiences. Institutional leaders should therefore exercise caution in selecting personnel on the basis of what they observe in an individual functioning in a time-limited group situation, although, by the same token, the group experience may dramatically highlight narcissistic and other types of character pathology.

The problem with the ascendence of the narcissistic personality in small and large group situations is that he may express, as part of his leadership function in regressive group processes, ideas acceptable to subgroups or the entire group because they are trivial, superficial, convincing, and easily understood. These ideas will be in response to and responsive to certain group actions, and will play right into the messianic or paranoid affect states that link the dependent-pairing or the fight-flight group constellations, or subgroups of the large group or even the large group *in toto*. The narcissistic personality constitutes an excellent instrument for transforming any ideology, regardless of its value, into a manageable system of immediately convincing slogans and clichés. Here, narcissistic leadership and the group's search for an ideology merge and reinforce each other.

Other Typical Observations in the Large Group

We observed patients' intolerance of individual thinking, the suspicion of original ideas, the envy of patients who seemed to preserve their autonomy. We were impressed by the facility with which primitive superego features distorted the perception of administrative decisions, and by the enormous amounts of time required for their resolution. We found dissociated sadism frequently expressed "by proxy." Individual members of subgroups incited one against the other, the other members becoming "innocent bystanders." The subtle ways in which the innocent bystanders influenced opposing "extremists" illustrate similar organizational problems in malfunctioning institutions. The masochistic rejection of sexuality, often reflecting a harsh and infantile conventional morality running counter to the simultaneous covert expression of primitive sexuality in destructive ways, was a continuing feature of group discussions. We found that the more that rational attitudes toward sexuality could be fostered in open discussions of these issues, the less such sadistically infiltrated "underground" sexual expression occurred. At times, patients became aware of the extent to which they colluded in a primitive, infantile, sadistically infiltrated sexualized ideology and how they projected equally sadistic prohibitions against it onto staff.

Group Processes Affecting Patients and Staff

It needs to be stressed that in our technique of conducting these large-group meetings, we never focused on individual patients' pathology per se, but only on the dynamic implications of "here and now" contents, emotional reactions, and behavior. However, patients spontaneously related these discussions to their own difficulties, in the same way that staff related large-group observations to the overall treatment atmosphere on the service and to the relation between patients' needs as a group, the availability of staff, and particular conflicts within the staff.

Each therapeutic community meeting was followed by a 45-minute discussion of it by staff only, again exploring group processes in the "here and now" among staff. What follows is an analysis of the positive and negative effects of these meetings for the treatment of patients and for the professional development of staff. Again, I highlight those findings that have relevance for the study of regression as a characteristic of group processes.

Staff was able to utilize the observations and self-observations within the large-group setting for better understanding of patients' transferences and emotional reactions, including countertransference, that patients were able to evoke in staff. For many residents, students, and staff members, the contents of the "dynamic unconscious," ordinarily repressed and only observable in derivative phenomena or in intensive individual treatment, emerged for the first time strongly and concretely in the content of the large-group meetings. Staff and patients could observe shared paranoid, hypomanic, depressive, and guilt-ridden group reactions, the manifestations of denial, projective identification, and the expression by individual patients of fantasies and actions that reflected immediately shared group "myths." The shifts in the various emotional constellations in the group provided an immediate learning experience for the residents about primitive emotional reality and prevalent defenses connected with it. Our psychiatric residents could transfer such learning into the understanding of the severe psychopathology of their patients as it emerged in individual psychotherapy sessions. Psychoanalytic theory, and a theory of technique of psychoanalytic psychotherapy became a more concrete, emotionally real experience.

The contamination of staff by group processes affecting patients was impressive. The staff's awareness of the universality of the regressive potential in group processes had a sobering effect. For example, a small group of patients started the rumor that I, who clearly have a German accent and whom they had observed speaking Spanish to some elevator operators was probably a Nazi who had first escaped to Argentina and had now been called to this institution because of my experiences with concentration camps. This rumor, embedded in a "fight-flight" group atmosphere and in the conflictual wish, vaguely shared by patients and staff alike, for a powerful authority which would control all expression of aggression in the social system of the service, finally became a shared fantasy that affected even staff members, one of whom actually approached me to assure me that he did not believe the rumor but, just in case, could I reassure him. . . .

Patients became aware of conflicts among staff, and this could sometimes be put to therapeutic use. As one example, patients became aware of administrative conflicts between the director and the associate director of the service; fantasies and rumors emerged in the large group that implied a life-and-death struggle, unending mutual envy, rivalry, and jealousy between those two staff members and their fantasied followers. In reality, the administrative conflicts were tolerated and resolved and expressed in a creative professional collaboration. Within the large group, however, we allowed these fantasies to emerge without prematurely reassuring the patients: Eventually, the patients could contrast them with the observable facts that two staff members could disagree with each other without having to abandon their collaboration in the large group. Tolerance of differences among staff led to a decrease of intolerance among patients.

Violent behavior between patients sometimes indirectly reflected conflicts between them and staff. In one instance, an impulsive, histrionic transvestite male patient who proclaimed his "femininity" in provocative behavior was hated by male patients, particularly those struggling against strong homosexual impulses. Female patients, in contrast, seemed to be mildly amused by him, but he evoked strong hostility in female staff. We finally diagnosed the unconscious collusion of both male and female patients in coaxing this patient into temporarily taking over the leadership and the focus of attention of the large group. It was the patients' way of attacking staff as "conventional and square," and a displacement of hatred for the — mostly female — nursing staff by subtle encouragement of what all the patients experienced as a hateful caricature of women.

This understanding, reached by the staff first and then ventilated in the large group, permitted the patient to become more aware of his hatred of women and to carry this awareness into his individual psychotherapy sessions.

One other positive effect of this work was to activate the staff to become highly motivated to participate and understand these group processes. In fact, staff was strongly tempted to participate in them as if they were patients — which leads to the dangers and negative effects of this method, my next point.

REGRESSIVE EFFECTS OF LARGE-GROUP PROCESSES ON STAFF FUNCTIONING

The "Messianic" Sense of Mission

All task groups develop "sentience" (a sense of emotional cohesion as a group) around the task, but the study of how group processes affect staff as well as patients brought about a particular activation of group sentience which had an exhilarating effect on all participants. The phenomenon was hard to diagnose at the time — indeed, some of the conclusions that follow were reached months and even years after the completion of the experience.

First, insofar as staff implicitly placed all the "sickness" within the patient group or within the administrative hierarchy of the institution, the staff members were tempted to see themselves as eminently reasonable, dedicated, intelligent, well-intentioned participants in serious and creative work which was difficult and sometimes not fully appreciated by people outside the system (and certainly not by the patients).

A subtle tendency to project aggression outside the staff group and to consolidate as an idealized group that satisfied both dependent and sexualized needs — Rice (1965) first pointed to the intimate connection between the pairing and the dependent groups — emerged gradually and could not be fully diagnosed and resolved. Even when conflicts occurred within the staff, the efforts to explore and resolve them reasonably implied that staff was imbued with a somewhat naïve, almost Pollyanna idea that all could be resolved by openness and reasonableness; the denial of ordinary ambivalence, aggression, and contradictory interests among staff was clearly exaggerated.

One might say that staff members managed, over a period of time, to collude in projecting their own aggression onto the patient group as well as the outgroup represented by the institution as a whole. A complementary development occurred in this context; hostile and envious reactions rose throughout the institution and were directed at this particular service, which was perceived as unduly privileged, self-centered, and haughty.

It would appear that groups that gather to learn about their own processes assume that there are no contradictory interests, no insoluble conflicts among them and that human beings, given a chance to discuss things reasonably with each other, will be able to work effectively and end up the better for it. This may be true of temporary groups such as a group-relation conference, but certainly does not correspond to all we know about group processes in general. In short, the examination of interpersonal reality implicitly activated a broadly shared idea of basic trust and confidence that had regressive features.

In this connection, there was a certain similarity between the staff experience and the effects of the short-term, small-group processes that occur in study groups, encounter groups, and various group-therapy methods, which promote "instant intimacy" and, with it, the easy activation of a sense of exhilaration, goodness, optimism, and self-satisfaction. The eroticized atmosphere of the pairing group (sometimes openly fostered in certain group-therapy methods by physical contacts and interactions) combined with a "total openness" about mutual fantasies and wishes in an atmosphere in which hostility, while tolerated, is "reasonably" resolved and explained away within a strong group cohesion, foster a sense of immediate oneness of the individual with the group, an acquisition of shared intimacy and power that causes the small group to resemble the mob intoxicated by identification with its leader.

The group's sense of oneness can be seen to parallel certain defensive operations found in hypomanic and in narcissistic personalities. The group's shared sexual excitement — uncomplicated by the intense ambivalence that would be found in a couple — together with its denial of aggression within the group correspond to the feelings of omnipotence, triumph, and contempt for those outside the magic circle brought on by introjection and self-idealization in hypomanic and narcissistic personalities.

Negative consequences of these developments on our service included denial of painful realities, deterioration of task performance, and an increase of the level of aspirations from work, which eventually brought about excessive frustration with the ordinary aspects of task performance.

Narcissistic Deteriorations

This heading covers several related phenomena. First, a pseudo-intimacy developed among the members of the staff group, a consequence of their open examination of psychological processes within a group setting, leading to a sense of closeness that related only to the task but was experienced as if it had profound human implications. The sense of closeness had a quality of emotional "stripping," but lacked differentiated concern for others. This is similar to what can so frequently be observed in encounter groups and group-relations conferences, where intense relationships over a brief period of time bring about a sense of great intimacy with persons whose names have been forgotten a few weeks later. The process seems particularly marked in narcissistic personalities, on whom this pseudo-intimacy has an exhilarating effect, replacing the more dangerous or unavailable relationships in depth with others by the easy, mutual acceptance that is automatically experienced within such groups.

The counterpart to pseudointimacy was a growing sense of physical and emotional exhaustion that we observed among staff over a period of time, particularly affecting the more mature members for whom the emotional engagement with other staff members required by our approach constituted an authentic effort. The intensity of their dedication, in a word, exhausted them. Students or residents with marked narcissistic features, however, throve on these intense experiences as fish do in water. While capacities for leadership in the field of group dynamics and the analytic study of group processes are not necessarily linked to narcissistic predispositions, narcissistic personalities may easily dominate group settings, with negative consequences for themselves and such settings.

One expression of this dominance was the transformation of language denoting intense emotional experiences into clichés and slogans. We observed that some members of the staff learned the language of regression without really experiencing the emotional implications of such terms as rage, persecution, or homosexual excitement.

An additional and related complication was the gradual increase of staff's concern with itself as a group; there was a natural tendency for the staff to spend more and more time discussing its own dynamics; indeed, one staff member complained, "If we just didn't have to take care of all these patients, we could resolve all the problems we have among ourselves." This concern was also reflected in the temptation for the administrative leadership of the service to neglect evaluating the total staff time spent in discussing group dynamics. Indeed, the establishment of therapeutic community models often seems to bring about an increasing absorption of staff in group meetings, a decrease of an effective utilization of time, and a loss of a sense of awareness of this process. By the same token, there were strong pressures on the leadership of the service to confirm the messianic sense of mission of the staff, and, particularly, for the director of the service to become a leader of either a dependent group or a sexualized pairing group, or else to establish rigidly bureaucratic norms of behavior as a protection against conflict and aggression. This illustrates the temptations that groups create to replace functional leadership by authoritarian or charismatic leadership or by a protective bureaucratization of the system.

*The Erosion of Decision-Making, Quality Control,
and of the Political Dimension of Boundary Control*

Insofar as an examination of group processes on the service required a functional administrative setting that would lend itself to
open examination of such processes, an extreme vigilance regarding
any development of excessive or distorted expressions of personal
power evolved. We were extremely sensitive to the possibility that
the development of the decision-making process might become
distorted, and were constantly concerned over preserving functional
leadership. The short-term effects of these policies favored functional decision-making. The long-term effects operated toward dilut-
ing functional authority, a growing tendency to transform functional
into democratic decision-making processes, and — retrospectively — a
striking innocence regarding the political dimension of boundary
control, that is, the influence of our service on other services, disci-
plines, and administrative structures within and outside the institution. All these are related processes: Because of the emotional
closeness that evolved within the staff group, once somebody was
accepted as part of the group, quality control slackened and there
was a tendency to replace administrative by therapeutic ways of
dealing with staff.

I must confess that I am afraid I was unduly influenced by the
hope and expectation that staff as well as patients would learn and
mature in this experience, and so I tended to neglect the differences
between individuals. My determination to avoid an authoritarian
attitude evolved into a reluctance to critically evaluate their progress
and to confront them with serious shortcomings when these existed.
All of which should not be construed as meaning that the negative
effects predominated over the positive. It is only because my principal focus has been on regression in groups, that I have highlighted
the regressive features of that particular experience.

The Dimension of Time

Because short-term study groups and encounter groups do not
provide a temporal dimension, they are not subject to certain group

processes that take time to develop. One such process is the activation of aggression, not only as a constituent of basic-assumption groups, but as an inevitable human attribute. The adaptive and defensive measures which the individual members have at their disposal to cope with aggression may contribute to controlling regressive group pressures by fostering, in the individuals, autonomous, responsible handling of ordinary human ambivalence.

The "messianic" developments in small-group processes under the combined effect of dependent and pairing assumptions tend to wear off rather quickly under ordinary organizational circumstances, thus destroying one regressive illusion triggered in short-term groups. By the same token, one of the reasons that what is learned from experiential group situations fails to be transposed into the work organization is the failure to fully analyze the messianic group spirit which many members carry with them to extragroup activities.

This is a particular application of the general observation made by Katz and Kahn (1966) to the effect that the learning of new attitudes on the part of an organization's staff, in the context of exploring the irrational aspects of group processes in an experiential setting, frequently fails because this learning neglects the analysis of the stable features of the organizational structure and the relation between that structure and the real (in contrast to fantasied or irrational) conflicts of interests that such organizational structures mediate.

Then too, short-term learning experiences in groups may neglect the importance of personality structures in members of organizations, particularly the personality of key leaders. Under the impact of the analysis of group processes, the irrational behavior of individuals and groups tends to be negotiated in terms of the immediate task, the "here and now," which neglects long-term dimensions of personality impact. The distortion in the organization's administrative structure derived from its leader's personality structure can be compensated for by structural arrangements in the organization which may not seem functional in a cross-sectional analysis, but which in the long run may be a very functional compromise between the optimal utilization of the leader's personality by the organization, on the one hand, and an effort to reduce or control his distortion of administrative structures, on the other. In more general terms, the ideal of the total coincidence between formal and informal structure of organizations may lead to an exhausting, time-consuming, ongoing revision of the decision-making process, which, in the long run, is more expensive than some distortion between formal and informal decision-making processes — such as derived from the leader's personality.

To conclude, unstructured group processes activate immediate strong regressive trends because unstructured small and large groups resonate with primitive ego organization, part-object relations, primitive defenses, and condensations of primitive aggression and sexuality. Unstructured group processes also foster regression because they tap profound longings for protective messianic and paranoid ideologies; they weaken ordinary time considerations, traditional organizational structures, and personality influences in terms of the reality of the task; they foster, instead, narcissistic leadership and ideological simplifications, and naturally neglect the influence of political action and its subtly controlling and distorting effect on boundaries.

Group processes permit expression of part-object relations that are unavailable in ordinary life situations — except for the characterologically determined lifestyle of borderline and narcissistic patients. They offer temptations to express part-object relations with idealized features that have an almost unreal quality and are protected from ambivalence and aggression — while the aggression is projected onto out-groups, the leadership, the group as a whole, or is rationalized in the prevailing ideology.

Chapter Twelve

Organizational Regression

Having considered the effects of group processes on members of the group, I now turn to the vicissitudes of the relations between the leader's personality, the organizational structure, group processes occurring in the organization, and organizational tasks. The focus again will be on psychiatric institutions.

Sometimes, the carrying out of treatment, research, and education seems to be limited by the leader's personality problems. Very often staff see the leader as arbitrary and authoritarian, as though he or she were misusing power to impose courses of action detrimental to commonly shared goals, a perception that may be a misperception. There is, too, often a shared conception — or fantasy — among staff that depicts the leader as not understanding, as arrogant and revengeful. Careful analysis of the total situation by outside consultants, however, particularly when modern approaches of organizational diagnosis are utilized, may reveal various and at times quite complex situations.

The effectiveness of leadership does not depend exclusively or primarily on the leader's personality. The first requirement for effective functioning of an organization — including its leadership — is an adequate relation between the organization's overall task and its administrative structure; the task has to be meaningful rather than trivial and, given the available resources, feasible rather than overwhelming. Psychiatric institutions operate within various kinds of environments, and their effectiveness in carrying out therapeutic, educational, and research tasks depends on the adequacy of their human and material resources as well as on the nature of their interaction with the environment. When any of these conditions is not met — when resources are insufficient for the tasks to be carried out or when the normal flow of resources and "products" across the boundaries of the institution breaks down, or when contradictory goals or failure to clarify priorities interfere with the functional relationship between task and administrative structure — the task-group structures in the organization deteriorate, morale breaks down, and the group processes within the organization regress; this regression, in turn, strongly affects the quality and effectiveness of leadership. The development of group fight-flight or dependency assumptions (Bion, 1961) moves or reduces the leadership of originally task-oriented groups into stands complementary to the emotional needs of their members or staff: A staff who expects a primitive kind of leadership from an omnipotent, giving figure (in the dependent group) or a powerful or dangerous, controlling authority (in the fight-flight group) tempts or provokes the task leader to regress. If these group processes remain undiagnosed, only their end product may be visible, in the form of what appears to be primitive, inadequate leadership and, more specifically, negative effects of the leader's personality on the organization.

The group processes occurring in psychiatric institutions are influenced, however, not only by the degree of task orientation and task appropriateness on the part of administrative and therapeutic structures. The very nature of the task carried out in psychiatric institutions, particularly those treating severely regressed patients, also exerts a strong influence on these group processes. I am referring here to the replication of the pathological internal world of object relations induced by borderline and psychotic patients in the group processes involving staff and these patients on each service, ward, or section. At certain times, severely regressed patients may provoke basic-assumption group processes in both formal and informal patient and staff groups on a service. This negatively affects leadership and, perhaps, the administrative structure of the entire service. One might say that the nature of the "product" handled by psychiatric institutions, namely, primitive and deep human conflict, strongly influences the functioning of such institutions.

Again, in this case, only the end product of a chain process may be visible, and the administrator of the service or of the hospital may appear as arbitrary, threatening, and irrational. Only a careful organizational analysis may bring to the surface the relation between problems of patients and of leadership.

It is, of course, possible that serious psychopathology in the leader is indeed responsible for the problems of morale, of breakdown of task groups, and the development of regressive group processes. The problem, then, is to differentiate the activation of emotional regression in the leader, reflecting problems in the institution, from the deterioration of organizational functioning, reflecting psychopathology of the leader.

The traditional analysis of institutional management has focused on the leader's personality, particularly such "inborn" characteristics as "charisma" and "authoritarian" qualities. Psychoanalytic thinking has focused on the distorted perception that staff may have of the administrator or leader as a function of the irrational relations with authority that stem from infantile conflicts, particularly from the oedipal situation. More recent sociological thinking has stressed the "role" aspects of leadership—that is, the activation of socially sanctioned and recognized functions in which leader and follower have mutually reinforcing perceptions and behavior (Adorno et al., 1950; Hodgson et al., 1965; Levinson, 1968). This sociological view focuses on the confusion that often develops in organizations between the leader's personality, his or her behavior in carrying out certain roles, and the perception of his behavior on the part of staff, who cannot easily differentiate role from personality (particularly, of course, when perception of the leader is distorted by unconscious conflicts).

More recently still, the application of psychoanalytic methods to the study of small-group processes (Bion, 1961; Rice, 1965; Rioch, 1970a, b) has revealed the activation in nonstructured and informal groups of primitive emotional contents and defensive operations that are ordinarily latent in all individuals and only become manifest in patients with severe regression, such as borderline conditions and the functional psychoses. These findings further complicate the study of the interaction of the leader's personality, behavior, the perception of that behavior by staff, and the mutual induction of regressive behavior in staff and leader under the influence of regressive group processes.

It is here that a systems approach may be helpful, not only in clarifying how the leader's personality, group processes, organizational structure, and organizational tasks influence each other, but also in pointing to the major origin of the distortions affecting all of these. A systems approach to organizations considers the institution as an overall system dynamically and hierarchically integrating various subsystems (such as the personality of leadership, the nature of group processes, the task systems, and administrative structures of the organization) and conceives of the environment of the organization as suprasystems affecting the institution in dynamically and hierarchically organized ways (Rice, 1963, 1969; Levinson and Klerman, 1967; Dolgoff, 1973).

A systems approach can have significant diagnostic and corrective impact on the work in psychiatric institutions. It is in contrast to linear and mechanical models, which attribute the sources of organizational disturbances to one or another of the sub- or suprasystems mentioned.

Sometimes it is the nature of the task that is overwhelming, and sometimes institutions are directed by leaders who are actually not good at their job. It is important to be able to differentiate this type of situation from the much more frequent one in which leadership problem represents a symptom rather than the cause. It can happen that most of the energy of an institution seems to be spent on "curing" its leader; it may well be that the astonishing capacity of so many people in so many places to tolerate an unsatisfactory situation over an extended period of time indicates how gratifying it is to attribute the cause of all problems to the administrator, rather than to focus upon the painful and complex interaction of the various systems involved in bringing about his behavior.

I have not yet mentioned the political dimension of conflicting interests between groups in institutions which influence their relation to the task as well as to the leadership. If we conceive of political strivings as the conscious or unconscious efforts of individuals or groups to defend their interests and expand their influence over other individuals and/or groups at their "boundaries," political action can be seen to be a normal aspect of institutional interactions. Insofar as group interests stem from the members' identifications with values of a social, cultural, or professional nature, conflicts develop between belonging to "task" or to "nontask" determined groups — "sentience" groups (Miller and Rice, 1967). Sentience here refers to the emotional bonds influencing group formation and cohesiveness; such emotional bonds may derive from the task performance itself or from past or present, real or fantasied things in common that link individuals in groups. Political strivings may reflect the efforts to bring about an optimal equilibrium between these conflicting identifications.

However, when political strivings evolve into an ideological commitment to establish an optimal equilibrium between politically opposite groups regardless of task requirements, a new complication for organizational functioning has arisen. The purpose of psychiatric institutions is basically professional and technical rather than political, and serious distortions in the task, in group processes, administrative structures, and leadership may evolve when political objectives replace task-oriented or functional ones. For example, "democratization" of an administrative structure may be perceived as an ideal solution to organizational conflicts, with consequent deterioration of task groups, special skills, and individual functions and responsibilities. It is an illusion that authoritarianism in institutions can be successfully overcome by democratization rather than by a functional analysis of task requirements and their corresponding functional administrative structures. There are dictatorships of groups as well as of individuals, and these can result as much from paralysis as from capriciousness at the top.

A few clinical examples of the preceding theoretical formulations might be helpful.

The activities department of a psychiatric hospital perceived its leader as inefficient, weak, and wavering; an organizational analysis of the functions of the department revealed that important changes had occurred (derived from the "unitization" or compartmentalization of the hospital) resulting in a contradiction between independent hospital units and an integrated organization of the activities department. This contradiction had brought about an unbearable complication in scheduling meetings, communications, and interdisciplinary work. A change in the administrative structure and functions of the activities department in consonance with the new developments of the hospital was achieved, with the result that the activities' functioning became flexibly integrated into the new units, while certain activities specialists were still available for the hospital. The consequent resolution of tensions within the hospital and the activities department itself brought about a fundamental change in how the activities department perceived its leadership. Their director and his associates were now seen as strong and reliable.

In another instance, an acute conflict erupted between a hospital service director, several senior consultants, the psychiatric resident in charge of the treatment of a very difficult case, and various other staff members taking positions in one of two feuding fields. An "in-group," led by the service director, considered that the patient had been treated "too leniently," that insufficient hospital-milieu structure had been provided, and that the resident's acting out of rebelliousness against authority figures had complicated the treatment situation: the patient was seen as acting out the resident's rebellion. An "out-group," consisting of various staff members, the psychiatric resident in charge of the case, and his supervisor, all felt that the patient's ego weakness had been underestimated, that more time and patience was needed — rather than consistent confrontation — and they experienced the service director as rather ruthless and domineering in his handling of the clinical conferences in which the case was discussed. Analysis of the situation showed that quite specific intrafamilial dynamics of the patient had been activated and projected onto the relationships among the staff and had intensified the potential conflicts around authority and power of all those involved in the patient's treatment. Once this was clarified and the split among staff was healed, better understanding of the patient's dynamics could be utilized in his psychotherapeutic and hospital-milieu treatment.

Conflicts which developed in a psychiatric hospital between the departments of rehabilitation, occupational therapy, and recreational therapy were first perceived as personal, having to do with power on the part of the leaders of two of these three groups; it later emerged that the leader of one of the groups had indeed been given some authority over the other two, but without a clear mandate over who controlled at the joint boundaries of all three departments. Insofar as the three departments continued to function autonomously and no clear coordination or integration of all these activities was possible, the leader who had been tentatively selected to direct the entire area projected an image of uncertainty and doubt.

The question arose: Where is the problem? In the personality of the leader who was not able to assert his authority over the entire department? In the nature of the administrative structure of these three departments, which were confusingly intermingled and spread over the entire hospital? In the nature of the task, which had become unclear as changes in the hospital philosophy and utilization of occupational, recreational, and rehabilitative services clashed with the traditional background of experience of these departments? In order to arrive at an answer, it is helpful to start by defining, first, the nature of the task and its constraints; second, the optimal administrative structure required for the task; third, the nature and amount of the authority functionally required by the leader; fourth, the leader's technical and conceptual skills and liabilities; and, finally, the leader's personality characteristics which might be involved in the problem.

For practical purposes, it is sometimes helpful to simply hire a new administrative leader, selecting a person with known and proven conceptual, technical, and personal skills (Katz, 1955) to diagnose the nature of the task and the required administrative structure for task performance, so that the selection of the leader precedes the adequate diagnosis of all other factors in the hope that a solution becomes available before the problem is fully diagnosed. An alternative method also exists: to first diagnose the nature of the task and the required administrative structure for that task, and only then to search for the "right person." This second method is slower, requires more input from the organization as a whole before a decision can be made regarding the required new leader, but it may be less risky than the first method. It is much easier to hire the right person when the nature of the task and its constraints have been clarified, although time considerations or political organizational constraints may make the first method preferable. In any case, the analysis of task priorities and administrative requirements should provide a safety margin against later problems which may reemerge — rightly or wrongly — under the mask of the new leader's personality difficulties. Hidden contradictions between the apparent expressed goals and the real underlying goals of organizations sometimes reveal themselves in the symptomatic act of selecting one incompetent or naïve leader after another for an impossible task.

Unresolved problems in the administrator's personality and unresolved problems within the nature of the specific tasks of the organization and its administrative structures are not the only sources of regressive pressures on the administrator's functioning. The executive administrator of a psychiatric institution occupies various boundaries. First, he occupies the boundaries between the organization and its social environment, and contradictions in and pressures from the social environment as well as those stemming from within the institution may affect his psychological functioning. Second, the leader is at the boundary between his professional background or convictions (his "sentience") and the nature of the task required within the organization. Third, he is also at the boundary between his personal value systems and ethical commitments and the task requirements of relating himself to a social organization. Conflicts of loyalty, regarding moral convictions, and other alternatives requiring courage may at times become prominent and create regressive pressures on the leader's functioning.

A major instrument permitting the administrator to evaluate the optimal functioning of his system is the exploration of group processes within his unit, ward, service, hospital, department, or institution. The technical utilization of his knowledge of group processes will permit him to evaluate the degree to which task groups are "work groups" or are being influenced by basic group assumptions (Bion, 1961). The analysis of the content of any regressive group processes may reveal the nature of the "hidden agenda" of the institution and therefore provide a test of the adequacy of task performance and of the administrative structure. At the same time, and insofar as patients are treated as individuals and/or as groups within the institution, the analysis of such regressive group processes will permit the carrying out of very important diagnostic work regarding the conflicts within the patients' internal world of object relations. Both kinds of regressive pressures — the organization's "hidden agendas" and the distortions of the social processes induced by regressed patients — will highlight the distorted way in which the administrator is viewed or the transferential reactions to him as he carries out his professional and administrative roles. The analysis of regressive group processes, in short, may reveal the effects of organizational and/or patients' conflicts, and thus help to evaluate, by elimination, to what extent the administrator's personality is complicating the situation.

REGRESSIVE PRESSURES ON LEADERS

Various aspects of administration or management place strong regressive pressures on the administrator's psychological functioning. Among these, the very loneliness of his position, the absence of the spontaneous and unconstrained feedback from peers, the uncertainty that is part of significant decision-making all may produce anxieties. Oedipal fears of failure or defeat, frustration of dependent needs, and general activation of conflicts around aggression in the administrator as a leader of and participant in various group processes all contribute to such a regressive pull. Nor is this all. Administrative concerns have a generally "invasive" nature — the invasion of the privacy of his thinking, around the clock, by pressing organizational issues for which no immediate solution can be found; the invasion of his life space as his public image infiltrates areas of privacy and reduces his time for careless leisure and freedom; the threat to the freedom of his fantasy life as his internal relations to people and nature, to art and leisure, all become contaminated by stress related to his responsibilities.

Aggression

In the realm of aggression, although creative administration may permit the expression of aggressive needs in sublimated form, there are also temptations for resolving such tensions by sudden exertion of authority. Groups only too readily tempt their leaders into impulsive action, but the leader must resist these temptations: he is usually aware that loss of control over his angry impulses might have devastating effects far beyond those occurring in ordinary situations. The role aspects of his functioning — the formal organizational authority he enacts — and the unavoidable transferential distortion of the perception of his behavior on the part of staff may amplify his expression of aggression dangerously and may bring about paranoid distortions in the minds of his staff.

The activation of primitive aggressive needs in the administrator ordinarily depends more upon the regressive pull of group processes in the organization than upon his personality characteristics. There certainly are leaders with strong sadistic trends, and, given the amplification of the leader's aggressive behavior by the staff's transferential perceptions and reactions, even relatively minor outbursts become major issues in the organization. But the influence of group processes triggering off and amplifying such reactions in the leader cannot be underestimated. For example, when a regressive group process corresponding to Bion's fight-flight assumption occurs, the leader of this basic assumption in the group — often representing "the voice of the opposition" — may provoke the administrative leader into a personal confrontation.

Often the most extreme paranoid oppositional member of the staff takes over group leadership at such junctures and now seems to control the group as well as the administrative leader himself, a development that may induce paranoid regressive processes in the administrator. The administrator may react with exaggerated fear, anger, and authoritarianism against the "challenger" and thereby miss the internal conflicts in the staff group, that is, the "silent support" for the challenge that exists in the group, and also miss the criticism of the violence among themselves on the part of other members of the staff. The administrator's awareness of group processes and of his own reactions to them may be very helpful to him in transforming such a potentially dangerous situation into a creative one.

The leader of any group or organization is constantly faced with the expression of aggression from various sources from those under him. The aggression directed at the parental images and its expression and/or projection onto the leader is an important aspect of group life: disappointment, rage, and rebellious hatred are the counterparts of idealization of and submission to the leader stemming from oedipal and preoedipal relations to the parents. Bion (1961) suggests that the inordinate expectations of the dependent group bring about hatred of the task leader, who frustrates the needs for total gratification and the groups' longings for unlimited dependency. The fight-flight group struggles with aggression against the task leader, who is perceived in distorted, paranoid ways as a vengeful, dangerous authority.

Because the leader does have limitations and does make mistakes, grounds can always be found for the staff's rationalizing the deeper levels of irrational hatred of him in terms of his human limitations. Therefore, hatred of authority usually seems logical enough, which compounds the actual distortions of leadership functions.

In any case, the various origins of hatred of leadership are usually condensed, and it is frequently hard to judge whether the leader is hated because the administrative structure is authoritarian, because he is incompetent, because he frustrates his followers' needs for idealization and unrealistic expectations, or because of individual psychopathology of all those involved, including the leader himself. Ideally, the answer to the question of the origin of the hatred of the leader should come from an analysis of the primary task of the organization, the adequacy of the administrative structure to that task, the adequacy of functional leadership to the task, etc.

Only after studying general morale problems within the organization and the task orientedness of the relations among groups within it may it be possible to conclude that regressive group phenomena are not the primary factor, and that the psychopathology of individuals—

particularly the leader — is involved. Distortions of organizations can be caused by individual psychopathology within crucial administrative points of the organizational structure, but this diagnosis can only be made after eliminating all other possible causes of emotional regression within the organization. This viewpoint is in contrast to the analysis of organizational conflicts exclusively in terms of individual psychopathology, or of group processes, organizational structure, or political factors.

If the leader appears reasonably adequate to his task and shows no significant personality disturbance, and if there are no major organizational problems evident at that point — that is, the administrative structure is adequate to task performance, and the external environment relatively stable — the question of "inappropriate" aggression of staff toward the leader can often be resolved in terms of the need for the leader to tolerate a certain amount of aggression without undue concern over it. In practice, when the leader is loved without reserve and nobody is ever angry with him, something must be wrong. Decisions — when they are meaningful decisions — always cause somebody pain. Naturally, those painfully affected blame the man on top, which the man on top must be able to tolerate. Such tolerance is required of a good leader; which is one reason why severely narcissistic and paranoid personalities make poor task leaders. The administrator's tolerance of temporary irrational staff outbursts may in itself often decrease the fears that underlie the expression of such anger and thus create an emotionally corrective experience for all concerned.

Sexuality

An increase of oedipal sexual temptations in the leader is the counterpart of the activation of oedipal aggressive rivalries around the issues of power and control within the hierarchy of the institution. While one genetic aspect of the drive for assuming positions of power is that of taking the place of father and becoming the domineering male of the social group, the staff's unconscious perception of the male leader as being the owner of all the women in the institution and the oedipal orientation of female staff toward him as a complement to this shared fantasy are additional potential sources for sexual temptations in leader and staff for acting out such oedipal wishes. The reverse situation develops when a woman is the leader of the organization, and in both cases—of male or female leadership—the prevalent social conventions and taboos regulating public and private interactions between the sexes exert a strong influence on these dynamics. The sexual politics of institutions—the political equilibrium reached in the power struggle and the sexual tensions involving men and women as complementary or opposite sentience groups—are often played out at the top of the institution, as in the proverbial relation between the boss and his secretary or between the chief doctor and head nurse.

Psychiatric institutions are mostly male dominated and reproduce the culturally dominant (apparent) control by "sadistic-controlling" men over "masochistic-subservient" women. Therefore, the political struggles between the sexes as expressed in regressive group phenomena often take the form of men (apparently) dominating the public decision-making process, and of women in (apparent) admiration of and subservience to male-made decisions, carrying out orders, while yet protesting in passive ways against such submission by means of making men feel guilty over the mistreatment to which they feel subjected. The conflicts between physicians and nurses concerning who in effect makes the final decisions on any psychiatric service is one illustration of this problem. The "sexual teasing" among staff, with unconscious efforts to make the other sex the first to cross the forbidden boundary from professional to sexual relations—in order to retaliate by making the offender feel massively guilty—is another aspect of the same problem. Behind the temptations and fears of crossing sexual boundaries are those of crossing hierarchical boundaries, with acting out of oedipal rebellion implicit in the process. Above all, because psychiatric institutions deal with patients who have not been able to satisfactorily resolve their oedipal problems outside the hospital, strong pressures derived from the nature of the task of treating such patients may exacerbate all these potential conflicts among staff.

The danger that the senior administrator's unresolved oedipal conflicts may trigger off a sharp increase of oedipal conflicts throughout the entire institution is often present. This situation becomes complicated by the frequent sexualization at the administrative level of conflicts actually related to the leader's frustrated dependency needs. Oedipal and preoedipal regressive pressures may combine to activate the administrator's sexualized dependent relationships, typically that of "the great man" who is "babied" by "mothering" — often admiring and subservient and yet dominating — women in his immediate "entourage."

In general, groups operating under the basic assumption of pairing experience intimacy and sexual developments as a potential protection against the dangers and conflicts around dependency and aggression. Sexual pairing may also represent a real or fantasied escape from the dangerous and/or controlling group pressures in the organization; it may symbolize a condensation of oedipal rebelliousness against the "established order" with the defensive sexualization of more primitive conflicts around aggression and dependency.

Thus, there may be sexually exciting and romanticized pressure around the administrator which fosters a sexualized bond between him and some administrative member of the other sex. Under optimal circumstances, this bond is expressed in a working relationship mildly infiltrated with sublimated erotic trends. Actually, a certain erotization of work relationships may be enhancing to the work group. But when regressive pressures lead to crossing the sexual boundaries, a couple's sexual intimacy may not only bring about an exaggerated condensation of sexualized sentience of the work group, with consequent distortions in ordinary work boundaries and relationships, but may also lead to a freeing of the aggressive components related to oedipal conflicts in such sexualized relations, with a general breakdown of interpersonal relations in the system. In organizational terms, it may be said that the sexualization of relationships among staff increases the level of aspiration to such an extent that ordinary gratifications at work will (sooner or later) fall disastrously short of such increased expectations, and a general breakdown of morale will ensue.

There is an obvious need that the administrator's sexual gratifications occur outside the boundaries of his administrative functions. This might seem too trivial to mention were the regressive pressures for sexualized relations within the administrative boundaries not so strong. At the same time, if and when a functional, mutually respectful, and open work-relationship between the sexes develops in an organization, eroticized perhaps, but still maintaining work boundaries, the exhilarating experience of men and women who work together as friends without necessarily having to become sexually engaged can be a most creative experience and indirectly foster a sexually mature and tolerant atmosphere which, in psychiatric institutions, will help in the treatment of patients.

General conflicts between the sexes within the social, cultural, and economic environment—for example, socially fostered and ritualized sadomasochistic relationships between women and men, sexual exploitation, and teasing—are automatically expressed as part of the sexual tension within organizations and threaten to distort task relationships. This is seen in the masochistic submission of nurses to doctors and in the manipulative exploitation of sexual seductiveness to reestablish a—real or fantasied—equilibrium between sadistically behaving men and masochistically behaving women. If political tensions between sentience groups and across task boundaries become sexualized, such sexual aggression, submission, and teasing acquire political significance and express sexual politics in an organization. Sexual politics reinforced by general sexual sentience may interfere with the task relationships and task structure. In order to bring sexual politics into the open, the extent to which sexual sentience and task sentience are related must be diagnosed, not with the intention of stripping away the barriers of privacy, but to avoid the misperceptions shared by groups of both sexes when sexual politics are operative. For example, the shared rebelliousness of young female nurses and male physicians against their respective female and male leaders may require diagnosis in order to avoid general distortions in the relations between nursing staff and medical staff.

All of this is not to be construed to mean that satisfactory sexual relationships cannot develop between individual staff members of organizations; on the contrary, people often establish lasting sexual and marital relations with those they meet at work. Usually, when this happens, the work relation between them shifts; one or both might even withdraw from work. Should a married couple or its equivalent continue in a work relation as well, there is a need to consolidate the sexual relation in terms other than that of the work relation proper; the couple that marries will have to establish a close relation in areas separate from those of the task. In turn, it will become particularly important that organizational leadership watch the maintenance of the task when a couple functions within a certain task system.

It is often not satisfactory when husband and wife work together as hierarchical leader and subordinate in the same task system, for this may have a deleterious effect on task relations with their peers. Couples are frequently perceived as powerful and even threatening alliances of power within organizations, so that even when task relations are scrupulously observed, groups do not so perceive them, and react to them with fear, aggression, resentment, and suspicion. This may reduce the couple's effectiveness even under ideal circumstances. Under less than optimal circumstances, the couple may be "sucked in" by the role-inducing shared fantasies and behavior of groups. Furthermore, the couple may be tempted to act out its own conflicts by projecting aggression onto the environment and by developing an idealized bond that tends to exploit its alliance to the disadvantage of others in the organization. Sometimes the stronger member of the couple controls the more subservient or masochistic one for his or her needs; when such a couple in fact occupies the position of leadership, distortion of exercise of authority may occur and typically authoritarian relations develop, which may become quite destructive. There is wisdom in the administrative principles within universities that are intended to prevent just such an eventuality. At the other extreme is the danger of unwarranted discrimination against couples because of the shared fantasies about them within the institution: it is unfortunate when two creative persons are limited in their development and/or contributions by such an organizational bias.

If "to work and to love" are the principal tasks in life, creative developments within organizations should permit the placing of Eros at the service of work, and the placing of work at the service of sublimated love. The main objective of an organization is not to satisfy the human needs of its members, but to carry out a task; one objective of intelligent leadership is to permit the gratification of human needs in carrying out that task.

Dependency

The major regressive pressure on the leader usually derives from the frustration of his dependency needs. There are many reasons for such frustration. For one thing, the potential activation of Bion's basic assumption of dependency is, at least to some extent, always present. Then, too, the administrator carries the burden of responsibility for the entire institution, for processes that to some extent are outside his control and boundaries. He is also confronted with a staff whose freedom of expression of their dependency needs is greater than his own. Subordinates who do well are often rewarded by the leader, but leaders usually receive few direct human rewards when they are effective.

There are, of course, important compensating aspects in the gratifications of the work as such. When the administrator truly knows that his job has been done well, that he has been able to introduce and carry out new ideas and programs, and that he has permitted and stimulated his staff to grow and become creative, important gratifications of his needs may occur. In general, creativity in administrative work may simultaneously gratify dependency needs (by projection), narcissistic needs (by success and approval), and oedipal strivings (by administrative victories). The administrator's immediate group of co-workers may, as part of their working relation with him, provide him with important gratification of his dependency needs.

Another important compensating factor for the frustration of the administrator's dependency needs is the availability of friendship and support outside his own administrative boundaries. Realistic gratification of all the administrator's instinctual needs in his daily life outside the work situation becomes very important in the long run. An excessive search for the gratification of dependency needs from his subordinates may distort the administrative structure and place too great a burden on the staff. A delicate balance exists between the administrator's being so reserved and self-contained that he feeds staff's dehumanizing distorted perceptions of him, or of his relying so much on gratification and support from staff that he overwhelms them and decreases their concentration on actual work. This delicate balance also raises the issue of the extent to which the administrator should or should not share with his staff his concerns and difficulties across the external boundaries of the organization.

The leader's openness about himself may increase staff's understanding of his own constraints, clarify distortions derived from their perception of his role (that is, from confusing his role with his personality), and increase staff moral. For the leader to excessively burden staff with his problems may, however, not only make them anxious about problems they cannot solve but also tremendously increase the expectation that "with openness and humanness all problems will get solved." In short, there is a danger that the supposedly "perfect" administrator fosters primitive idealizations related to the dependency assumptions of staff, and such idealizations necessarily lead to disappointment reactions.

Chapter Thirteen

Regression in Leaders

In the previous chapter I described the effects on administrators of institutions of regressive pressure from the organization. I turn now to consider regressive pressures stemming from the character pathology in the administrators themselves. Although my focus has been on psychiatric institutions (because they are where I have made my observations), the findings, apart from the factors resulting from the special nature of the population of such institutions, can be applied as well to organizations of all kinds—corporate, political, etc.

There are two opposing approaches to the question of leadership: the traditional one according to which it is "inborn" and the more recent one which views it as derived mostly or exclusively from learned skills and understanding. My own approach is intermediate between the two, based on the findings of various investigators (Stantón and Schwartz, 1954; Sanford, 1956; Main, 1957; Bion, 1961; Rice, 1963, 1965, 1969; Hodgson et al., 1965; Miller and Rice, 1967; Dalton et al., 1968; Levinson, 1958; Rioch, 1970a; Emory and Trist, 1973) in combination with a psychoanalytic focus on the leader's personality features and on regressive group processes. Because individuals, groups, and the organization interact dynamically, the origin of failure or breakdown may lie in any one or more of these areas, necessitating an open-systems-theory view of organizational functioning.

THE AUTHORITARIAN LEADER

Adorno and his co-workers (1950) have described the "authoritarian personality" as follows: He tends to be very conventional, rigorously adhering to middle-class values and unduly sensitive to external social pressures; he is inappropriately submissive to authority and at the same time extremely punitive to those who oppose such authority, and to those under him; he is generally opposed to feelings, fantasies, and introspection, and tends to shift responsibility from the individual onto outside forces; he is stereotyped, thinks in terms of black and white; he tends to exercise power for its own sake and admires power in others; he is destructive and cynical, rationalizing his aggression toward others; he tends to project onto others — particularly "out-groups" — his own unacceptable impulses; and finally, he is rigid with regard to sexual morality.

While Adorno and his co-workers applied psychoanalytic concepts to study the metapsychological determinants of such a personality structure, in their methods and clinical analyses they combined both personality and sociological criteria: their authoritarian personality structure seems to me a composite formation, which reflects various types of character pathology exacerbated by authoritarian pressures exerted by social, political, and cultural systems. In my view, within the restricted frame of reference of the study of leadership of psychiatric institutions, the social, cultural, and political issues may be relatively less important than the mutual reinforcement of authoritarian pressures derived from the institutional structure and from various types of character pathology that contribute to authoritarian leadership behavior. In what follows, I explore the pathological contributions of the leader's specific personality characteristics to the development of authoritarian pressures throughout the organizational structure. However, I wish to emphasize again that a leader's authoritarian behavior may stem from features of the organizational structure and not necessarily from his personality.

Sanford (1956) has pointed out the need to distinguish between authoritarian behavior in leadership roles and authoritarianism in the personality, and that the two do not necessarily go together. An authoritarian administrative structure is one that is invested with more power than is necessary to carry out its functions, whereas a functional structure is one where persons and groups in positions of authority are invested with adequate but not excessive power.

The adequate power invested in the leadership in a functional structure usually receives reinforcement from social and/or legal sanctions. Authoritarian behavior that exceeds functional needs must be differentiated from authoritative behavior that does not. In practice, authority — the right and capacity to carry out task leadership — stems from various sources (Rogers, 1973). Managerial authority refers to that part of the leader's authority which has been delegated to him by the institution he works in; leadership authority refers to the aspect derived from the recognition his followers have of his capacity to carry out the task. Managerial and leadership authority reinforce each other; both are in turn dependent upon other sources of authority, such as the leader's technical knowledge, his personality characteristics, his human skills, the social tasks and responsibilities he assumes outside the institution. The administrator is responsible not only to his institution but also to his staff, to his professional and ethical values, to the immediate community, and to society: responsibility and accountability represent the reciprocal function of the administrator to the sources of his delegated authority. In addition, because of his personality characteristics or because he belongs to special groups or to political structures that invest him with power unrelated to his strictly technical functions, the leader may accumulate power beyond that required by his functional authority — the excessive power that constitutes the basis for an authoritarian structure.

In contrasting an authoritarian administrative structure with a functional administrative structure, I am emphasizing the opposition between authoritarian and functional structure, not that between authoritarian and democratic structure. This point is important both theoretically and practically. A tendency exists in some professional institutions — and psychiatric institutions are no exception — to attempt to modify, correct, or resolve by means of democratic political processes problems created by an authoritarian structure. Insofar as those involved in actual tasks should indeed participate in the decision-making process, such "democratization" is helpful; but where decision-making veers toward being determined on a political rather than on a task-oriented basis, distortions of the task structure and of the entire administrative structure may occur. These are extremely detrimental to the work being carried out, and eventually may even reinforce the authoritarian structure they are intended to correct.

PATHOLOGICAL CHARACTER STRUCTURES IN THE ADMINISTRATOR

Schizoid Personality Features

Schizoid personality features may in themselves protect the leader against excessive regression — his emotional isolation makes him less pervious to regressive group processes. However, the proliferation of distorted fantasies about him is hard to correct because of his distance and unavailability. An excessively schizoid leader may also frustrate the appropriate dependency needs of his staff; usually, however, the warmth and extroversion of managerial figures at the intermediate level tend to compensate for his remoteness.

A very schizoid head of one department of psychiatry conveyed the impression that "no one was running the place." Most authority for daily operations had been delegated to the director of clinical services, who was seen as the actual leader of staff and who, because of his excellent capacity for carrying out the boundary functions between the department head and the staff, did indeed fulfill important leadership functions. However, the needs of the senior staff for support, warmth, and understanding were not met, and the atmosphere of each being on his own was transmitted throughout the entire institution. Although this department was considered a place with ample room for independent, autonomous growth of staff "if one had it within oneself," a considerable number of staff members were not able to work in this relative human isolation, and decided to leave.

In another institution, a markedly schizoid hospital director was insufficiently explicit and direct in making decisions, which created ambiguity with regard to delegation of authority. Not knowing of sure how much authority was vested in any particular person, nobody cared to commit himself to anything without repeated consultations with the director. This produced excessive cautiousness and concern for political considerations in making decisions throughout the organization. Eventually, the message was conveyed that one had to become a very skilled and tactful manipulator to get ahead in that department and that direct emotional expression was very risky. Thus, the leader's personality characteristics, through group interactions, filtered down and became characteristic of the entire organization.

Obsessive Personality Features

Obsessive personality features in top leadership are quite frequent. On the positive side, the focus on orderliness, precision, clarity, and control may foster good, stable delegation of authority and clarity in the decision-making process. Contrary to what one would expect, there is usually very little doubtfulness in obsessive personalities in leadership positions; severely obsessive personalities who are full of doubt and hesitation usually don't reach top positions. Chronic indecisiveness in the administrator may have obsessive origins, but is most frequently really a consequence of his narcissistic problems. Obsessive personalities, then, usually function rather efficiently from an organizational viewpoint. Their clear stand on issues and commitment to values have important creative functions for the institution.

On the negative side, some dangers are the leader's excessive need for order and precision, to be in control, and the expression of the sadistic components that often go with an obsessive personality. An inordinate need for orderliness and control may reinforce the bureaucratic components of the organization—that is, encourage decision-making on the basis of rules and regulations, all of which may interfere with the creativeness of staff and with appropriate autonomy in the decision-making process at points of rapid change or crises. Excessive bureaucratization may sometimes protect the organization from political struggle, but it reinforces passive resistance in the negotiations across boundaries and fosters misuse of resources.

Because pathological defense mechanisms and, particularly, pathological character traits of the leader tend to be activated in times of stress, an increase in obsessive perfectionism and pedantic style may characterize the obsessive leader at critical moments. This may create additional stress for the organization at a time when rapid and effective decision-making is required. An educated awareness in the staff that under such conditions it is necessary to protect the security system of the leader in order to get the work done may be very helpful. This, of course, is true for the effects of pathological character features of any kind in the leader; to know how to help him in times of crises is a basic skill demanded of intermediate management.

A major problem created by some obsessive personalities in leadership positions is that of severe unresolved sadism. The need to sadistically control subordinates may have devastating effects on the organization's functional structure. Whenever there is strong opposition among staff to a certain move by the administrator, he may become obstinate and controlling, revengefully "rubbing the message in," and forcing his "opponents" again and again into submission. Such behavior reinforces irrational fears of authority and the distortion of role-perception in the staff; it also fosters a submissiveness to hierarchical superiors, which reduces effective feedback and creative participation from the entire staff.

The result may be the development of chronic passivity, a pseudo-dependency derived from fear of authority rather than from an authentic "dependent" group, and a transmission of authoritarian, dictatorial ways of dealing with staff and patients in the whole institution. The appointment of an obsessive and sadistic director to a department of psychiatry drove the most creative members of the senior professional leadership away from the institution within a year and brought about consolidation around the leader of a group of rather weak, inhibited, or mediocre professionals who were willing to pay the price of sacrificing their autonomous professional development for the security and stability afforded them by submission to the leader. The repetition of these conflicts approximately a year later at the next lower level of organizational hierarchy, however, created such "fight-flight" grouping and general breakdown in carrying out organizational tasks that the staff finally united and brought about the removal of the administrator.

Paranoid Personalities

Paranoid personalities always present a serious potential danger for the functional relationships administrators must establish with their staff. The development of "fight-flight" conditions in the group processes throughout the organization—which may occur even in the most efficiently functioning organization from time to time—may propel into the foreground a "leader of the opposition." With the silent tolerance or unconscious collusion of the majority of staff, a violent attack on the administration by this opposition leader may cause the leader to regress into paranoid attitudes even if he does not have any particularly paranoid traits. In other words, there is always a potential—particularly in large organizations with several levels of hierarchy—for suspiciousness, for temptations to exert sadistic control, and for the projection of the administrator's rage onto staff. When the administrator also has strong paranoid character features, the danger of paranoid reactions to "fight-flight" conditions is intensified, and he may perceive even ordinary discussions or minor opposition as dangerous rebelliousness and potential hidden attacks. The need to suppress and control the opposition, which we saw in the obsessive leader with sadistic trends, becomes paramount in the paranoid leader. Because of the ease with which the leader may interpret what "they say" as lack of respect, mistreatment, and hidden hostility toward him, staff now may become afraid of speaking up. Staff's fearfulness, in turn, may increase the administrator's suspiciousness, thus generating a vicious circle.

Because paranoid personalities are particularly suitable to take on the leadership of basic assumptions groups in a "fight-flight" position, the "leader of the opposition" is often a person with strong paranoid tendencies. I do not mean to imply that all leaders of revolutions are paranoid personalities, but that because of the nature of their psychopathology paranoid personalities may function much more appropriately under such revolutionary conditions. The fighting "in-group" that they represent becomes "all good," and the external groups or the general environment they fight becomes "all bad." The successful projection of all aggression outside the boundaries of the group he controls permits the paranoid oppositional leader to function more effectively within the boundaries of his group, even though at the cost of an important degree of distortion of perception of external reality. But when such a paranoid leader succeeds in occupying power and takes over control of the organization, the very characteristics that helped him gain leadership of the "fight-flight" group may become very damaging to the institution. The tendency to project all hostility outside may temporarily help to protect the good relations between the leader and his followers; in the long run, however, the price paid for this is institutionalization of paranoid distortions of perceptions of external reality, distortions in the boundary negotiations between the institution and its environment, and the possibility that the leader's capacity to carry out his organizational tasks will break down. Within the organization, the revengeful persecution of those the paranoid leader suspects of being potential enemies may eliminate creative criticism to a much larger extent than in the case of obsessive personalities with sadistic features.

The director of a psychiatric institution that functioned closely with several other psychiatric institutions felt chronically endangered by what he saw as the power plays against him of the directors of the other institutions. At first he appealed to his own staff for help and support, and temporarily morale improved as all felt united against the external enemy. Eventually, however, by constantly antagonizing leaders and representatives of the other institutions, the director became less able to carry out his functions in representation of his own institution, and started to blame subordinates within his own system for his difficulties in obtaining the necessary space, staff, funding, and community influence. He began to suspect some of the members of intermediate management of his own institution of having "sold out to the enemy," further reducing the effectiveness of his institution vis-à-vis its professional environment.

The following example, in contrast, illustrates the resolution of paranoid regression induced by "fight-flight" conditions in an organizational leader without paranoid personality characteristics. The director of a hospital was very suspicious and upset over a senior member of his staff, Dr. B., who seemed to challenge him at all professional meetings. The director saw Dr. B. as a severely paranoid character whose group behavior was splitting staff and potentially damaging the organization and who perhaps should not continue on the staff. He nevertheless accepted other staff members' judgment that Dr. B. was a good clinician and was providing valuable services to the hospital. A consultant recommended to the director that he meet privately with Dr. B. and discuss his group behavior. The director did so and discovered that Dr. B. was much more open and flexible in individual meetings than in group situations. But the challenging behavior continued in groups, and the director now concluded that regardless of the personality characteristics of the "leader of the opposition" a group process must be fostering his contentious behavior and that a study of this particular organizational area was indicated. In the course of the ensuing study, it became apparent that there were serious conflicts within the institution that had reduced the effectiveness of the professional group to which Dr. B. belonged, so that "fight-flight" assumptions chronically prevailed among them and drew Dr. B. into the role of their leader. Analysis of the organizational problem involved led to resolution of the conflicts concerning the entire professional group; Dr. B., finding himself no longer supported by the "silent consensus" and actively discouraged by the group itself, finally stopped dominating group discussions.

Narcissistic Personality Features

Of the dangers to institutions stemming from the leader's character pathology, narcissistic personality features are perhaps the most serious of all. The inordinate self-centeredness and grandiosity of these persons is in dramatic contrast to their chronic potential for envy of others. Their inability to evaluate themselves and others in depth brings about a lack of capacity for empathy and for sophisticated discrimination of other people, all of which may become very damaging when they occupy leadership positions. In addition, when external gratifications fail to come forth, or under conditions of severe frustration or failure, they may develop paranoid trends rather than depression and a sense of personal failure. Such paranoid tendencies reinforce even further the damaging impact on the organization of the leader's narcissistic character structure.

Because narcissistic personalities are often driven by intense needs for power and prestige to assume positions of authority and leadership, individuals with such characteristics are found rather frequently in top leadership positions. They are often men of high intelligence, hardworking and eminently talented or capable in their field, but with narcissistic needs that dramatically neutralize or destroy their creative potential for the organization.

Pathologically narcissistic people aspire to positions of leadership more for their power and prestige than because of commitment to a certain task or ideal represented by the functions carried out by the institution. As a consequence, they may neglect the functional requirements of leadership, the human needs and constraints involved in the work, and the value systems that constitute one of the important boundaries against which administrative and technical responsibilities have to be measured. Leaders with narcissistic personalities are unaware of the pathological human relations they foster around themselves and throughout the entire organization. In contrast to leaders with pathological obsessive and paranoid features, the narcissistic leader not only requires submission from staff, but also wants them to love him. He not only fosters but artificially increases the staff's normal tendency to depend on and idealize the leader: as staff become aware how important it is for the administrator to receive their unconditional, repetitive expression or demonstration of love and admiration, adulation and flattery become constant features of the process of communication with him.

Before proceeding further, it must be emphasized that the negative influence of pathological narcissism has to be differentiated from the normal narcissistic manifestations that are part of the gratifications of any position of responsibility and leadership, gratifications that may be the source of increased effectiveness in leadership as well as a compensation for administrative frustrations. Striving for a position of leadership may involve idealism and altruism intimately linked with normal narcissism.

With pathological narcissism, however, the leader's aspirations center around primitive power over others, inordinate reception of admiration and awe, and the wish to be admired for personal attractiveness, charm, and brilliance, rather than for mature human qualities, moral integrity, and creativity in providing task-oriented professional and administrative leadership. His tolerance for the normal unavoidable frustrations that go with his position is low, and a number of pathological developments take place within him, in his interactions with staff, and throughout the entire organizational structure.

Above all, the preeminence of unconscious and conscious envy has very detrimental consequences for the relations between him and his staff. Insofar as he cannot tolerate the success and gratification that others obtain from their work, and cannot accept others' professional success, which he sees as overshadowing or threatening his own, he may become very resentful of the most creative members of his staff. Narcissistic personalities may often be very helpful to trainees or junior members of the staff, whose development they foster because they unconsciously represent extensions of the leader's own grandiose self. When these younger colleagues become autonomous and independent, however, the leader's previous support may shift into devaluation and relentless undermining of their work.

It is part of normal narcissism to be able to enjoy the happiness and triumph of those one has helped to develop. Enjoyment of the work and success of others — a general characteristic of the normal overcoming of infantile envy and jealousy — is an important function that is missing in the narcissistic personality. The narcissistic administrator may also envy some on his staff for the strength of their professional convictions; it is one of the tragedies of narcissistic personalities that the very superficiality of their values results in a chronic deterioration of those they do have.

Another consequence of pathological narcissism stems from the encouragement of submissiveness in staff. Since narcissistic leaders tend to surround themselves with "yes men" and shrewd manipulators who play into their narcissistic needs, more honest and therefore occasionally critical members of the staff are pushed onto the periphery and eventually may constitute a relatively silent but dissatisfied and critical opposition. The dependent group of admirers further corrodes the administrator's self-awareness and fosters in him additional narcissistic deterioration.

The narcissistic leader might depreciate those he perceives as adulating him, but he cannot do without them; and his respect for the integrity of those who criticize him gradually erodes into paranoid fears. In terms of internalized object relations, it is as if the narcissistic leader evokes in the network of the organization a replication of his internal world of objects populated only by devalued, shadowy images of others and by images of dangerous potential enemies.

The narcissistic leader's inability to judge people with any degree of penetration is a consequence of the pathology of his internalized object relations—of his failure to achieve total-object relations (Kernberg, 1975, Chapters 1 and 8) and of his lack of commitment to professional values and to value systems in general. The inability to judge people in depth and the reliance on people who play into his needs for admiration reinforce each other so that eventually he may be surrounded by people similar to himself, people suffering from serious behavior disorders or cynically exploiting their awareness of his psychological needs.

Paradoxically, in large institutions the worse the distortion of the administrative structure by the leader's narcissistic pathology, the more may compensating mechanisms develop in the form of breakdown of boundary control and boundary negotiations, so that some institutional functions may actually go "underground," or become split off from the rest of the organization. It is as if a parallel existed here to what happens in some cases of severe psychopathology, when splitting or primitive dissociation of the ego permits the patient to maintain some semblance of adaptation to external reality at the price of fragmentation of his ego identity. However, the general thesis still stands that the overall creativity of the organization suffers severely under such excessively narcissistic leadership. Although in the short run the grandiosity and expansiveness of the narcissistic leader may transmit itself throughout the organization as a pressure to work or as "charismatic" excitement, and bring about a spurt of productivity, in the long run the deteriorating effects of pathological narcissism tend to drown creativity in sweeping dependency or in the cynicism that develops among those in the organization with the greatest knowledge and strongest convictions.

When the institution directed by a narcissistic leader is small, the negative effects may be overwhelming from the beginning, for everybody is directly affected by his problems. The development of understanding is hampered by the leader's constant doubts and uncertainty over everything—doubts derived from unconscious envy, devaluation, and lack of conviction—and by his need to constantly change his interests as he loses the enthusiasm for what is no longer new and exciting. The narcissistic leader's incapacity to provide gratification of realistic dependency needs of staff—in a word, his incapacity really to listen—frustrates staff's basic emotional needs and at the same time strengthens the negative consequences of the distortions in group processes: the submissive and dependent in-group and the depressed and angry out-group mentioned before.

Severely narcissistic leaders whose ambition is frustrated by the external reality of the organization may require so much additional support from their staff that most energy is spent in attempts to restore the leader's emotional equilibrium. In one department of psychiatry, the chairman had reached this position at an early stage of his career, when he seemingly was one of the promising members of his generation; however, he had progressively lost his professional leadership functions and had become chronically embittered and depressed. After a number of years, those senior staff members who remained saw it as their principal organizational task to protect the leader from unnecessary stress and narcissistic lesions and to stimulate his capacities by ongoing applause and rewards. As a result, the general productivity of the department decreased noticeably.

At times, it is amazing and truly encouraging to observe how staff members of institutions directed by a narcissistic leader maintain their personal integrity, autonomy, and independence in spite of the corrupting influence of their immediate environment. These isolated members may provide an outside consultant with the most meaningful information about the organization's "hidden agendas" and preserve the hope for change in the midst of general despondency. It is as if the social situation of the institution were reflecting the intra-psychic life of narcissistic personalities—with fragments of healthy ego floating in the midst of a sea of deteriorated internalized object relations.

Although narcissistic leaders often irradiate a quality of personal prominence and of messianic suggestibility, and have the capacity to stimulate the group's identification with the leader's confidence in himself, not all narcissistic leaders are charismatic and not all charismatic leaders are narcissistic. Personal charisma may stem from a combination of various personality traits and may be imbedded in strength of technical, moral, and human convictions. Staff sometimes accuse a strong and committed leader of being "narcissistic" when in reality they are projecting onto him their own frustrated narcissistic aims and expressing envy of the successful man. The "consensus" leader—whom Zaleznik (1974) has contrasted with the "charismatic" one—may also present either severe narcissistic or normal personality characteristics. One has to differentiate the mature "consensus" leader, who has the capacity to explore the thinking of his staff and to use creatively the understanding and skills of his administrative group for carrying out the task, from the power-oriented, smoothly functioning, politically opportunistic, narcissistic "consensus" leader, who shrewdly exploits groups phenomena for his narcissistic aims.

There is a special kind of narcissistic leader whose gratifications come mostly from keeping himself in the center of everybody's love, and at the same time in the center of the decision-making process, while he coolly sacrifices any considerations regarding value systems or the organization's functional needs to what is politically expedient. The typical example is the leader who is a "nice guy" with no enemies, who seems slightly insecure and easily changeable, and who at the time is extremely expert in turning all conflicts among his staff into fights that do not involve himself. The general narcissistic qualities of shallowness, inability to judge people sensitively, inability to commit oneself to any values are dramatically evident in his case, but what seems to be missing is the direct expression of grandiosity and the need to obtain immediate gratification from other people's admiration. This kind of leader obtains gratification from his position by using it as a source of power and prestige beyond the organization itself. He may let the organization run its own course, trying to keep things smooth, so long as his power base is stable.

A somewhat similar outcome may stem from a different type of personality structure — that of individuals with strong reaction formations against primitive sadistic trends. Here the friendliness of the leader with his immediate subordinates is in contrast to violent conflicts in the next level below. Still another type of consensus leader has achieved his position on the basis of his technical or professional skills and has been willing to accept the position without ever fully assuming the responsibilities it entails. This is one of the conditions leading to an essentially leaderless organization: the man at the top is really more interested in a particular work of his own than in developing authentic leadership and, for that reason, stays away from the painful process of making hard decisions. In summary, both charismatic and consensus leadership may stem from various normal and pathological sources.

One major question that can be affected by pathological narcissism is the perennial one of when to compromise and when to hold to one's convictions in any particular conflict. At one extreme, the rigid, self-righteous person who has to have his own way and cannot accept any compromise may reflect pathological narcissism; at the other extreme, the person willing to sell his convictions — and his staff — down the river for any opportunistic reason may equally reflect severe pathological narcissism. Somewhere in between are the realistic compromises by which the leader's essential convictions are respected and effective boundary negotiation is carried out to achieve a creative balance among conflicting priorities, tasks, and constraints. In other words, intelligent political maneuvering may protect the task and distinguish between what is essential and what is not. Sometimes it takes very long-range vision indeed to separate the immediate political implications of a certain move from its value in terms of the overall, long-range organizational tasks and goals. Pathological narcissism dramatically interferes with the leadership function which differentiates the expedient from the constructive.

THE PSYCHOANALYTICALLY TRAINED CONSULTANT

Consultants are usually called at times of crisis, but the nature of their task is not always clear: an organization may use a consultant to escape from full awareness and resolution of a problem as much as to realistically diagnose the problem and its potential solutions (Rogers, 1973). The consultant's first task is to clarify the nature of his contract, and to assure himself that the resources to carry it out are adequate. This means not only sufficient time and financial support but necessary authority to examine problems at all levels of the organizational structure.

It goes almost without saying that support from the leader of the organization is essential. At the same time the consultant needs to be sufficiently independent from the organization to be able to reach his conclusions without excessive fears of antagonizing the leader; he must therefore be alert to maintaining his autonomy.

One question to be formulated is whether a certain conflict within the organization represents a problem stemming from: "personality" issues, the nature of the task of the organization and its constraints, or "morale"—that is, group processes within the organization. The nature of the problem is often described in such confused and confusing terms that a translation into these three domains is difficult.

It is helpful to focus first on the nature of the organizational tasks and their constraints, for only after task definition has been achieved, the respective constraints have been outlined, and priorities have been set up regarding primary and secondary tasks and constraints is it possible to evaluate whether the administrative structure does indeed fit with the nature of the tasks, and, if not, how it should be modified. This analysis requires the clarification of the organization's real tasks in contrast to its apparent ones. In one psychiatric hospital, the apparent task was to treat patients and to carry out research, but the real task seemed to be to provide the owners of the institution with an adequate return on their investment.

Once tasks and constraints have been defined, questions regarding the administrative structure required for task performance can be examined. Does the organization have effective control over its boundaries, and, if not, what administrative compensating mechanisms can be established to restore it? A psychiatric organization depended on one institution for its administrative-support funding, and on another for its funding for professional staffing. Chronic conflicts between administrators and professionals throughout the entire organization reflected the lack of resolution of boundary control at the top. The consultant's recommendation that all funding be channeled into a central hospital administration directed by a professional with administrative expertise became acceptable to both funding institutions and to the staff, and provided the organizational solution to the "morale" problem that had prompted the request for consultation.

Once boundary control seems adequate, the nature of delegation of authority in the institution and each task system can be studied. Inadequate, fluctuating, ambiguous, or nonexisting delegation, on the one hand, and excessive, chaotic delegation, on the other, are problems that have to be solved as part of the redefinition of the administrative structure in terms of task requirements.

Having diagnosed the overall task and its constraints, and, it is hoped, corrected the respective administrative structures, it becomes possible to focus on the nature of the leadership and, more concretely, on the qualities of the leader himself. The consultant should attempt to diagnose the personality qualities of the administrator that influence the organizational functioning, the regressive pulls that the leader is subjected to from group processes in the organization, and his own contributions to such regressive group processes. What kind of intermediate management has the leader assembled? How much understanding in depth does he have for people, their assets and liabilities? How much tolerance of criticism does he have, how much strength and yet warmth, flexibility and yet firmness and clarity, in his relation to staff? The accuracy and quality of the leader's judgment of those around him is a crucial indicator, not only of his administrative skills, but of his total personality. What are his reactions under stress? In which direction does his personality regress under critical conditions? The strength of his convictions, the presence or absence of his envy of staff, the extent of his moral integrity and courage — these are usually surprisingly well known through the organization.

The psychoanalytic exploration of group processes in the organization may become a crucial instrument for evaluating problems in both the administrative structure and the personality of the leader. The regressive nature of group processes in psychiatric organizations — "morale" — may reflect conflicts in the organizational structure, the impact of the leader's personality, the regressive pull directly induced by the pressure of patients' conflicts, or combinations of these factors. The closer the observed group processes are to the actual work with patients, the more the patients' conflicts will directly influence the development of regressive group processes within staff and the staff-patient community generally. The closer the observed staff groups are to the final decision-making authority at the top, the more the conflicts of top leadership and of organizational structure will dominate. However, it is impressive how the conflicts affecting the total organization are reflected in actual group processes at all levels. Therefore, the careful observation of group processes at various administrative levels constitutes a kind of "organizational projective test battery," which may give the direct information needed to clarify problems at the levels of task definition and constraints, patients, administrative structure, and leadership, all in one stroke.

For practical purposes, the consultant usually obtains this most helpful information from senior and intermediate management in a free and open discussion of issues within a group atmosphere which permits some exploration of group processes as well as of the actual content of the administrative problems.

When the conclusion reached is that the leader's personality problems or his general incompetence resulting from lack of technical knowledge, conceptual limitations, or administrative inadequacies are involved, the question arises whether he can be helped to change, or whether he should be helped to leave his job. Improvement in task definition, task performance, boundary controls, and the administrative structure as a whole may bring out the leader's positive assets and reduce the negative impact of his personality characteristics. At other times, the best solution seems to be to help him step down by either changing his professional functions or moving him geographically within the organization — if such alternatives are available. Although the recommendation that he resign is always a serious narcissistic blow, it often happens that deep down the administrator knows he has not been able to do his job well and he may feel relieved when someone from outside confronts him with that reality. On the other hand, when the consultant concludes that the organization has a poor leader, the consultant might discreetly withdraw (or discreetly be asked to withdraw).

The situation is different, of course, when the problem involves an administrator at some lower hierarchical level. Here the leader needs to be helped in understanding that firmness in eliminating bad situations is indispensable for the health of the organization. To help a man who cannot do his job to leave may seem aggressive or even sadistic to his superior; but it is usually more sadistic to leave an inefficient leader in charge of an organization than to ask him to change his functions. The suffering he causes in staff should be of primary concern to him. Optimal leadership sometimes requires hard decisions, and, unfortunately, there are times when the leader must be able to be very firm and decisive with somebody who may be a close personal friend.

Sometimes the problem can be diagnosed but for some reason cannot be resolved. Some organizations function as if they were geared to self-destruction, unable and unwilling to accept positive change. This is a dramatic situation for a consultant and, of course, much more dramatic for the staff. One important use of an understanding of organizational structure and conflict may be the possibility for staff, particularly senior staff who are able to obtain an overview of the situation, to diagnose the organizational conflicts and even their sources and reach realistic conclusions about the prognosis and, therefore, their personal future.

Certain situations can be so bad that the only solution is for self-respecting staff to leave; in other words, there is such a thing as a "poisonous" organizational environment that is bad for everybody in it. It is impressive how often staff developing within such a destructive environment deny the insoluble nature of the problems of the organization and obtain gratification of pathological dependency needs by such denial and failure to admit the need to move on. Understanding organizations in depth can be painful; such awareness sometimes does not improve the effectiveness of staff members; but understanding always makes it possible to gain a more realistic even if painful grasp of what the future probably will be. The situation is parallel to the painful learning about some aspects of one's unconscious in a psychoanalytic situation: there are pathological defenses against becoming aware of what the reality is about the place where one works. At some point, the individual has a responsibility to himself which transcends his responsibility to the organization; and knowledge of organizational conflicts may permit him to reach more quickly an understanding of what that point is and where his personal boundaries are threatened by an organization from which he should withdraw.

Under less extreme circumstances, there is much that an educated, task-oriented staff can do to help its leadership correct or undo distorted administrative structures and reduce the effects of pathology at the top. The staff in positions of intermediate management may be of particular help to the organization and the top administrator in preserving functional administrative relationships by open sharing of communication and of analysis of the situation. In this regard, the responsibility of followers in not perpetuating and exacerbating the problems of the leader cannot be overemphasized.

Disruption of functional administration always brings about regression to "basic group assumptions" (Bion, 1961). Such regressive phenomena in groups involving intermediate leadership and staff may reinforce the personality difficulties of individual staff members and reduce their awareness of the need for change or their willingness to fight for it. For individual staff members to courageously spell out the situation may have a positive therapeutic effect in increasing rational behavior throughout the organization; in such instances, helpfulness emerges from a functional attitude of criticism based not upon fight-flight assumptions but upon a genuine interest in helping the leader and staff generally to improve their understanding and functioning in the organization. Open communication among the intermediate management group may also help reduce their mutual suspicion and distrust and their fear of speaking up. An alliance for the sake of the functional needs of the organization is a good example of political struggle in terms of the task, rather than in terms of perpetuating the distortions in the distribution of authority and power.

For the leader, particularly at a time of crisis when uncertainty is increased for him and everyone else, the availability of senior staff who are willing to speak up openly and responsibly without excessive distortion by fear or anger can be very reassuring. A mutual reinforcement between staff who are able and willing to provide new information to the leader and a leader who encourages such staff action may strengthen the task group throughout.

"Participatory management" as a general principle is an important protection against regressive effects of the leader's personality on the administrative structure. A variety of factors affect the general question of what degree of participatory management or what degree of centralized decision-making is required. When a distortion of the administrative structure has occurred under the impact of regressive pulls on top leadership from whatever source, increasing participative management is indicated. Such an emphasis on participatory decision-making does not mean a replacement of a functional by a "democratic" structure. Flexibility is necessary regarding the extent to which the organization shifts back and forth from centralized to participatory management; at periods of rapid environmental change, of crisis or "turbulence" in the external environment, there may be a need for increased centralized decision-making (Emery and Trist, 1973). At times of external stability, increased decentralization and participatory management may be helpful. Internal change often requires participatory management, especially in the preparatory or early stages of change. A centralized, simplified administrative structure may become functional in times of internal consolidation or stability.

Part Four

LOVE, THE COUPLE, AND THE GROUP

Chapter Fourteen

Boundaries and Structure in Love Relations

The study of regressive features in group processes and organizations and their interaction with regressive pressures within the individual has paved the way for an examination of the relations between two people who join together to form a sexual couple. For the couple, as we have seen, while consisting of two individuals is also an entity vis-à-vis the group. And insofar as the couple is united — or is assumed to unite — because of sexual needs, an examination of its dynamics will require a discussion of love. Just as I have found object relations theory helpful in offering new insights on the unconscious forces that determine the vicissitudes of love relations, so I find it offers new insight into the relations between the couple and the group. The couple stands at the crossroads where individual unconscious conflicts intersect with the expression of these conflicts in the external world. Before describing the relations between the couple and the group, I shall present an extension of my previous contributions on sexual love (Kernberg, 1976a, Chapters 7 and 8). A brief résumé of that work would probably be the best way to begin.

I have concluded that in order to fall and remain in love two developmental tasks must have been achieved. First, the capacity for establishing a total object relation must have been integrated with a previously established capacity for experiencing sensuous stimulation of erotogenic zones. Second, full genital enjoyment can incorporate early body-surface erotism in the context of a total object relation, including a complementary sexual identification. The first task requires, in essence, that primitive dissociation of the self- and object representations be overcome so that ego identity and the capacity for total- in contrast to part-object relations are established. The second task requires the successful overcoming of oedipal conflicts and the related unconscious prohibitions against a full sexual relation.

I also traced a continuum of character constellations on the basis of the capacity — or rather, the incapacity — to fall and remain in love: (1) narcissistic personalities who are socially isolated and who express their sexual urges only in polymorphous perverse masturbatory fantasies; (2) narcissistic personalities who are sexually promiscuous; (3) the ordinary borderline patient who engages in chaotic, polymorphous perverse activity. (Paradoxically, disturbed, inappropriate, and immature as the ordinary borderline patients' falling in love, primitive idealization, and sexual promiscuity may appear, these patients do have a much better prognosis for further development than the descriptive pathology of their love relations would initially suggest. In contrast to narcissistic patients, they have a better capacity for investment in others, or a less active deterioration of their object relations.) These three configurations represent the pathology of "stage one," that is, before the achievement of an integrated self-concept and an integrated conceptualization of others and the concomitant capacity for relations in depth with significant others, in short, the achievement of libidinal object constancy. (4) Next along the continuum is the neurotic patient and those with less severe character pathology. With these patients we find present various sexual inhibitions, masochistic love relations, a greater capacity for romantic idealization and tenderness coupled with sexual inhibition. Here the chief etiological conflicts are in the triadic, oedipal realm. (5) Finally we have the normal person who has the capacity to integrate genitality with tenderness and a stable, mature object relation.

I also attempted to redefine the normal capacity for falling and remaining in love, stressing that, in addition to the general capacity for a normal integration of genitality with the capacity for tenderness and a stable, deep object relation with a person of the other sex (Balint, 1948), normal love relations include other factors in the sexual experience and behavior, in the object relation with a sexual partner, and in superego development. All I have said so far certainly suggests that, as Lichtenstein (1970) and Ross (1970) have suggested, the concept of "genital primacy" as simply the capacity to achieve orgasm in sexual intercourse badly needs revision (see also Kernberg, 1976a, Chapter 8).

In summary, it seems to me that for normal love relations one must have developed, first — at the level of actual sexual behavior — the capacity for broadening and deepening the experience of sexual intercourse and orgasm with sexual eroticism derived from the integration of aggression and bisexuality (sublimatory homosexual identification); second, an object relation in depth, which includes the general transmutation of pregenital strivings and conflicts in the form of tenderness, concern, and gratitude, and the capacity for genital identification with the partner, coupled with a sublimatory identification with (and yet leaving behind) the parental figure of the same sex; third, depersonification, abstraction, and individualization — that is, maturation — in the superego so that infantile morality has been transformed into adult ethical values, and a sense of responsibility and moral commitment which reinforces the couple's emotional commitment to each other.

The study of pathological love relations led me to postulate an orderly sequence of psychological developments culminating in the capacity for mature love relations. I emphasized a continuity between the normal states of falling and remaining in love, a continuity leading to the couple's having a stable, affectionate relationship. The achievement of the capacity for relating in depth to one's own self as well as to others seemed the basic precondition for a mature and lasting relationship between two people who love each other. But I was also forced to conclude that emotional maturity is no guarantee that the couple will be stable and conflict-free. The very capacity to love and to realistically appreciate — and evaluate — another person over the years, and to be committed to the values and experiences of a life lived together, may reconfirm the relationship or lead to its termination. The complication is that both individuals and couples change, and neurotic reasons for remaining together may be resolved (with or without treatment), or they may intensify and create stress on the marriage; or increasing maturity may open new areas of freedom and cause the couple to reexamine realistically the basis of the marriage. The resolution of pathological dependency, for example, may dissolve the marriage or permit its re-creation on a new basis. Maturity, with its acceptance of the imperfection and frailty of life and human relationships and of the inevitable decline and renunciation that time will demand, may either terminate or perpetuate the relationship, as may the neurotic refusal to accept this reality.

As an illustration: a woman who had completed her psycho-analysis, which had sufficiently resolved oedipal conflicts related to a severe depression and had brought about fundamental changes in her character structure and symptoms, achieved a more realistic vision of herself, of the motivations for her marriage, and of her husband. After she had been married for many years, she realized that in the past she had needed to identify herself with an idealized husband, whom she now perceived as a quite selfish and arrogant man. She then had to face the painful question of whether, or under what conditions, she was willing to continue her marriage. One might, of course, say that in this case only one of the partners had been able to achieve change, thus threatening a previous equilib-rium, and that under ideal circumstances change and growth in both partners may reinforce and renovate the relationship. This certainly happens in many cases; however, the assumption that change and growth will develop in the direction of reconfirming the couple can be wishful thinking: children grow up and leave home, education and professional developments take place which change the couple's life space and style, and external challenges and stress may bring about circumstances under which individual growth and the couple's growth do not necessarily coincide. Then too, a couple's sexual identifications and conflicts may change over the years, especially under the impact of the growth of their children. Certain identi-fications and past conflicts with their own parents emerge dramat-ically when the children reach adolescence, a time when old battles are fought over again — but this time with the roles reversed. All of this creates new stress, opportunities, challenges, and dangers for the couple.

The observation of patients in later stages of their psychoanalysis, the follow-up of patients who have successfully completed psychoanalytic treatment, and also the knowledge about colleagues and friends that one acquires in the course of a professional life, and self-analysis, all led me to a sense of the instability of the equilibrium reached at the end of the road of the developmental sequences I have mentioned, and seemed to justify further study of what constitutes normality in love relations.

SOME RECENT PSYCHOANALYTIC STUDIES OF PSYCHOSEXUAL DEVELOPMENT AND LOVE RELATIONS

In agreement with Altman (1977), it seems to me that, subsequent to Freud, psychoanalytic contributions have dealt more with the psychology and psychopathology of sexual life than with the psychology and psychopathology of love relations. Some more recent psychoanalytic writings about love have been approaching this problem more from the philosophical (and particularly existential) than from the clinical psychoanalytic standpoint (Fromm, 1956; van den Haag, 1964; May, 1969). Not too long ago, a group of French psychoanalysts—J. Chasseguet-Smirgel and her co-workers (1970, 1973), David (1971), and Braunschweig and Fain (1971)—made a concerted effort to focus on this problem. The following review of psychoanalytic studies of the development of love relations from this country and abroad will focus particularly on these still mostly untranslated French contributions.

The state of being in love enriches the self. David (1971) and Chasseguet-Smirgel (1973) say that, when one is in love, the libidinal investment of the self increases because an ideal state of the self is fulfilled and because the exalted relation of the self to the object reproduces a relation between the self and ego ideal. Van der Waals (1965) had earlier pointed to a simultaneous increase of object and narcissistic libidinal investment in normal love. (I think that love, even if unfulfilled, increases normal narcissism simultaneously with the capacity for object love.)

Chasseguet-Smirgel (1973) suggests that in mature love, in contrast to transitory adolescent falling in love, there is a limited projection of a toned-down ego ideal onto the idealized love object and a simultaneous enhancement of narcissistic (self-) investment from the sexual gratification provided by the loved object. Her observations are, I believe, compatible with my thinking that normal (as against primitive) idealization constitutes an advanced developmental level of this mechanism, wherein infantile and childhood morality are transformed into adult ethical systems. Idealization, thus conceived, is a normal function of love relations, and establishes a continuity between "romantic" adolescent and mature love. Under normal circumstances, it is not the ego ideal that is projected, but ideals that stem from advanced structural development within the superego (including the ego ideal).

I believe there is a natural continuity of the early narcissistic function of establishing an ideal relationship with the loved object — in the last resort, the normal resolution of the rapprochement subphase of separation-individuation that leads to libidinal object constancy, which in turn symbolically replaces the earlier symbiosis with mother (Mahler and Furer, 1968; Bergmann, 1971; Mahler, 1972b) — and the later functions of narcissistic gratification in the primitive oedipal relationship. It is only under conditions of pathological narcissism that narcissistic needs run counter to the capacity for oedipal investments in love relations; and, even under conditions of excessive fixation at normal infantile narcissism as a defense against oedipal relations, one finds the continuity and complementarity of narcissistic and oedipal features in love relations. Which leads us to the centrality of the oedipal situation in the ability to fall and remain in love.

David (1971) calls attention to the very early arousal of oedipal longings in children of both sexes, their intuition of an exciting, gratifying, and forbidden relationship which links the parents and excludes the child, and their longing for and excitement about forbidden knowledge — particularly sexual knowledge — as a crucial precondition for and part of the quality of being in love. Stoller (1974) also emphasizes the importance of mystery in sexual excitement and mentions various anatomical and physiological factors which, in their interaction with oedipal desires and dangers, contribute to the exciting and frustrating qualities that are so much a part of mystery. Mystery both induces and is part of sexual fantasy, which is an essential aspect of sexual excitement in human beings.

David says that the prolonged state of infantile dependency in both sexes is linked with the establishment of firm boundaries separating the generational identity of parents and children and the sexual identity of male and female. In both sexes, this longing, envy, jealousy, and curiosity finally lead to the active search for the idealized oedipal object. What is new in this formulation (and these concepts are developed further by Braunschweig and Fain [1971]) is the longing for the unavailable and forbidden object which energizes the sexual developments in both sexes, but which may also activate guilt which opposes this development, thus undermining the future capacity for establishing satisfactory love relations.

Braunschweig and Fain (1971) suggest that the little boy and the little girl have different developmental tasks, tasks which, together with the developmental constraints associated with them, create later potential conflicts. (In summarizing some of their salient conclusions, I shall try to remain as close as possible to their language.) For the boy, the pregenital relation with mother already involves a special sexual orientation of her toward him, which stimulates his sexual awareness and the narcissistic investment of his penis. The danger is that the mother's excessive pregenital gratifications of the boy's narcissistic needs may stimulate him to fantasize that his small penis is fully satisfactory to her, and thus contribute to his denial of the difference between his and his father's powerful penis. Under these circumstances, narcissistic fixation may later result in a kind of infantile, playful sexual seductiveness toward women without full identification with the "penetrating power" of the paternal penis. This fixation will interfere with full genital identity, with the internalization of the father into the ego ideal, and will foster the repression of excessive castration anxiety. The unresolved competition with father and the defensive denial of castration anxiety are expressed in the narcissistic enjoyment of infantile dependent relations with women who represent mother images. This constellation, for these authors as well as for Chasseguet-Smirgel (1973, 1974), is an important source of narcissistic fixation (I would say fixation at a level of normal infantile narcissism) and for failure to resolve the oedipal complex in boys, and is fostered by those aspects of mother's behavior through which she rebels against the "dominance" of the paternal penis and the "paternal law" in general. Hence, an unconscious collusion exists between eternally little boys — Don Juans — and seductive maternal women who utilize the rebelliousness of the Don Juan against father's "law and order" to express their own competitiveness with and rebelliousness against the father. Braunschweig and Fain state that, normally, mother's periodically turning away from the male child to return to the father as a woman who is sexually committed to him frustrates the little boy's narcissism and stimulates him to identify competitively with father, thus initiating or reinforcing the positive oedipal constellation in boys. One consequence is the boy's heightened feeling of frustration at being sexually rejected by mother so that his orally derived — and projected — aggression toward her is reinforced by early oedipally determined aggression. This development will crucially influence the love life of men who, unconsciously, do not change their first sexual object.

Chasseguet-Smirgel et al. (1970) and Braunschweig and Fain also stress the existence of the little girl's vaginal excitability and of her feminine sexuality in general. In this regard, the French group's observations are similar to those of Horney (1967), Jones (1948), and Klein (1945), and to recent investigators in this country, indicating early vaginal masturbatory activities of little girls and the intimate connection between clitoral and vaginal erotic responsiveness in the female (Barnett, 1966; Galenson and Roiphe, 1976). These studies suggest that a very early vaginal awareness exists in the little girl, and that this vaginal awareness and sexual response is inhibited and later repressed under the influences of various factors.

The French authors stress that evidence seems to be accumulating indicating that the parental, particularly the mothers' attitude toward the infants of both sexes varies and has a strong influence on gender identity (see also Stoller, 1973). The French group think that the mother, in contrast to her early stimulation of the little boys' genitality, does not particularly invest the little girls' genitals because she maintains her own sexual life, her "vaginal sexuality," as part of her separate domain as a woman relating to father. Even when mother narcissistically invests her little daughter, her narcissism has mostly pregenital features (except when the mother has strong homosexual inclinations). Also, mother's failure to invest her daughter's genitals would be in response to the culturally determined pressures and shared inhibitions regarding the female genitals which stem from male castration anxiety.

Blum (1976) has stressed the importance of oedipal rivalry and of conflicts around self-esteem as a woman that the little girl arouses in her mother: if the mother has devalued herself as a woman, she will devalue her daughter; the mother's self-esteem will have a strong influence on her daughter's self-esteem. The mother's unresolved conflicts about her own genitality and her admiration of her little boy's penis will induce in her daughter a merging of penis envy with sibling rivalry. Normally, the little girl turns to her father not only from disappointment in, but in identification with, her mother.

A general implication of the French writers' line of thought is that castration anxiety is not a primary determinant of the little girl's turning away from the mother toward father, but a secondary complication reinforcing the primary inhibition and/or repression of vaginal genitality under the influence of mother's implicit denial that her daughter has genitals. The intensity of castration anxiety in women would depend largely upon a three-step displacement of pre-genital aggression: first projected onto mother, then reinforced by oedipal competitiveness with her, and finally displaced upon father. Penis envy in little girls would in large part reflect reinforcement of oedipal conflicts under the effect of the displacement of pregenital aggression and envy onto the penis.

By the same token, Chasseguet-Smirgel (1974) has suggested that the little boy's fantasy of a phallic mother may serve as a reassurance against, or denial of,perceiving the female genitals as a product of castration, and also against the awareness of the adult vagina, which would prove his little genitals highly inadequate. Chasseguet-Smirgel here follows Horney (1967).

The little girl and the little boy thus have to pass through various developmental stages as part of their road to identifying with adult genitality. For the boy, the identification with father implies that he has overcome his pregenital envy of women, the projection of this envy in the form of primitive fears of women (Kernberg, 1976a, Chapter 7), and his fears of inadequacy regarding the feminine genitals. The French writers quoted consider Don Juan halfway between the inhibition of sexual drive in men toward women who represent the oedipal mother, on the one hand, and the adult identification of a man with father and the paternal penis in an adult sexual relation with a woman, on the other: Don Juan, Braunschweig and Fain suggest, affirms genitality without paternity.

I do not think there is a unitary etiology of the Don Juan syndrome in men. In ways similar to promiscuity in women, the cause of which may range from severely narcissistic character pathology to relatively mild, masochistically or hysterically determined pathology, male promiscuity exists along a continuum. The promiscuous narcissistic personality is a much more severe type of Don Juan than the infantile, dependent, rebellious but effeminate type of Don Juan the French authors described.

I think that the next step toward normal sexual identification with father on the part of boys is the conflict-ridden identification with the primitive, controlling, and sadistic male who represents the fantasied, jealous and restrictive father of the early oedipal period. The final overcoming of the oedipal complex in men is characterized by a man's identification with a "generous father" (Braunschweig and Fain, 1971) who no longer operates by means of repressive laws against the sons. The capacity to enjoy the growth of a son without having to submit him to punishing initiation rites reflecting unconscious envy of him is a landmark of the definite overcoming of oedipal inhibitions in the father. The practical implication of these formulations is that one important source of instability of love relations of adult men derives from incomplete identification with the paternal function, with various fixations along these developmental stages.

For the little girl, the lack of direct stimulation of her genital erotism in the early relation with mother, and, above all, the mother's conflicts over the value of her own genitals and genital functions in the broadest sense would bring about an inhibited psychosexual development which is then secondarily reinforced by the development of penis envy and the repression of sexual competitiveness with the oedipal mother. However, the mother's depreciation of men and her little boy's genitals may radically alter the sexual perceptions and conflicts of her children of both sexes.

For the French authors, the little girls' genitality, in contrast to the socially reinforced "public display" of male genitality in little boys' pride in their penis, is private — she is alone in the realm of her sexual development. Under these circumstances, her silent and secret unconscious hope resides in turning from mother to father and in her intuitive longing for the paternal penis, which, in penetrating the vagina, would eventually recreate the affirmation of vaginal genitality and of female sexuality in general. Braunschweig and Fain suggest that, because the road of female sexual development is lonelier and more secretive, it is more courageous than the little boy's, whose genitality is for various reasons stimulated by both parents. Perhaps because under optimal circumstances the little girl has had to change the first erotic object in turning from mother to father, and in the process has had to move from pregenital to genital developments earlier more definitely and in a lonely way, the adult woman has a potentially greater courage and capacity for heterosexual commitment than the adult man.

In a different context, Altman (1977) has pointed out that, in contrast to the permanence of the first object in men, the change of object in women may be one important source of the generally greater ease women have in committing themselves to a stable love relation. Men would be inclined to eternally search for the ideal mother and would be more prone to reactivate pregenital and genital fears and conflicts in their relations with women, which predisposes them to escape from abiding commitments. Women, having already renounced their first object, would be more able to commit themselves to a man who is willing to establish a full genital and "paternal" relationship with them. An additional crucial factor in women's capacity for commitment may be their concern for the stability of care and protection of their young, involving biological, and psychosocial determinants, mostly the identification with maternal functions and related sublimatory superego values (Blum, 1976).

SEXUAL PASSION AND THE CROSSING
OF BOUNDARIES IN LOVE RELATIONS

A central issue in the study of the psychology and psychopathology of love relations is that of sexual passion, an issue which seems related in many ways to the question of stability or instability of love relations. The very term "passion" as I am using it implies a combination of meanings that defies the dictionaries' tendency to divide up these meanings. Passion derives from the Latin *passio* — a translation from the Greek *pathos* — meaning to suffer or endure. Its archaic meaning of suffering, of martyrdom, reflects that origin. Passion also means strong love, affection, feeling or emotion of any kind, rage, hatred, and intense sexual desire. I think, precisely because it encompasses all these meanings, this word is well suited to describe a special quality of sexual love that includes intensity of feeling and a painful and yet highly pleasurable subjective experience of transformation and longing. Therefore, in spite of the multiple meanings of passion, I shall use the term sexual passion as the embodiment of a fundamental quality of love.

Sexual passion is not simply a characteristic of romantic falling in love or of the early stages of love relations, which gradually disappears and is replaced by a more toned-down, "affectionate" relationship. Sexual passion is a basic ingredient of what keeps couples together, an expression of (as well as guarantee of) the active, creative functions of love. And sexual passion, a precondition for the couple's stability is also a potential source of threat to it, so that a most viable, creative love relation is by implication also more threatened than one characterized by a relatively quiet harmony and feeling of security. Sexual passion is not limited to, although it is typically expressed in, sexual intercourse with orgasm. To the contrary, sexual passion expands from the core intuitive awareness of intercourse and orgasm as its final liberating, consuming, and reconfirming aim into the broad field of sexual longing for the object, of sexual excitement heightened by the appreciation of the physical, emotional, and ethical aspects of the sexual object. Sexual passion is, therefore, expressed as passionate excitement and human longing. But sexual passion cannot be equated with its external, behavioral manifestations, nor with the quality of overwhelming ecstatic mood characteristic of idealization in adolescence. The subtle yet deep, self-constrained and self-critical awareness of love for another person, together with the awareness of the final mystery separating one person from any other person, and the acceptance of unfulfillable longings as part of the price to pay for facing reality are also essential ingredients of sexual passion.

I concluded earlier (1976a, Chapters 7 and 8) that being in love is a complex emotional disposition which integrates sexual excitement, tenderness, genital identification, a mature form of idealization, and the commitment to an object relation in depth.

I would now add that this commitment is passionate, and that sexual passion itself is an emotional state that characterizes the love relation at all three levels: sexual excitement, object relation, and superego investment. Passion in the realm of sexual love, I propose, is an emotional state that expresses the crossing of boundaries in the sense of bridging intrapsychic structures which are separated by dynamically or conflictually determined limits.

The concept of boundary as employed in this formulation is related to but not synonymous with its use in systems theory. In what follows, I use the term boundary in the restricted sense of boundaries of the self, except where explicit reference is made to a broader use of the term as the active, dynamic interface of hierarchically related systems (particularly social systems). The most important boundaries crossed in sexual passion are those of the self. In contrast to regressive merger phenomena which blur self-nonself differentiation, concurring with the crossing of boundaries of the self—a step in the direction of identification with structures beyond the self—is the persistent experience of a discrete self. In this process, there is a basic creation of meaning, of a subjective ordering of the world outside the self, which actualizes the potential structuring of human experience in terms of biological, interpersonal, and value systems. Crossing the boundaries of self, thus defined, is the basis

for the subjective experience of transcendence. Psychotic identifications (Jacobson, 1964) with their dissolution of self-object boundaries interfere with the capacity for passion thus defined; madness,
in other words, is not in continuity with passion.

Norman Brown (1968) has pointed out a paradoxical feature of
the boundary between the self and the object: This boundary both
establishes and conforms to the reality principle and yet brings about
alienation because it artificially splits "me" from "non-me," "good"
from "bad." In his words: "Dionysus, the mad god, breaks down the
boundaries; releases the prisoners; abolishes repression; and abolishes the *principium individuationis,* substituting for it the unity of man
and the unity of man with nature" (p. 161). Brown proposes the
abolition of boundaries; I think, however, that there can be no
meaningful love relation without the persistence of the self, without
firm boundaries of the self, which generate a sense of identity.

There is a basic intrinsic contradiction in the combination of these
two crucial features of sexual love: the precondition of firm boundaries of the self with the constant awareness of the indissoluble
separateness of individuals, and the sense of transcendence, of
becoming one with the loved person. The separateness brings about
loneliness and longing and fear for the frailty of all relations; the
transcendence in the couple's union brings about the sense of oneness with the world, of permanence and new creation. Loneliness,
one might say, is a precondition for transcendence.

To remain within the boundaries of the self while transcending
them in the identification with the loved object is an exciting, moving, and yet painful condition of love. The Mexican poet Octavio
Paz (1974) describes this aspect of love with an almost overwhelming
conciseness: Love is a point of intersection between desire and reality. Love, he says, reveals reality to desire and creates the transition
from the erotic object to the beloved person. This revelation is
almost always painful because the existence of the other person presents itself simultaneously as a body which is penetrated and a
consciousness which is impenetrable. Love is the revelation of the
other person's freedom and brings about the contradictory nature of
love in that desire aspires to be fulfilled by the destruction of the

desired object while love discovers that this object is indestructible and cannot be substituted.

A clinical illustration may be helpful at this point. The illustration is of the quality of a maturing capacity for the experience of sexual passion, the development of a romantic longing in a previously inhibited, obsessive man in psychoanalytic treatment. I am by-passing the dynamic and structural preconditions of this change and mentioning only the relevant subjective experience of the patient's integration of eroticism, object relations, and value systems. The patient, a college professor in his late thirties, shortly before setting out on a professional trip to Europe had become engaged to a woman he felt very much in love with. On his return, he described an experience he had when visiting the Louvre and seeing there, for the first time, Mesopotamian miniature sculptures from the third millennium before our era. At one point, he had the uncanny experience that one of these diminutive sculptures, the body of a woman whose nipples and navel were marked by tiny precious stones, resembled the body of the woman he loved. He had been thinking about her, longing for her as he walked through the practically deserted halls, and while he was gazing raptly at the sculpture, a wave of erotic feeling seized him, together with an intense feeling of being close to her. He also was very moved by what he considered the extreme simplicity and beauty of the sculpture, and he felt that he could empathize with the unknown artist who had died over four thousand years ago. He had a sense of humility and yet of reassuring communication with the past, and felt as if he had been allowed to share the understanding of the eternal mystery of love as expressed silently in that work of art. The sense of sexual excitement had become fused with the sense of oneness, of longing for and yet close-ness to the woman he loved, and through that oneness and love he had been permitted entrance into the transcendent world of beauty. At the same time, he had a strong sense of his own individuality, and of a feeling of gratitude for being permitted to share the experience of this work of art and of humility in being faced with it.

The central dynamic expression of sexual passion and the poten-tial core of its culmination is the experience of orgasm in intercourse; in the experience of orgasm, gradually mounting sexual excitement culminates in an automatic, biologically determined response with a primitive, ecstatic affect, which requires for its full experience a temporary abandonment of the boundaries of the self, or rather, an expansion — or an invasion — of the boundaries of the self into the awareness of the subjectively diffuse biological roots of existence.

I have elsewhere (1973, 1976a, Chapter 3) explored the relation between biological instincts, affects, and drives. Here I would like to stress the key function of affects as subjective experiences at the boundary (in general-systems terms) between the biological and the intrapsychic realms and their crucial function in organizing internalized object relations and drives and, thus, secondarily, psychic structure in general.

The experience of orgasm does not by itself constitute sexual passion. Sexual passion implies a simultaneous crossing of the boundary of the self into awareness of biological functioning beyond the control of the self and a crossing of boundaries in a sophisticated identification with the loved object while yet maintaining a sense of separate identity. The shared experience of sexual orgasm also includes, in addition to the temporary identification with the sexual partner, the feeling that one is transcending the experience of the self and experiencing the fantasied union of the oedipal parents and, beyond that, is abandoning that union in a new object relation which reconfirms one's separate identity and autonomy. One crosses time-determined boundaries of the self in sexual passion, transcending the past world of object relations and creating a new, personal one. In this connection, orgasm as part of sexual passion also may represent symbolically the experience of dying, of still maintaining self-awareness while being swept into passive acceptance of neuro-vegetative sequences involving excitement, ecstasy, and ending. And the transcendence from self to a passionate union with another person and the values for which both stand also is a challenge to death, to the transitory nature of individual existence.

Dissolving the protective barriers against primitive diffuse affects while still remaining separate — that is, aware of one's self — and leaving behind the oedipal objects also implies the acceptance of danger, not only of losing one's identity, but of liberating aggression against internal and external objects, and of their retaliation. Sexual passion, therefore, also implies the acceptance of risks in abandoning oneself fully in the relation to the other person, in contrast to the fear of the dangers from many sources that threaten when amalgamating with another person; but there is also the basic hope in the sense of giving and receiving love and thus being reconfirmed in one's own goodness, in contrast to guilt and fear over the danger of one's aggression toward loved objects. And sexual passion also includes a crossing of time boundaries of the self in the commitment to the future, to the loved object as an ideal which provides personal meaning to life. In sum, sexual passion is a basic experience of simultaneous forms of transcendence beyond the boundaries of the self.

Sexual passion reactivates and normally contains the entire sequence of emotional states which assure the individual of his own, his parents', the entire world of objects' "goodness" and the hope of fulfillment of love in the face of frustration, hostility, and normal ambivalence. To experience sexual passion assumes the capacity for continued empathy with — but not merger into — a primitive state of symbiotic fusion (the "oceanic feeling" [Freud, 1930]); the exciting reunion or closeness with mother at a stage of self-object differentiation; and the gratification of oedipal longings in the context of overcoming feelings of inferiority, fear, and guilt regarding sexual functioning. Sexual passion is the facilitating core of a sense of oneness with a loved person as part of adolescent romanticism and, later, mature commitments to the beloved partner in the face of the realistic limitations of human life, the unavoidability of illness, decay, deterioration, and death. It is an important source of empathy with the loved person. So that the crossing of boundaries and the reconfirmation of a basic sense of goodness in the face of many risks link biology, the emotional world, and the world of values in one system.

Crossing the boundaries of the self in sexual passion, the integration of love and aggression, of homosexuality and heterosexuality in the internal relation to the loved person is illustrated eloquently in the declaration of love of Hans Castorp to Clawdia Chauchat in Thomas Mann's *Magic Mountain* (1924). Breaking away from his humanist, rational, and mature "mentor," Settembrini, Hans Castorp declares his love to Madame Chauchat (in French, which becomes an almost private and intimate language in the German context of the book). Excited and liberated by her warm though slightly ironical response, Hans Castorp tells her that he has always loved her and hints at a past homosexual relation with a friend of his youth who resembled her and whom he had asked for a pencil in the same way he had asked Madame Chauchat for one earlier in the evening. He tells her that love is nothing if it is not madness, something senseless, forbidden, and an adventure in evil. He tells her that the body, love, and death — all three are but one thing. He talks about the miracle of organic life and about physical beauty, which is composed of life and corruptible matter.

But crossing the boundaries of the self implies certain preconditions: As mentioned before, there has to be an awareness of and a capacity for empathy with the existence of a psychological field outside the self, hence, the erotically tinged states of manic excitement and grandiosity of psychotic patients cannot be called sexual passion; and the unconscious destruction of object representations and external objects that are so prominent in narcissistic personalities destroys their capacity for transcending into intimate union with another human being, therefore eroding and eventually destroying the capacity for sexual passion in such patients. Sexual excitement and orgasm also lose their function of boundary-crossing into biology when mechanical, repetitive sexual excitement and orgasm are built into the self experience dissociated from the deepening of internalized object relations. Here is where sexual excitement becomes differentiated from sexual passion; basically, masturbatory activity may (and usually does) express an object relation, typically the various aspects of oedipal relations from early childhood on. But masturbation as a compulsive, repetitive activity, functioning defensively against forbidden sexual impulses and other unconscious conflicts in the context of a regressive dissociation from conflicted object relations, loses its transcendent function. I am suggesting that it is not the endless, compulsively repetitive gratification of instinctual urges that brings about a deterioration of the excitement, pleasure, and satisfaction derived from them, but the loss of the crucial function of crossing self-object boundaries, which is guaranteed by the normal investment in the world of object relations. In other words, it is the world of internalized and external object relations that keeps sexuality alive and provides the potential for "eternal" sexual gratification.

The integration of loving and hating self-images and object images and affects in the transformation of part- into total-object relations — or object constancy—is a basic precondition for the capacity to establish a stable object relation. It is essential for crossing the boundary of an integrated self and identifying with the loved object.

But the establishment of object relations in depth also liberates primitive aggression in the relationship, for repressed or dissociated pathogenic object relations from the infancy and childhood of both partners are reactivated in the context of intimacy throughout time. The more pathological and aggressively determined a person's repressed or dissociated internalized object relations, the more primitive are the corresponding defense mechanisms; these, particularly projective identification, may evoke experiences or reactions in the partner that reproduce these threatening object relations. Reactivation of these processes in one partner will reactivate them in the other. Idealized and devaluated, mourned-for and persecutory object representations are superimposed on the perception and interaction with the loved object and may threaten—as well as strengthen—the relationship.

As both partners become increasingly aware of the effects of distortions in their perceptions of and behavior toward each other, they may become painfully aware of mutual aggression without necessarily being able to resolve their interactional patterns, so that the unconscious cement of the relationship may also endanger it. It is at this point that superego integration and maturation, expressed in the transformation of primitive prohibitions and guilt feelings over aggression into concern for the object—and the self—protect the object relation and the capacity for crossing the boundaries toward the loved object. The mature superego fosters love and commitment to the loved object.

But, by the same token, superego functions that include prohibitions against the remnants of oedipal conflicts may threaten the capacity for sexual love by prohibitions directed against oedipal genital impulses and the underlying prohibitions against genitalized aggressive impulses. So the superego may guarantee the lasting capacity for sexual passion, or it may destroy it. And at a certain intensity of primitive superego pathology, sadistic superego forerunners coincide with aspects of primitive dissociated object relations activated in the couple's relationship. Here the psychopathology of the individuals becomes a psychopathology of the couple.

Obviously, we expect mature superego functioning to tolerate sublimated oedipal strivings in the context of mature object relations, and thus trust the mature superego to be protective, in contrast to inhibiting, with regard to the capacity for sexual love. However, insofar as all crossing of boundaries (in the broader sense of systems theory) implies a defiance of prohibitions against entering forbidden territory — and particularly defiance of prohibitions against sexual and generational barriers, which are so deep a component of human life — there is an implicit intrinsic quality to sexual passion that directs it almost by definition against superego functioning.

The activation of superego functions in both partners creates the danger of mutual inhibition or a "freezing" of the relationship: each projects guilt feelings onto the other in the form of fantasied prohibitions and accusations. But there is also the protective function of the gratification of their sexual and human needs by the very activation of the "repetition compulsion" in expressing repressed internalized object relations in the context of the breakthrough of renewed passion after internal distancing from each other. Under optimal circumstances, both the mature and the neurotic aspects of the object relationship neutralize repressive superego features. By feeling "guilty" because of projected self-accusations attributed to the partner, each partner may unwittingly reinforce mutual suspicions of guilt, and, by rebelling against the "accusing" partner, free him/herself from neurotic inhibitions. This represents a creative use of aggression in the service of love. In more general terms, the neurotically determined unconscious bonds reflecting the activation of repressed or dissociated reciprocally reinforcing past object relations may, paradoxically, add intensity and richness to the couple's life, and foster stability in spite of the conflictual nature of the relationship.

One general implication of the definition of sexual passion proposed is that it constitutes a permanent feature of love relations rather than an initial or temporary expression of the more "romantic" qualities of idealization processes of adolescence and early adulthood; that it has a function of providing intensity, consolidation, and renovation to love relations throughout life; and that it provides a quality of permanence to sexual excitement by linking it with the couple's total emotional experience. This leads us to the quality of the erotic aspects of stable sexual relations; I think that clinical evidence clearly indicates the intimate link between sexual excitement and enjoyment and the quality of the couple's total relationship. Although statistical studies of large populations (Kinsey et al. 1953) show a decrease of frequency of sexual intercourse and orgasm over the decades, clinical study of couples indicates the significant effect of the nature of their total relationship on their sexual experiences: the frequency of intercourse, the intensity of its erotic quality, the excitement related to the enactment and sharing of sexual fantasies — all depend on the quality of the couple's object relationship. The sexual experience remains a constant central aspect of love relations and marital life throughout. Under optimal circumstances, the intensity of sexual enjoyment has an ongoing renovative quality which does not depend on the mechanical features of sexual gymnastics but on the couple's intuitive capacity to weave changing personal needs and experiences into the complex net of heterosexual and homosexual, loving and aggressive, aspects of the total relationship expressed in unconscious and conscious fantasies and their enactment in sexual relations.

THE OEDIPAL SITUATION AS SUBJECTIVE EXPERIENCE AND STRUCTURE

I agree with David (1971) that the quality of longing for the unavailable and forbidden oedipal object which energizes sexual development in both sexes is a crucial component of sexual passion and love relations. In this regard, the oedipal constellation may be considered a permanent feature of human relations, and it may be important to stress that neurotic solutions to the oedipal conflicts have to be differentiated from the normal manifestations of oedipal structuring of intrapsychic as well as interpersonal and social situations.

In terms of crossing the boundaries of sexual and generational prohibitions, this might be formulated as the active reconstruction, on the part of the individual in love, of his past history of oedipal relations (including the defensive and sublimatory fantasies that recreate the encounter with oedipal figures, and, in the process, also reenact the leaving and mourning the loss of the oedipal parents) in the new longing for and encounter with the love object. Crossing of generational and sexual boundaries transforms unconscious fantasies into subjective experience, and the couple, in reciprocally activating the world of internal object relations, reactivates the oedipal myth as a social structure (Arlow, 1974).

In both sexes, oedipal longings, the need to overcome fantasies of oedipal prohibitions and to satisfy curiosity about the mysterious relations between the parents stimulate sexual passion. Because of the factors mentioned earlier, it seems likely that women are earlier to cross the final boundary of an identification with the oedipal mother, affirming their female sexuality in the change of erotic object from mother to father. Men have to cross the final boundary of the identification with the oedipal father, not only in their capacity to establish a sexual relation with a loved woman, but to carry out the functions of paternity and "generosity" (Braunschweig and Fain, 1971) in this context. In this connection, clinical experience reveals how guilt-ridden men feel when they decide to terminate a relationship with a woman, whereas women usually feel free in letting a man know when they do not love him. This difference most probably reflects the deep-seated guilt over aggression toward mother which is reenacted so frequently in men's relationships with women (Jacobson, personal communication). But, in women, unconscious guilt connected with the rebellion against the pregenital and genital mother's fantasied prohibitions against vaginal genitality requires the additional carrying out of a full genital affirmation in the sexual relationship with a man. One factor contributing to the great frequency of genital inhibitions in women may be that the sadistic superego forerunners related to the introjected primitive preoedipal mother are condensed with the later prohibitive aspects of the oedipal mother. This may also be an important element in the prevalence of "female masochism."

There has been a growing questioning of assumptions regarding inborn dispositions to masochism in women, and an increasing awareness of the various psychological and social factors contributing to women's masochistic tendencies and sexual inhibitions. Person (1974) and Blum (1976) have recently reviewed the pertinent literature and stressed the psychosocial determinants of feminine masochism. Blum concludes that there is no evidence that the human female has a greater endowment than the male to derive pleasure from pain, and that the girl's earliest identifications and object relationships are of crucial importance in determining her later sexual identity, feminine role, and maternal attitudes: Masochism is more likely to be a maladaptive solution to feminine functions.

Stoller (1974) has suggested that, because of the original merging with mother, the sense of femininity is in fact more firmly established in women than the sense of maleness in men. Men, because of their original merger with a female may be more vulnerable regarding their bisexuality and more prone to the development of perversion.

It seems to me that after the full analysis of a woman's pregenital and genital sources of penis envy and the loathing of her own genitals, one regularly encounters an earlier capacity for a full enjoyment of vaginal eroticism, an affirmation of the full value of her own body simultaneously with the capacity to love her man's genitality without envy. I do not think that normal female sexuality implies the need to renounce the penis as the most appreciated genital, and I think there is good evidence that the fear of female genitals in men is not only secondary to oedipal castration anxiety but, in most severe cases, has profound pregenital roots. In short, overcoming fear and envy of the other sex represents in both sexes an exhilarating experience of fully crossing the boundaries of prohibitions against sexuality.

From a broader perspective, the couple's discovery vis-à-vis each other of the enjoyment of full genitality may cause it to change radically from submitting to cultural conventions and ritualized prohibitions and superstitions that erect barriers against expressing mature genitality in both sexes. This degree of sexual freedom, together with the final overcoming of oedipal inhibitions may constitute the

ultimate potential for sexual enjoyment in love relations and reinforce passion by creating a new mystery of sexual secrets shared by
the couple which frees it from the surrounding social group. In other
words, crossing the sexual boundaries so strongly impelled by the
mystery of oedipal longings from early childhood on may result in
the couple's establishing a new common social boundary which protects the secret and the mystery of its sexual communion. From a
developmental point of view, the elements of secrecy and opposition
in sexual passion derive from the oedipal constellation as a basic
quality of human sexuality.

The tragic incapacity to identify with the paternal function, so
that all love relations are doomed to failure in spite of "genital primacy," and the rationalization of this failure in terms of the myth of a
male-dominated culture are dramatically illustrated in Henri de
Montherlant's *Les Jeunes Filles* (1936). Speaking ambiguously for his
young hero (or antihero) Pierre Costals, Montherlant bitterly
resents the pressures derived from the desire that brings men and
women together in an eternal misunderstanding. For women, he
says (pp. 1010–1012), love begins with sexual gratification, whereas
for men, love ends with sex; women are made for one man, man is
made for life and for all women. Vanity is the dominant passion of
man, while the intensity of feelings related to the love for a man
represents a major source of happiness for women. The happiness of
women comes from man, but that of man comes from himself. The
sexual act is surrounded by dangers, prohibitions, frustrations, and
disgusting physiology.

It would be easy and perhaps tempting to dismiss Montherlant's
description of the aesthetically oriented, anguished, proud, old-
fashioned, cruel, and self-destructive Costals as the product of a
paternalistic ideology; such a conclusion would miss the deeper
sources of the intensity of the longing, and the fear and hatred of
women that underlie this rationalization in terms of a certain
cultural style of life.

For both sexes, the principal interferences with a stable, fully
gratifying relationship with a member of the opposite sex are caused
by pathological narcissism and by unresolved oedipal conflicts, especially the failure to achieve full genital identification with the parental

figure of the same sex. Narcissistic pathology in men and in women has relatively similar or complementary features; in contrast, and for the various reasons mentioned here and in my earlier work on love relations (1976a, Chapters 7 and 8), pathology derived from oedipal conflicts has different features in men and women. In women, unresolved oedipal conflicts show most frequently in various masochistic patterns, such as a stable attachment to unsatisfactory men and an incapacity to fully enjoy or maintain a relationship with a man who could be fully satisfactory to them. Men also attach themselves to unsatisfactory women; but, culturally, in the past they were freer to dissolve such unsatisfactory relationships. And women's value systems, their concern and sense of responsibility for their children, may reinforce whatever masochistic tendency they have. However, the natural ego ideal and maternal concerns are not masochistic goals (Blum, 1976) in the "ordinary devoted mother." In men, the principal pathology of love relations derived from oedipal conflicts takes the form of fear of and insecurity vis-à-vis women and reaction formations against such insecurity in the form of reactive and/or projected hostility toward them which combines in various ways with pregenital hostility and guilt toward the maternal figure. Pregenital conflicts, particularly conflicts around pregenital aggression, are intimately condensed with genital conflicts. In women, this condensation appears typically in the exacerbation of conflicts around penis envy; the orally determined envy of the pregenital mother is displaced onto the idealized genital father, his penis, and onto the oedipal rivalry with mother. In men, pregenital aggression and envy and fear of women reinforce oedipal fears and feelings of inferiority toward them: the pregenital envy of mother reinforces the oedipally determined insecurity of men regarding idealized women.

The universal nature of the oedipal constellation, the fact that oedipal features — if not neurotic oedipal conflicts — color the entire life span of the couple, make for the reemergence of oedipal conflicts in various stages of the relationship so that social circumstances may sometimes induce in the couple and at other times protect it from the reactivation of neurotic expression of oedipal conflicts.

For example, a woman's consistent, dedicated commitment to her husband's studies or professional development may reflect an adaptive expression of her ego ideal, but it may also compensate adaptively for masochistic tendencies related to unconscious guilt at taking the place of the oedipal mother. When the husband no longer depends on her, and the economic and social relationship within the couple changes, no longer requiring or warranting her "sacrifice," unconscious guilt from unresolved oedipal conflicts may no longer be compensated; it may trigger various conflicts, perhaps unconscious needs to destroy the relationship out of guilt, or unresolved penis envy and related resentment of male success. Or, a man's failure at work may decompensate his previous sources of narcissistic affirmation, which have protected him from oedipal insecurity vis-à-vis women and pathological rivalries with men, and bring about a regression toward sexual inhibition and conflictual dependency on his wife, which further reactivates his oedipal conflicts and neurotic solutions of them.

The social, cultural, and professional development and success of women in our society, then, may threaten traditional, culturally sanctioned and reinforced protection of men against their oedipal insecurity and fears, and against their envy of women in the broadest sense; and the changing reality of their life faces both participants with the potential reactivation of conscious and unconscious envy, jealousy, and resentment, which dangerously increase the aggressive components of the love relation.

These sociocultural dimensions of the couple's unconscious conflicts are subtly but dramatically illustrated in the series of films, *Six Moral Tales,* dealing with love and marriage, by Eric Rohmer, particularly *My Night with Maude* (Rohmer, 1968; Mellen, 1973). Jean-Louis, an intelligent, sensitive but conventional young Catholic, is afraid of responding to the equally intelligent but warm, vivacious divorcée, Maude. He prefers to remain "faithful" to and marry the secretive, submissive, and rather insipid girl he has met in church and idealized (before meeting Maude). Jean-Louis appears to be a man of commitment and consistency, but he is afraid to commit himself to a full although uncertain relationship with a woman who is his equal. And Maude, in spite of her charm and talent and her capacity for personal fulfillment, cannot understand that Jean-Louis will not give her anything because he is afraid and unable to do so.

She rejects Jean-Louis' friend Vidal, who loves her, and we leave her on the verge of embarking on yet another unsatisfactory marriage to still another man. The sadness of lost opportunities and the tragic cruelty of the unconscious destruction of opportunities which have been achieved in a love relationship or marriage are the counterparts to the potential happiness and fulfillment of a stable love relation or a marriage within which the couple is able to transcend the dangers which have been mentioned.

SOME CONSEQUENCES OF MATURE LOVE RELATIONS

Overcoming the fears and inhibitions connected with genital eroticism brings about a sexual freedom which enhances the couple's relations with an ongoing renewal of sexual life. The potential for variety in human sexual behavior increases the experience of personal freedom and enjoyment and adds to the uniqueness and complexity of human sexuality, as Eissler (1975a) has pointed out. This freedom, which integrates partial sexual drives, aggressively derived impulses, as well as sublimated homosexual identifications into libidinal eroticism, is in contrast to the restricting rigidity of sexual perversions and to the deteriorating quality of sexual excitement in narcissistic pathology.

The capacity for the development of total object relations protects and expands the continuing renewal of genital eroticism. But sexual freedom may also threaten the stability of the couple when disturbances in the realm of its object relations or mutual induction of superego pathology distort and inhibit the love relations and defensively reactivate the search for new sexual experiences in order to escape from the no-longer-tolerable relationship. Under optimal circumstances, the increased sexual temptations that go with increased sexual freedom are redirected into the couple's sexual life; the combination of creative innovation and relaxed intimacy in its sexual behavior cements its stability even when conflicts threaten in the realm of human relationships in other areas.

The couple's emotional relationship permits an intimacy which gratifies many human needs; but intimacy also threatens the release of aggression. The danger of uncontrolled intimacy, of "complete openness," is compensated for by the ongoing re-creation of areas of secrecy and mystery. Shared secrets and mystery increase the couple's freedom from the surrounding social world; and each partner's secrets and mystery maintain and create new boundaries in the couple's relationship. Secrecy and mystery are maintained as new tasks, challenges, and crises reactivate conflicts and needs from the past and bring about subtle changes and actualization of unknown potentials, which may bring the couple closer together or further apart.

The capacity for development of object relations in depth protects the couple's stability, but also creates the possibility of establishing a new relationship with another person, who correctly may be perceived as promising a more satisfactory human relationship at a different stage of life (Kernberg 1976a, Chapter 8). Under optimal circumstances, such intuitively perceived, longed-for, and tempting possibilities may be redirected to the life of the couple and add to the dimension of mystery and secret enrichment of its love life. The values of a life lived together and of a past created jointly, the difficult challenges of later life, separation, and death also cement the couple.

The maturation of the superego is a very strong element in providing the capacity for concern, loyalty, and commitment to the loved object, for the mature idealization of the relationship which, together with the satisfaction of a deep human relation, elevates sexual excitement into sexual passion and love. But, insofar as primitive remnants of the superego always remain active, and their persistence is almost a necessary price to pay for superego integration, the mutual induction of guilt or superego projections may inhibit the couple, decrease the tolerance of unavoidable aggression, and eventually restrict its emotional, particularly its sexual, life. This may foster the temptation to break out of the relationship, to again cross new boundaries, in this case, the barriers of conventional limitations the couple has unwittingly created for itself. However, the presence of such superego functions also increases the couple's moral commitment to a life lived together and protects the couple's relation in times of stress and conflict. Mature love implies concern, and concern is expressed in commitment. Under optimal circumstances, superego functions are strong enough to reinforce the commitment of the couple while yet mature and flexible enough to protect it against excessive primitive guilt, recrimination, and inhibition derived from primitive superego functions.

To conclude, maturation in the sexual realm, in the realm of object relations, and in superego development jointly determines the capacity for mature love and for the couple's stability, but it also creates potential conditions for its dissolution. Sexual passion as the ongoing crossing of boundaries in the realm of self-experience both protects the couple and creates new conditions for it, with consequences that cannot be fully foreseen. I think that mature love relations are not "postambivalent," but remain ambivalent with love prevailing over hatred; and they remain ambiguous, with a combination of intimacy and secrecy, growing freedom in sexual experience, and a persistent mystery of the ever-changing nature of private fantasy life. Intimacy and discretion are two essential ingredients of mature love relations; they permit a uniting of the optimal expression of sex and love and the optimal absorption and neutralization of aggression in the relationship.

The awareness, tolerance, and integration of the many complex aspects of one's own sexuality reinforce the capacity for mutual empathy, another dimension of the growth of the couple. And empathy, in turn, reinforces intimacy, discretion, and love.

Chapter Fifteen

The Couple and the Group

The description of the regression that occurs in groups and the regression that occurs within the intimacy of the couple brings me to an exploration of the relations between the couple and the group. My thesis is that the couple has its own dynamics—dynamics that interact with group dynamics. Freud hinted at this in his Postscript to *Group Psychology and the Analysis of the Ego* (1921) when he wrote: "Two people coming together for the purpose of sexual satisfaction, insofar as they seek for solitude, are making a demonstration against the herd instinct, the group feeling. The more they are in love, the more completely they suffice for each other" (p. 140). Freud (1921) also stressed the intolerance of crowds to sexuality, citing the Church and the Army as institutions that could not tolerate sexual relations between men and women. He saw this intolerance as a derivative of the original danger facing the primitive horde, namely, the rivalry among the sons in the context of their competition for their mothers and sisters. Freud proposed that totemic exogamy protected the social structure at the cost of repressing sexual urges within it.

Bion (1961) showed the small group's need for the couple; his pairing-assumption group protected the group against preoedipal conflicts and expressed derivatives of the oedipal conflict. I have already explored the conventional and antagonistic attitudes of the large group toward sexuality. In general terms, while the small group needs the couple, the large group tolerates it only within the limits of stereotyped convention, and the mob does not tolerate it at all. Jointly, all these group processes indicate the projection onto the couple of oedipal longings, and the expression of jealousy, envy, and destructiveness. The couple, in turn, projects its shared oedipal and preoedipal conflicts onto the groups surrounding it, and attempts thus to discharge intolerable sexual and aggressive drive derivatives. A couple may provocatively display its closeness and intimacy to tease the group or to provoke it into retaliatory action (an expression of the couple's oedipal guilt). It is my belief that, because of these unconscious pressures, the couple needs the group. Just as the individual uses the group to project early dissociated or repressed aggression, sexuality, and superego-determined prohibitions against these, so does the couple.

From here on, unless otherwise specified, I am using the term group in a global sense, to denote the informal network of couples and individuals of the same generation that constitutes a couple's social environment. This informal social group combines the dynamics of small and large group processes in varying, ever-shifting ways. Group formation of this type begins in latency, expands in early adolescence, reaches maximum intensity in late adolescence, and persists into and through adulthood. I have already suggested that the stability of the couple is determined by both partners' capacity for tolerating aggression and the crossing of oedipal boundaries, and that this capacity carries with it the potential for breaking down. I am now suggesting that when a breakdown occurs, the couple turns again to the group from which it emerged.

There is a built-in, complex, and fateful relationship between the couple and the group. Because the couple's stability depends upon the successful establishment of its autonomy within the group setting, it cannot escape from its relation to the group. Because the couple enacts and maintains the group's hope for sexual union and love in the face of the potential destructiveness activated by ever-available large-group processes, the group needs the couple. However, the group cannot escape from the internal sources of hostility and envy toward the couple that derive from envy of the happy and secret union of the parents and from the deep unconscious guilt over forbidden oedipal strivings.

Leadership of task groups, large and small, requires power, but power granted for authoritative leadership almost inevitably leads to the group's according excessive powers to the leader, transforming it from authoritative to authoritarian. The idealization of the leader, stemming from oedipal sources, brings about projection onto the leader of the preoedipal superego, with its infantile features and regression from adult to childhood morality. Authoritarian leadership, operating through projected, primitive superego activity, while it protects the group — and thus the couple — from aggression, brings in its wake an infantile attitude toward the couple: they may love each other, but they should not indulge in any sort of "forbidden" erotic activity. In larger, more informal group situations, such as in politically organized or institutional settings, this infantile attitude toward sexuality determines a "bureaucratization" of love relations that is reflected in the restrictions of socially sanctioned, stereotyped notions of love and marriage and in the development of restrictive norms and concept of normality. The couple can protect itself against this only by privately and secretly crossing the boundaries demanded by the group.

In social organizations, one task of the members of informal groups is to struggle against the regressive group pressures that foster the development of authoritarian leadership. Authoritarianism and sexual suppression usually go hand in hand. As Braunschweig and Fain (1971), to whom I have already referred in other connections, have pointed out, there is a difference between the fantasied harsh father of the early oedipal constellation, who has to control the rebellious son, and the mature, generous father who personifies not only genitality and paternity, but also the generative and creative aspects of the father as provider of rationality, encouragement, and love. The image of the father who tolerates and understands the rebellion of the sons without being internally destroyed or corrupted by it and without retaliating is reflected in the concept of tolerant leadership and in the related acceptance of the existence of erotic

love relations in couples within the social group. Similar considerations apply to organizations directed by women.

In light of the observations stemming from small groups and large
groups I am suggesting that the individual's need for social control —
in the form of an idealized leader or of ritualized suppressive social
structures — stems first from the need to defend himself or herself
against the emergence of primitive aggression in the context of loss of
ego identity, and second, from the aspiration for — and envy directed
against — the sexual couple who symbolize a new identity and a
transcendence into the freedom of sexual love. Thus, both the wish for
the young couple's oedipal triumph and the hatred and envy of it
foster the group member's need for social control and for an idealized leader, that is, for the symbolically oedipal father and his law.

Insofar as the struggles and contradictions that evolve within
group processes reflect the intrapsychic struggles of each of the members of the group, the fights between factions in the group are an
expression of intrapsychic conflicts that the individual cannot fully
tolerate and integrate. The temptation to identify with the oedipal
father perceived as the guardian of the law, the owner of all women,
and the dangerous punisher of rebellion, and related tendencies
toward authoritarian structuring of social reality, sexual repressive-
ness, and the idealization of autocratic leaders are present in all the
members of the group. At the same time, the oedipal wish to
dethrone and kill the father, conquer all the women, and establish a
mythical era of sexual freedom is also a powerful shared emotional
force in the group, which requires and supports the myth of the
young hero and the romantic struggle of the ideal couple against a
repressive social organization.

ROMEO AND JULIET

Shakespeare's play *Romeo and Juliet* may serve to illustrate my
thesis. At the risk of forcing the structure of the play into a direction
that was far from the playwright's intention, I shall attempt to let it
speak for what seems to me to be relevant issues linking the love life
of the couple with the couple's surrounding social group.

Romeo's family, the Montagues, have been feuding for generations with Juliet's family, the Capulets, a feud carried on by the followers of the heads of the two aristocratic families. Viewed in terms
of group processes, the play depicts a large-group process evolving
within the unstructured setting of the streets of Verona and demonstrates the expression of ever-lurking violence and loss of personal
identity characteristic of such large-group processes (as described by
Turquet [1975]).

Romeo and Juliet find each other, rebel against the restrictions
and prohibitions of their parents, and resolve adolescent oedipal
conflicts by dissociating themselves from their parents and turning
to a newly idealized love object of the opposite sex. In so doing, they
integrate their romantic idealization of one another with an actual
sexual encounter which cements their relationship. This brings
about a unity that liberates the couple internally from the biases and
feuds of its surrounding social group, that allows it to dare to identify
with the secret relationship of the oedipal couple, and facilitates its
almost miraculous maturation (particularly in Juliet), which transforms it from two adolescent individuals into an adult couple. (This
of course is a classical psychoanalytic interpretation.)

But I think the relation of Romeo and Juliet to the large group, to
the clans of the Montagues and the Capulets, is more complex than
the romantic encounter of two lovers in a sea of indifferent — and
even potentially hostile — people. This finding of each other, of a
man and a woman who meet in the middle of an indifferent and
unknowing crowd, and whose love removes them from participating
in the meaningless, endless, timeless feuding of the crowd and transforms them into a couple with a personal history and meaning, also
corresponds to the longing of every member of the crowd — of every
member of the large group. It corresponds, in fact, to universal longings, to which the story of Romeo and Juliet speaks so movingly.

In another respect, the couple, which by virtue of its love overcomes the aggression of the group, fulfills an ideal of the group itself.
It satisfies the "messianic" hopes of the group (Bion, 1961) for a
savior from the internal destructive forces that threaten the group's
existence. In Shakespeare's play, three individual members of
the surrounding group express that hope, and, although they

demonstrate varying degrees of ineffectiveness and failure, try to help the couple.

Mercutio, the poet and lover of dreams and Romeo's close friend, tries to protect Romeo from getting lost in illusions. At the very moment he is fighting—for Romeo—with Juliet's cousin Tybalt, Romeo, in conscious innocence, shall we say, attempts to interpose himself between Mercutio and Tybalt and thus causes Mercutio's death. Romeo's action, consciously intended to avoid bloodshed, brings it about, initiating a vicious cycle of increasing retaliations, which, in the end, lead to his own and Juliet's death. Romeo's deadly naïvete appears to result from his denial of aggression while caught in the idealization produced by love.

Friar Laurence consciously seeks to aid Romeo and Juliet, in the hope that by helping them he will be able to mitigate the animosity between the two feuding houses. But he too fails. His opposition to the aggression in the large group is secret and, for this reason, represents an attempt to find only an escape, not a true solution.

The efforts of Escalus, the Prince of Verona, to maintain the law by means of stern prohibitions and punishments also fails because his interventions are too few, too uninformed, too late, and, I would suggest, too indiscriminate and general. The Prince and the power of rational control for which he stands symbolize the efforts to reduce aggression in the large group by providing structure, rationality, and justice. But rationality, even when coupled with moral intent and integrity, requires the exercise of power over the large unstructured group. And when morality is combined with power it easily deteriorates into a morality contaminated by the effects of the group's collective projection onto the leader of superego features of childhood morality. Firm, consistent social structure, as we know from the treatment of adolescents, prevents as well as controls violence, but what might be optimal for the large group as a whole can stifle individuality in its members.

I am suggesting that group morality may protect a couple against the aggression of the large group of which it is a part, but at the cost of impoverishing "permissible" sexuality for the couple. This conflicts with the couple's search for liberation and meaning in a sexual relation that is unconsciously experienced as the breaking down of oedipal barriers and prohibitions.

Capulet's and Lady Capulet's belief that Juliet will obey them and marry the young Count Paris conforms with society's expectation that children will submit to the social order as expressed to them through their parents. The Capulets' expectation that Juliet will yield to their wishes is the counterpart of the imposition of social control and regulation via the law of the Prince. The correspondence between the law of the Prince and the law of the father reflects the attempt of the large group to establish control over adolescent couples by offering them protection and "legitimate" forms of sexual expression while suppressing their wishes for freedom to pursue sexual intimacy in their own way.

The Poet, the Friar, and the Prince, however, also represent societal functions that support the aspirations and longings for beauty, belief systems, and rational thinking, which exist in each of the individuals who are part of a large group. Thus, Romeo and Juliet, in their encounter (and in what those who support them represent) express the unspoken hopes and wishes of everyone, and this is their function for the group. When the play opens, both are ready for love, and we suspect that just about anybody would do. We may assume that the healthier the individual, the wider and more open is the potential for falling in love with one of the anonymous strangers in the crowd. Chance brings lovers together. It is their capacity to transform chance into a voluntary act and a commitment that liberates them from both dependence upon chance and from the group that actualizes their potentials. When they transform the capacity to fall in love to actually being in love, they acquire a new freedom. By doing so, they enact for everyone the emotional reality underlying the romantic myth of lovers who find themselves under the threat of potential destruction as a result of the hatred, envy, and jealousy they evoke in the group. The group's reaction to the couple is basically ambivalent: the idealization, hope, and longing that the couple evokes in the group is balanced by envy, resentment, and the wish to destroy the couple's union.

However, I believe that, just as innumerable Romeos and Juliets remain stillborn within the large group, the aggression of the large group is present in every one of its members, including Romeo and Juliet. Here my focus is on the dialectic of the management of aggression in the interaction of couple and group. Romeo's naïvete in separating Tybalt and Mercutio, his sudden access of benevolence — as though everyone else's world should be as full of love and free from hatred as his own — reflects a tragic denial of his awareness of the universality and intensity of aggression. His attitude is incomprehensible to his friend Mercutio and is despised by his enemy Tybalt. After Romeo unwittingly contributes to Mercutio's death, he is overwhelmed by a resurgence of aggression and kills Tybalt. In this sudden reencounter with his own aggression, he temporarily succumbs to the pressure of the group and, in so doing, seals his own fate. It is Juliet's maturity, her capacity to continue to love Romeo in spite of knowing that he killed her cousin, that consolidates her determination to sever her relationship with her family, including her corrupt nurse, and consolidates the union of the couple as well.

In their final encounter, after a night of love which takes place despite the danger of aggression against them, the lovers reveal their awareness of their predicament in their final dialogue before sunrise. Both of them struggle with the temptation not to separate again, despite the danger of death if they are together at sunrise. The point I wish to make is that the couple, while overcoming the aggression, meaninglessness, and anonymity of the large group by means of its love, must also be prepared to find in the midst of its intimacy precisely what it is attempting to escape from. Both Romeo and Juliet commit suicide. They die in innocence — not ignorant of but denying aggression even as they perpetrate it upon themselves.

The story of Romeo and Juliet seems to express the dynamics of the couple within the group processes I have described. The lovers' longing is the secret longing of everyone in the group or crowd. Their capacity to establish a perfect relation that unites tenderness, passion, and sensual eroticism within a secret union that transcends the hatred of their respective clans represents the realization of the wish to cross the boundaries of oedipal prohibitions and to overcome primitive aggression through sexual love. But, insofar as those who admire them are caught up in group processes, they are unconsciously pleased with the lovers' death: preoedipal envy and oedipal jealousy combine into hatred for those who fulfill their own deepest aspirations and defy the prohibitions and fears that inhibit them from realizing those aspirations themselves.

The Prince in *Romeo and Juliet* can be seen as representing both the idealized leader of the mob and the father figure who controls violence by providing rational structure to the social group. There are dangers emanating from the ambivalent roots of social control, however, and the rigidity of his laws contributes to the death of the young lovers.

ON "ROMANTIC" LOVE

The romantic love of adolescence is a normal, indeed essential, prelude to adult sexual love—a precondition for the gradual development of the capacity for a stable love relation. In romantic love, the normal idealization of the sexual partner, the experience of transcendence in the context of sexual passion, and the liberation from the surrounding social group are maximal.

That there is a difference between romantic love and romantic sentimentalism should be stressed; in the latter, libido is dissociated into idealized, desexualized love, on the one hand, and depreciated, purely genital arousal and eroticism, on the other. The dissociation results from the activation of oedipal longings in the context of the awakening of strong sexual drive and defense against it, in conformity with an infantile superego, all of which is characteristic of early adolescence.

My thesis is that the romantic element in the relationship of the couple is permanent and does not end with adolescence. On the contrary, I believe that the traditional distinction between "romantic love" and "marital affection" that permeates so much of the writing on the subject of love reflects the ongoing conflict between the couple and the group, namely, the suspicion with which the social group views love and sexual relationships that escape its total control. The insistence on this distinction also reflects denial of aggression within the couple's relationship, a denial which often transforms a deep love relation into a superficial and conventional one that lacks the very essence of love. This romantic love relation, I propose, is always in open or secret opposition to the group; it is by nature nonconventional; it frees the couple from participation in the restrictions imposed by the sanctioned sexual norms of its social group, creates an experience of sexual intimacy that is eminently private and secret, and lays down the setting in which mutual ambivalences will be integrated into the love relation, enriching it and at the same time threatening it; finally, it permits a certain amount of aggression to be redirected toward the social environment surrounding the couple.

What I am calling the nonconventional quality of romantic love corresponds to a deep conviction and attitude shared by the couple regarding its freedom from submission to the pressures of its surrounding social group. Its autonomy as a couple must be differentiated from "unconventional" (in the usual sense) behavior, for example, the rebelliousness of certain adolescent subgroups or exhibitionistic behavior reflecting various kinds of pathology. I am describing an internal attitude that cements the couple, often in very subtle ways, and that may be masked by surface adaptation to the social environment. The mature couple's nonconventionality, therefore, and its inclusion of infantile features into its sex life, is, paradoxically, more mature than the repressive and regressive group pressures that attempt to restrict sexuality under the influence of infantile superego remnants. The immature couple, in contrast, loses its opposition to the group—indeed, it returns to the group.

It is helpful to keep in mind that there is a phase-specific, normal search for a "romantic" road to sexual intimacy in the context of a full and intense relationship. If this road is not successfully traversed in adolescence, it will remain to compromise the success of future commitments. Adolescent love relations can become solid and deep, but for them to become stable depends upon personality features that require time to develop, making the outcome unpredictable. An adolescent couple's commitment to each other must remain an uncertainty, an adventure, to some extent, but this is also true for the adult couple.

I think that the violent and sudden ending so common in legends of romantic love gives evidence of a collectively shared sense of impotence to resolve the contradiction between infantile morality, with its demands for perfection at the cost of repressing sexual and aggressive drives, and adult morality, with its replacement of guilt and demands for perfection by a new sense of responsibility and concern, but with demands for new freedom in love and integration of aggression. The stable relation of the couple, particularly in marriage, implies a commitment to each other, to paternity and maternity, in the context of uncertainty; it is always a "bet," as Pascal has said.

The sentimental dilution of romantic legends by their — never fully specified — "happy ending" also reflects, by its unreal character, protection against the unconscious envy of the group toward the couple. The "official" love stories in totalitarian regimes (boy gets girl and both live happily working for the state) as well as the conventional assumptions made about married couples in all societies bespeak the need to domesticate the couple's relationship. The man and woman who in reality dare to overcome oedipal prohibitions by courting sex and tenderness by the same token also separate out from the collective fantasies that infiltrate the sexuality of their surrounding group. This process can be seen with maximum intensity in adolescence, but persists throughout life in the subtle but important interactions of the married couple and the social group within which the relationship of the couple evolves.

Romantic love stories do not necessarily end in the death of both lovers, but the death of one member of the couple is fairly common. Perhaps the most characteristic mark of romances is the closure of the story before the element of time penetrates the love relationship. In actual life, the development of the relations between two people over time gradually exposes the hidden presence of ambivalence and aggression. They must struggle to maintain their relationship by containing the aggression and by displacing part of the aggression outward, back onto the social group that surrounds them. Most conveniently at hand for this purpose is the social group by which they are surrounded — another facet to the interaction of couples and groups.

THE ADULT COUPLE

Love and aggression, as I have suggested in earlier work (1976a, Chapters 7, 8), are intimately linked in several ways. First, they are linked in the integration of loving and hating self-representations and of loving and hating object representations, which is a precondition for establishing ego identity and an internal world of object relations in depth. Second, they are joined together in that sexual love binds the sensual excitement of aggression with the sensual excitement of erotic gratification. Third, love and aggression are linked in that the aggression that enters into the consolidation of the mature superego transforms the infantile sense of guilt and shame into an adult sense of concern, responsibility, and commitment. Aggression is thus a key component of object relations, sexual encounters, and value systems that provide intensity, depth, and continuity to love relations.

Paradoxically, the consolidation of the couple's union reinforces its efforts to deny aggression in its idealized love relation and also increases the opportunities and temptations for the freeing of aggression in its relationship. The normal idealization of the loved person, reflecting a partial reprojection of idealized superego functions, easily regresses into a more immature idealization which reflects a reaction formation against unconscious ambivalence and aggression toward the idealized object. Under the impact of ongoing intimacy, reprojection of superego functions onto the sexual partner may bring about inhibitions through the projection of guilt feelings and fantasied expectations of perfection. The experience of intimacy also activates whatever potential there is for dissociated or repressed past object relations which become condensed with the couple's actual interaction, thus reproducing conflict-laden and aggressively infiltrated early object relations. The excitement, the search for sexual merger, and the longing for total liberation in sexual exploration and fulfillment also threaten to activate primitive aggression.

The need to release this aggression is what most endangers the couple. It is here that the interaction of couple and group becomes crucial. A couple in isolation can destroy itself because it has no outlet for aggression other than itself; the couple, which created itself in opposition to the group, needs the group for survival. To the isolated couple, marriage may feel like a prison from which breaking away and entering into a group situation may feel like an escape into freedom. The sexual promiscuity that immediately follows many separations and divorces illustrates such an escape into the freedom and anarchy of the group. On the other hand, the group may become a prison for those of its members who cannot or dare not become attached to someone else and thus become part of a stable couple. The couple's relationship offers a liberation from the loss of identity and primitive aggression that is inherent in the large group. Engagement in group sex represents an extreme form of dissociation of object relations from sexual activity, which masks the reality of that imprisonment from those who participate in it.

An ongoing excitement exists within the informal group of adult couples regarding the private lives of the couples composing it. At the same time, each partner is tempted to express rage in aggressive behavior toward the other within the relative intimacy of being with close friends. Unable to contain the aggression within the privacy of its relationship, a couple may thus use the group as a channel for its discharge as well as a theater for its display. That the bond between some couples who quarrel chronically in public may be deep and lasting should not come as a surprise. The danger, of course, beautifully illustrated in Albee's play *Who's Afraid of Virginia Woolf?* (1962), is that so much aggression will be expressed that the remnants of the couple's shared intimacy, particularly its sexual bonds, will be destroyed. The friends within the immediate social group who witness the combatants obtain vicarious gratification from the other people's quarrels and a reaffirmation of the security of their own relationship via reassurance that aggression is prevalent and can be handled by proxy.

Frequently, severe psychopathology in one or both participants may bring about the activation of repressed or dissociated, conflict-laden, internalized object relations that are reenacted by the couple through projective experiencing of the unconscious past, and rupture the couple's union. Both participants return to the group in a final desperate quest for individual freedom. When the psychopathology is less serious, unconscious efforts by one or both partners to blend or dissolve into the group, particularly by breaching the barrier of the sexual exclusiveness, may be a way of preserving the couple's existence at the risk of invading its intimacy and leading to its deterioration.

In sum, by asserting its independence of the group, the couple establishes its identity. Dissolution back into the group represents the final haven of freedom for the survivors of a couple that has destroyed itself.

There are times when an individual's submerging within a group may reflect a search for new aspects of his own identity precisely because of the loss of stable social roles and the derived transitory reactivation of older identity features — a temporary loosening of ego identity — that groups permit to individuals. Groups are usually much more tolerant of individual deviance than of couples' deviance, for reasons already spelled out (see Chapter 11).

Most adult social networks consist of a limited number of couples in voluntary association as a group. Because the members of this group presumably like each other, oedipal longings and rivalries are easily activated among them. The stability of each couple and a shared morality and sense of responsibility protect the couples, while the intensification of real likings and longings, together with social opportunities, activate the temptations to transform oedipal fantasies into action.

The conventional assumption that sexual boredom in marriage is a cause for dissolution of marital love is based on a misunderstanding of the way in which inhibitions of preoedipal and pregenital eroticism together with oedipal anxiety and guilt can interfere with sexual fulfillment. One would, according to my thesis, have to explore the development of boredom and indifference in marital relations as a consequence of denial of very intense and ambivalent aspects of the relation, similar to the function that boredom has clinically as a chronic experience with patients having severe psychopathology.

Polymorphous perverse infantile impulses, which are part of normal foreplay and of eroticism in general, are linked to early part-object relations or dissociated, split-off self- and object representations. Sadistic, masochistic, exhibitionistic, and voyeuristic impulses allow deep levels of aggressive and homosexual impulses to be integrated into a heterosexual relationship, permitting the regressive enjoyment in intimate sexual encounters of ordinarily inhibited sexual needs. Singer (1973), studying the differences between sensuous and what I am calling passionate aspects of sexual relations, described sexual encounters that are of either one or the other variety or that blend the two. Sexual eroticism that permits a full and playful enjoyment of each other's bodies is an important aspect of the enrichment of sexual relations and reflects the freedom to treat each other and to be treated as "sex objects." Such freedom can permit the gratification of sadomasochistic needs in a relationship enveloped or contained by love. The sharing of sexual fantasies (oedipally derived fantasies including third parties in the sexual experience in the context of jealousy and teasing are probably the most frequent types of fantasies during intercourse) and the real or symbolic enactment of them in the sexual relation may enrich the couple's sexual experience, but may also increase the danger of liberating aggression.

However, the effort to artificially manipulate such erotic components of sexuality, as in the currently fashionable assumption that the mechanical learning of sexual techniques will by itself enrich a couple's long-term relationship, leads to results that are, at best, temporary. This is not surprising, since erotic pleasure depends more upon the reenactment of internalized object relations than upon mechanical techniques. It is the unconscious fantasy of primitive object relations enacted in erotic play, combined with actual and symbolic physical intimacy, that gives intensity to the erotic relationship.

Group sex is the ultimate effort to enact this erotic fantasy life in external reality. At the same time, group sex is the ultimate destroyer of eroticism. In this connection, Freud's (1921, p. 140) penetrating comments regarding the relation between the couple and the group are most pertinent: "It is only when the affectionate, that is, personal, factor of a love relation gives place entirely to the sensual one, that it is possible for two people to have sexual intercourse in the presence of others or for there to be simultaneous sexual acts in a group, as occurs in an orgy."

The connection between sensuous eroticism and early oedipal and preoedipal impulses also accounts for the most fantastic, exciting, and frightening aspects of primal-scene fantasies. Unconscious prohibitions against such fantasies are reflected in the conventional prohibitions against, or restrictions of, polymorphous perverse aspects of sexuality. These fantasies are the deep source that feeds into the eroticism of pornography and the sharp contradictions between conventional and private attitudes that exist about it.

INTERACTION OF COUPLE AND GROUP

As relations between partners deteriorate, the couple maintains a pathological equilibrium as it turns to and is in turn invaded by the group. The equilibrium may take one of several forms. Triangular relationships with obvious oedipal implications are one type; entering into an open marriage, with loss of the couple's sexual boundaries is another; and the total loss of sexual intimacy as both partners enter into group sexual behavior is a third. Here, pregenital conflicts frequently predominate in the couple, and the relationship is more seriously damaged by what they resort to than it is in the two other types.

One means of regressively maintaining some sort of equilibrium is for one partner to establish a relationship with a third party; here we must distinguish between cases in which an affair is preliminary to the destruction of the couple and those in which the marriage seems to stabilize with the presence of a third party. In the latter instance, various outcomes can materialize. Frequently, the affair permits the stabilizing expression of unresolved oedipal conflicts. A woman who is frigid with her husband and sexually satisfied by her lover may experience a conscious sense of thrill and satisfaction which sustains the marriage while unconsciously she enjoys her husband as a hated transference representative of her oedipal father. In the dual relationship, she experiences the satisfaction of an unconscious triumph over the father who had had both her mother and herself under his control, whereas now she is the one who has two men under hers. The wish for the affair may also stem from unconscious guilt over experiencing her marital relationship as an oedipal triumph, while not daring to establish a total identification with the oedipal mother; a conflict between desire and guilt is acted out by playing Russian roulette with the marriage.

Paradoxically, the deeper and fuller these parallel (marital and extramarital) relationships become, the more they tend toward self-destruction because, in the long run, the splitting of the object representation attained through the triangular situation tends to be lost. The film *Captain in Paradise* illustrated how parallel relationships tend to become more and more identical with time, imposing an increasingly impossible psychological burden. Whether such relationships are maintained secretly or accepted openly depends of course upon other factors, such as the extent to which sadomasochistic conflicts play a role in the marital interaction. Open acceptance regarding extramarital affairs more often than not represents aggression, sadomasochism, and a defense against guilt feelings.

These situations should be differentiated from those in which the couple's actual relationship is obscured by the parallel maintenance of a liaison established in response to social, political, or economic pressures. Here a very meaningful, often secret relationship can exist parallel to a merely formal one such as a marriage of convenience. There are other instances in which both parallel relationships in a triangular situation are basically formalistic and ritualized, such as in subcultures in which having a mistress is a status symbol expected of a man of a certain social stratum.

What I wish to stress is that triangular situations, especially those that include a long-term, stable extramarital relationship, may have varying effects upon the relation of the primary couple, usually reflecting different types of compromise formations of unresolved oedipal conflicts. They may protect a couple against some types of aggression being directly expressed between them, but in most cases there is a loss in the capacity for real depth and intimacy as the price exacted for the protection that is provided against aggression.

Bartell (1971) richly documented some of the dominant social characteristics of promiscuous sexuality in an open group situation. He found that the idea that group sex protects and renews the marital relationship by creating new, shared sexual stimuli and experiences is actually an illusion. Typically, the "swinging" scene involves a minimum of interpersonal relationships other than those linked to the preparation and carrying out of sexual get-togethers. While the marital couples profess to being freed from their chronic boredom by their exciting secretive participation in the swinging social group, actually the social relationships, both within the swinging group and within the traditional group from which the participants derive, deteriorate even further over a relatively brief period of time, usually in less than two years. Sex then becomes boring once again, only even more so. Although Bartell remained faithful to a descriptive, sociopsychological approach and avoided a study in depth of individual or group psychology, he hinted at the discrepancy that exists between the exciting fantasies with which members approach group sex and the actual mechanical aspect of the interactions.

What group sex represents is a pale reflection of the stimulus pornography provides to individual masturbatory fantasy, namely, the full expression of pregenital, erotic and aggressive partial drives in the context of part-object relations. Albee's assertion in *The Zoo Story* (1958) that in childhood masturbation fantasy is a substitute for the "real thing" while in adulthood actual sex is a substitute for fantasy seems to have particular relevance to group sex, with all of the failure that is implicit in the substitution.

Bartell found that group sex liberates polymorphous perverse sexuality, especially female homosexuality, but at the same time there exists a strong inhibition against male homosexuality. This finding may be an indirect confirmation that women have a stronger core gender identity (Stoller, 1968) than men because of the differences between the sexes in early identifications; the boy must shift from mother to father whereas the girl can condense pregenital and genital identifications with mother. A stronger core gender identity would result in less fear of homosexual urges in the group situation. In short, women would be less threatened by homosexuality than men would be. However, one could raise the question to what extent social pressures, i.e., the greater social tolerance for female homosexuality, may also be playing a role.

The extreme instability of the group that gathers for group sex and an orgy illustrates the deteriorating and self-eliminating effects of unrestricted sex upon a social group. This brings us back to the liberation of aggression in group situations without any limiting social structure and to the activation of aggression by regressive expression of pregenital drives. Underlying sadistic trends are camouflaged in group sexual encounters by a studiously impersonal friendliness; tenderness and mutual concern do not provide a limiting boundary to the sexual experience.

The rapid self-dissolution of the sexually promiscuous group protects the shared illusion of eroticism from which aggression has been dissociated. I have had the opportunity to study the masturbatory fantasies of participants in group sex when they were getting progressively bored with the group activities: sadistic and masochistic fantasies were the only stimuli remaining that could kindle sexual arousal within group sex.

"Open marriage" as described by O'Neill and O'Neill (1973) and the so-called new lifestyle described, for example, in *Beyond Monogamy* (Smith and Smith, 1974) have among their professed goals the preservation of marital stability by opening channels for more or less casual or more or less permanent extramarital experiences. What is lacking in discussions of new lifestyles and open marriage is that, as is customary with sexual utopias, sexuality is discussed in terms of erotic and loving emotional experiences, whereas the importance of aggressive components in all intimate human relations is almost totally neglected.

Returning to the types of conflicts that seem to be associated with different ways of maintaining an equilibrium as a couple, the conflicts of couples who turn to open marriages usually fall somewhere between the oedipal and the pregenital. When one of the participants engages in more or less frequent extramarital affairs and the other partner displays marked masochistic features, the stability may be maintained by the acting out of a sadomasochistic relationship which reflects unconscious needs in both participants.

When both partners engage in multiple relationships, in the long run the situation is strikingly close to participating in group sex. The various lovers seem to belong to different social groups, and it is the marriage that becomes the impersonal railroad station that gathers occasional strangers under the common roof of a fixed point of reference. Some couples maintain a façade of conventional marital stability while their emotional relationships actually are in different arenas. A stable relationship by each of the marriage partners with another person outside of the marriage over an extended period of time implies a mutual acceptance of severe restriction in personal intimacy within the couple. This may provide for very polite, smooth social functioning, but it is a far cry from what can be provided by a full sexual and emotional relationship.

In short, the degree of invasion of the couple by the group or the dissolution of the couple into a group situation is reflected by the extent to which a purely formal marriage or a true emotional relationship is maintained. The more open, indiscriminate, and promiscuous the sexual behavior, the more likely it is that the psychopathology of the couple contains preoedipal features with a predominance of aggression and polymorphous perverse infantile sexual needs. Unless these are resolved, the result is a progressive deterioration of internalized object relations and of sexual enjoyment between the two members of the couple.

CLINICAL ILLUSTRATION

An artist in his early forties, whose transformation of a regional artistic style into an original, personally expressive style had gained him significant recognition, came for treatment after a brief hospitalization because of depression, chronic dissatisfaction with his life, and marital conflicts. In terms of diagnosis, he impressed me as having a narcissistic personality. In the analysis, his inability to present any real picture of his wife or of the various women with whom he carried on affairs was most conspicuous; they came across as shadowy, unreal figures.

His childhood history included a controlling but distant father and a rather conventional, guilt-inducing, dishonest and manipulative, subtly controlling and resentful mother. He sought dependent relationships with protective men which at times had homosexual undertones combined with intense rivalry, envy, and eventual devaluation of them. He perceived these men as distant from him and felt incapable of bringing them around to his side in order to obtain something from them. He viewed women as uniformly exploitative and dangerous. He constantly sought out women with perfect bodies and extreme beauty who would provide him with so much gratification by giving themselves to him that he would not need to be concerned about their exploiting him. Indeed, he saw any woman with a physical "defect" as a potential danger because it made her needy and greedy and therefore exploitative.

He married his wife when he was already a well-known artist. She had come from his home town, but from a lower socioeconomic stratum, which made him think that he could count on her gratitude and dedication to him. The sexual inhibition he discovered in her seemed to be an insult and an attack, and he quickly established an almost open pattern of sexual involvement with other women who catered to his sexual and personal needs while his wife took care of his home and his children. When his wife developed serious depression, however, and entered psychotherapy, she began to confront him with his sexual promiscuity. He told her he would not change his pattern of life as long as she was not fully satisfactory to him sexually; they then agreed to carry out an open marriage. The patient's fantasy, however, was that his wife would never become involved with another man so long as he was available to her. In the course of her own treatment, however, his wife became sexually freer, and for a time they had fully satisfactory sexual relations. But the patient continued his extramarital affairs and suggested to his wife that they try group sex. He did not understand his interest in group sex, but in the analysis it eventually became clear that his unconscious envy and hatred of his wife, displaced from his frustrating and overprotective mother, had increased when his wife became sexually responsive.

Active participation in group sex over a period of several months, requiring rather extensive travel by the couple, apparently led to a decrease in mutual recriminations and brought about a more distant but tolerable relationship. But the sexual pleasure they derived from having intercourse steadily diminished to the point that they were able to enjoy sex fully only with the heavy use of marijuana, which made them experience each other's bodies as disconnected from any emotional relationship between them. This facilitated the "use" of each other's bodies without apparent concern for the emotional deterioration of their relationship. The patient gradually became depressed, dissatisfied, and unhappy, without knowing why, and he now resented what he saw as the self-satisfied life of his wife, who had become successful in a new profession.

In the course of the analysis, the patient's unconscious resentment and hatred of women contributed to the development of a rather typical narcissistic transference, which also included thinly veiled homosexual yearnings. At one point, he became aware that he was denying his wife's sexual involvement with other men. She had mentioned to him that she was dating a certain man whom he had actually met with her. As usual, she was making plans so that her dating would not interfere with their jointly planned social activities. In turn, the patient usually let his wife know which nights he was going to meet with other women. When I asked what made him so sure that she would not go to bed with that man, given her enjoyment of sexual activities with many other men in his presence during "swinging" parties, the patient first angrily accused me of wanting to make him feel jealous and then reacted with intense anger toward both me and her. Before we could analyze his warding off his unconscious wish that his wife go to bed with other men, the patient impulsively suggested to her that they resume swinging. She immediately acceded, and they went to a party at which she became involved sexually with three men simultaneously. The patient's intense sexual excitement while watching that scene confirmed the homosexual component of his interest in group sex.

The depression for which he had originally entered treatment reappeared after the party. He was convinced that he had definitely lost his wife. He did not feel guilty for having brought about his and his wife's participation in the perverse sexual activity, although he felt that it had destroyed any remnant of intimacy between them. He was astonished, however, to find himself without any satisfaction in their relationship. Even the illusion of intimacy and sexual freedom he had earlier felt under the influence of "pot" was no longer available to him.

Later, analysis made it clearer to him that his deep rage against women as representatives of the early mother had led him to an almost premeditated effort to destroy anything valuable in his relationship with his wife. Unconsciously, sex at swinging parties implied to him a dismemberment and fragmentation of women and their bodies.

The patient's core pathology stemmed from an early preoedipal stage of pregenital eroticism that predates the capacity for a total-object relationship to differentiated objects. Although some superego integration was maintained, it was insufficient to sustain the ordinary social and sexual boundaries of marriage. His object relations were so disturbed that he was unable to have any real picture of, let alone deep emotional relationship with his wife. Even the minimal emotional relation necessary to gratify the couple's apparently free but actually polymorphous perverse sexual wishes was almost impossible, except under the influence of marijuana.

Discussion

Let us review this example of deterioration in the relationship of a married couple in light of the three areas contributing to what I have called sexual passion: the nature of the sexual experience, the level of object relations, and the degree of superego integration.

Neurotic patients with a predominance of oedipal conflicts and excessive superego pressures manifested by unconscious prohibitions against genital sexuality usually present sexual inhibition in the context of stable, deep object relations and maintenance of moral commitments and concern in the marital relationship.

In cases of more severe character pathology with regressive activation of dissociated and/or repressed pathological object relations in the marital interaction, lack of normal integration of superego functions, and condensation of genital and pregenital aims, there is, paradoxically, less sexual inhibition and more direct expression of polymorphous perverse infantile trends in the sexual relation. Partial dissolution of the marital relation in the form of extramarital affairs is more prevalent and the relations of the couple more disturbed, but its sexual bonds may be strong and satisfactory.

The case presented illustrates extreme deterioration of object relations and the way in which the quality of object relations and superego integration correlate with one another: the two usually deteriorate in parallel. Superego failure permits an increased *apparent* sexual freedom which contains the seeds for further disintegration of the couple's object relation. This disintegration further erodes the capacity for sexual enjoyment. Hence we find, paradoxically, the severest sexual inhibitions in patients and couples with the best-integrated (although infantile prohibitive) superego and a correspondingly high level of object relations — the typical neurotic case — and also in the severest types of psychopathology of individuals and couples where sexual experience is destroyed by the deterioration of object relations and superego functions. The failure of the superego to protect the couple's boundaries with the group, the need to escape from the intolerable activation of aggression activated by the part-object relations dominant in these couples, and the subsequent deterioration of sexual experiences — the mechanization of sex — all lead to the couple's dissolution into the group.

In contrast, a mature superego of the individuals forming the couple, which frees it from infantile prohibitions against a full sexual experience — including pregenital aggressive and homosexual components — also solidifies the bond protecting it from invasion by the group: Concern and responsibility for each other combine with a set of ethical values that reinforce the boundaries created by the couple's object relations. An object relation in depth lends maximum intensity to the sexual experience, and all three — superego functions, object relations, and sexual experience — strengthen the couple's boundary, separating it from the group.

Psychoanalytic object relations theory throws new light on the dynamics of the interaction of couples and groups. Early object relations are organizers of human development and subsequent behavior. Primitive, part-object relations lie dormant in the psyche, waiting to be activated both in the intense, intimate, long-term relations of a couple, and in groups with their ever-present proclivity for regressive processes. Regression in groups encourages regression in the individuals who constitute them; regression in groups threatens the couple because of the envy and idealization the couple evokes and because of the restrictions the group's primitive superego places on the couple. Couples need the group to project aggression activated in their relationship and to protect themselves from disintegration. The group is

a theatre for sublimations of the couple, and the couple may insti-
gate the activation of aggression in the group. Thus, couples and
groups need each other for survival and may endanger each other's
basic existence.

In the last resort, the conflict between love and hatred—between
libido and aggression—evolves within the individual, within the
couple, and within the group. I have attempted to explore the normal and pathological vicissitudes of this conflict from the vantage
point of the encompassing framework of psychoanalytic object
relations theory.

REFERENCES

Abadi, M. (1960). *Renacimiento de Edipo.* Buenos Aires: Editorial Nova.

Abenheimer, K. M. (1955). Critical observations on Fairbairn's theory of object relations. *British Journal of Medical Psychology* 28: 29–41.

Abraham, K. (1911). Notes on the psycho-analytic investigation and treatment of manic-depressive insanity and allied conditions. In: *Selected Papers on Psycho-analysis.* New York: Basic Books, 1953, pp. 137–156.

———(1916). The first pregenital stage of the libido. In: *Selected Papers on Psycho-analysis.* New York: Basic Books, 1953, pp. 248–279.

———(1924). A short study of the development of the libido, viewed in the light of mental disorders. In: *Selected Papers on Psycho-analysis.* New York: Basic Books, 1953, pp. 418–501.

Adorno, T. W. et al. (1950). *The Authoritarian Personality.* New York: Harper.

Albee, E. (1962). *Who's Afraid of Virginia Woolf?* New York: Simon and Schuster Pocketbook, 1964.

———(1958). *The Zoo Story.* New York: New American Library, Signet Book, 1959.

Altman, L. L. (1977). Some vicissitudes of Love. *Journal of the American Psychoanalytic Association* 25: 35–52.

Anzieu, D., Pontalis, J.-B. and Rosolato, G. (1977). A propos du texte de Guntrip. In: *Memoires: Nouvelle Revue de Psychanalyse* 15: 29–37. Paris: Gallimard.

333

Arlow, J. A. (1974). Dreams and myths. Presented on the occasion of the founding of the St. Louis Psychoanalytic Institute, October. Unpublished.

Balint, M. (1948). On genital love. In: *Primary Love and Psychoanalytic Technique*. London: Hogarth Press, 1952, pp. 128–140.

———(1956a). Criticism of Fairbairn's generalisation about object-relations. *British Journal of the Philosophy of Science* 7: 323–327.

———(1956b). Pleasure, object and libido: Some reflexions on Fairbairn's modifications of psychoanalytic theory. *British Journal of Medical Psychology* 29: 162–167.

———(1965). *Primary Love and Psychoanalytic Technique*. New York: Liveright.

———(1968). *The Basic Fault: Therapeutic Aspects of Regression*. London: Tavistock Publications.

———, Ornstein, P. H., and Balint, E. (1972). *Focal Psychotherapy: An Example of Applied Psychoanalysis*. London: Tavistock Publications.

Barnett, M. (1966). Vaginal awareness in the infancy and childhood of girls. *Journal of the American Psychoanalytic Association* 14: 129–141.

Bartell, G. D. (1971). *Group Sex*. New York: Signet Books.

Beres, D. and Arlow, J. A. (1974). Fantasy and identification in empathy. *Psychoanalytic Quarterly* 43: 26–50.

Bergmann, M. S. (1971). Psychoanalytic observations on the capacity to love. In: *Separation-Individuation*, ed. J. B. McDevitt and C. F. Settlage. New York: International Universities Press, pp. 15–40.

Bibring, E. (1953). The mechanism of depression. In: *Affective Disorders*, ed. P. Greenacre. New York: International Universities Press, pp. 13–48.

———(1954). Psychoanalysis and the dynamic psychotherapies. *Journal of the American Psychoanalytic Association* 2: 745–770.

Bion, W. R. (1961). *Experiences in Groups*. New York: Basic Books.

———(1962). *Learning from Experience*. New York: Basic Books.

———(1963). *Elements of Psycho-Analysis*. New York: Basic Books.

———(1967). *Second Thoughts. Selected Papers on Psycho-Analysis*. New York: Basic Books, 1968.

———(1970). *Attention and Interpretation*. New York: Basic Books.

———(1973). *Brazilian Lectures 1, Sao Paulo, 1973*, ed. J. Salomao. Rio de Janiero: Imago Editora Ltda.

———(1975). *Brazilian Lectures 2, Rio/Sao Paulo, 1974*. Rio de Janiero: Imago Editora Ltda.

———(1977a). *Two Papers: The Grid and Caesura*, ed. J. Salomao. Rio de Janiero: Imago Editora Ltda.

Bion, W. R. (1977b). Emotional Turbulence. In: *Borderline Personality Disorders,* ed. P. Hartocollis. New York: International Universities Press, pp. 3–13.

Blanck, G. and Blanck, R. (1974). *Ego Psychology: Theory and Practice.* New York: Columbia University Press, pp. 61–73.

Blum, H. P. (1976). Masochism, the ego ideal, and the psychology of women. *Journal of the American Psychoanalytic Association* 24 (suppl.): 157–191.

———(1977). The prototype of preoedipal reconstruction. *Journal of the American Psychoanalytic Association* 25: 757–785.

Bowlby, J. (1969). *Attachment & Loss, vol. I: Attachment.* New York: Basic Books.

Braunschweig, D. and Fain, M. (1971). *Eros et Anteros.* Paris: Petite Bibliotheque Payot.

Brierley, M. (1937). Affects in theory and practice. In: *Trends in Psychoanalysis.* London: Hogarth Press, 1951, pp. 43–56.

Brown, N. O. (1968). *Love's Body.* New York: Vintage Books.

Cath, S. H. (1962). Grief, loss, and emotional disorders in the aging process. In: *Geriatric Psychiatry,* ed. M. Berezin, and S. H. Cath. New York: International Universities Press, 21–72.

Chasseguet-Smirgel, J., ed. (1970). *Female Sexuality.* Ann Arbor: University of Michigan.

———(1973). *Essai sur L'ideal du Moi.* Paris: Presses Universitaires de France.

———(1974). Perversion, idealisation and sublimation. *International Journal of Psycho-Analysis* 55: 349–357.

Dalton, G. W. et al. (1968). *The Distribution of Authority in Formal Organizations.* Cambridge: Harvard University Press.

David, C. (1971). *L'État Amoureux.* Paris: Petite Bibliotheque Payot.

Devereux, G. (1953). Why Oedipus killed Laius: A note on the complementary Oedipus complex in Greek drama. *International Journal of Psycho-Analysis* 34: 132–141.

Dewald, P. (1969). *Psychotherapy: A Dynamic Approach.* Second edition. New York: Basic Books.

Dolgoff, T. (1973). Organizations as sociotechnical systems. *Bulletin of the Menninger Clinic* 37: 232–257.

Eissler, K. R. (1953). The effects of the structure of the ego on psychoanalytic technique. *Journal of the American Psychoanalytic Association* 1: 104–143.

Eissler, K. R. (1975a). The fall of man. *Psychoanalytic Study of the Child* 30: 589–646. New Haven: Yale University Press.

————(1975b). On possible effects of aging on the practice of psychoanalysis: An essay. *Journal of the Philadelphia Association of Psychoanalysis* 2: 138–152.

Emery, F. E. and Trist, E. L. (1973). *Towards a Social Ecology.* New York: Plenum Press.

Erikson, E. H. (1950). Growth and crises of the healthy personality. In: *Identity and the Life Cycle.* New York: International Universities Press, 1959, pp. 50–100.

————(1956). The problem of ego identity. In: *Identity and the Life Cycle.* New York: International Universities Press, pp. 101–164.

————(1959). *Identity and the Life Cycle. Psychological Issues,* Monograph 1: 1–171. New York: International Universities Press.

————(1963). *Childhood and Society.* Second Edition. New York: Norton.

Fairbairn, W. R. D. (1931). Features in the analysis of a patient with a physical genital abnormality. In: *An Object-Relations Theory of the Personality.* New York: Basic Books, 1954, pp. 197–222.

————(1940). Schizoid factors in the personality. In: *An Object-Relations Theory of the Personality.* New York: Basic Books, 1954, pp. 3–27.

————(1941). A revised psychopathology of the psychoses and psychoneuroses. In: *An Object-Relations Theory of the Personality.* New York: Basic Books, 1954, pp. 28–58.

————(1943). The repression and the return of bad objects (with special reference to the 'war neuroses'). *British Journal of Medical Psychology* 19: 327–341.

————(1944). Endopsychic structure considered in terms of object-relationships, with an addendum (1951). In: *An Object-Relations Theory of the Personality.* New York: Basic Books, 1954, pp. 82–156.

————(1946). Object-relationships and dynamic structure. In: *An Object-Relations Theory of the Personality.* New York: Basic Books, 1954, pp. 137–151.

————(1949). Steps in the development of an object-relations theory of the personality. *British Journal of Medical Psychology* 22: 26–31.

————(1951). A synopsis of the development of the author's views regarding the structure of the personality. In: *An Object-Relations Theory of the Personality.* New York: Basic Books, 1954, pp. 162–179.

————(1952). Theoretical and experimental aspects of psycho-analysis. *British Journal of Medical Psychology* 25: 122–127.

Fairbairn, W. R. D. (1954a). *An Object-Relations Theory of the Personality.* New York: Basic Books.

———(1954b). Observations on the nature of hysterical states. *British Journal of Medical Psychology* 27: 105–125.

———(1955). Observations in defence of the object-relations theory of the personality. *British Journal of Medical Psychology* 28: 144–156.

———(1957). Freud, the psycho-analytical method and mental health. *British Journal of Medical Psychology* 30: 53–62.

———(1958). On the nature and aims of psychoanalytic treatment. *International Journal of Psycho-Analysis* 39: 374–385.

———(1963). Synopsis of an object-relations theory of the personality. *International Journal of Psycho-Analysis* 44: 224–255.

Fenichel, O. (1941). Problems of psychoanalytic technique. Albany: Psychoanalytic Quarterly, Inc.

Freud, S. (1894). The neuro-psychoses of defence. *Standard Edition* 3: 41–61.

———(1910). A special type of choice of object made by men (Contributions to the psychology of love, 1). *Standard Edition* 11: 164–175.

———(1913). Totem and taboo. *Standard Edition* 13: 1–162.

———(1914). On narcissism. *Standard Edition* 14: 69–102.

———(1915). Repression. *Standard Edition* 14: 143–158.

———(1917). Mourning and melancholia. *Standard Edition* 14: 239–258.

———(1920). Beyond the pleasure principle. *Standard Edition* 18: 3–64.

———(1921). Group psychology and the analysis of the ego. *Standard Edition* 18: 67–143.

———(1923). The ego and the id. *Standard Edition* 19: 3–66.

———(1926). Inhibitions, symptoms and anxiety. *Standard Edition* 20: 77–174.

———(1930). Civilization and its discontents. *Standard Edition* 21: 59–145.

Fromm, E. (1956). *The Art of Loving.* New York: Bantam Books.

Frosch, J. (1964). The psychotic character: Clinical psychiatric considerations. *Psychiatric Quarterly* 38: 81–96.

———(1970). Psychoanalytic considerations of the psychotic character. *Journal of the American Psychoanalytic Association* 18: 24–50.

———(1971). Technique in regard to some specific ego defects in the treatment of borderline patients. *Psychiatric Quarterly* 45: 216–220.

Furer, M. (1977). Personality organization during the recovery of a severely disturbed young child. In: *Borderline Personality Disorders,* ed. P. Hartocollis. New York: International Universities Press, pp. 457–473.

Galenson, E. and Roiphe, H. (1976). Some suggested revisions concerning early female development. *Journal of the American Psychoanalytic Association* 24 (suppl.): 29–57.

Gill, M. M. (1951). Ego psychology and psychotherapy. *Psychoanalytic Quarterly* 20: 62–71.

————(1954). Psychoanalysis and exploratory psychotherapy. *Journal of the American Psychoanalytic Association* 2: 771–797.

————(1978). Psychoanalysis and psychoanalytic psychotherapy. Unpublished.

Glatzer, H. and Evans, W. N. (1977). On Guntrip's analysis with Fairbairn and Winnicott. *International Journal of Psychoanalytic Psychotherapy* 6: 81–98.

Glover, E. (1955). *The Technique of Psycho-Analysis*. New York: International Universities Press.

Goethe, J. W. (1807). *Die Wahlverwandtschaften* (Elective Affinities), *Goethes Werke*, vol. 8, p. 111. Berlin: Bibliographische Anstalt.

Greenson, R. R. (1954). The struggle against identification. In: *Explorations in Psychoanalysis*. New York: International Universities Press, 1978, pp. 75–92.

————(1958). On screen defenses, screen hunger, and screen identity. In: *Explorations in Psychoanalysis*. New York: International Universities Press, 1978, pp. 111–132.

————(1974). Transference: Freud or Klein. In: *Explorations in Psychoanalysis*. New York: International Universities Press, 1978, pp. 519–539.

Guntrip, H. (1961). *Personality Structure and Human Interaction*. New York: International Universities Press.

————(1975). My experience of analysis with Fairbairn and Winnicott. *International Review of Psycho-Analysis* 2: 145–156.

Hartmann, H. (1948). Comments on the psychoanalytic theory of instinctual drives. In: *Essays on Ego Psychology*. New York: International Universities Press, pp. 69–89.

————(1950). Comments on the psychoanalytic theory of the ego. In: *Essays on Ego Psychology*. New York: International Universities Press, 1964, pp. 113–141.

————(1952). The mutual influences on the development of ego and id. In: *Essays on Ego Psychology*. New York: International Universities Press, 1964, pp. 155–181.

————(1955). Notes on the theory of sublimation. In: *Essays on Ego Psychology*. New York: International Universities Press, 1964, pp. 215–240.

Hartmann, H., Kris, E., and Loewenstein, R. M. (1946). Comments on the formation of psychic structure. In: *Papers on Psychoanalytic Psychology. Psychological Issues,* Monograph 14. New York: International Universities Press, 1964, pp. 27–55.

————, Kris, E., and Loewenstein, R. M. (1949). Notes on the theory of aggression. In: *Papers on Psychoanalytic Psychology. Psychological Issues,* Monograph 14. New York: International Universities Press, 1964, pp. 56–85.

———— and Loewenstein, R. M. (1962). Notes on the superego. In: *Papers on Psychoanalytic Psychology. Psychological Issues,* Monograph 14. New York: International Universities Press, 1964, pp. 144–181.

Hoch, P. and Cattell, J. P. (1959). The diagnosis of pseudoneurotic schizophrenia. *Psychiatric Quarterly* 33: 17–43.

———— and Polatin, P. (1949). Pseudoneurotic forms of schizophrenia. *Psychiatric Quarterly* 23: 248–276.

Hodgson, R. C., Levinson, D. J., and Zaleznik, A. (1965). *The Executive Role Constellation: An Analysis of Personality and Role-Relations in Management.* Cambridge: Harvard University Press.

Horney, K. (1967). *Feminine Psychology.* New York: Norton.

Isaacs, S. (1948). The nature and function of phantasy. *International Journal of Psycho-Analysis* 29: 73–97.

Jacobson, E. (1937). Wege der weiblichen Über-Ich-Bildung. *Int. Zeitschrift fur Psychoanalyse,* 23: 402–412.

————(1943). Depression: The Oedipus conflict in the development of depressive mechanisms. *Psychoanalytic Quarterly* 12: 541–560.

————(1946). The effect of disappointment on ego and superego formation in normal and depressive development. *Psychoanalytic Review* 33: 129–147.

————(1952). The speed pace in psychic discharge processes and its influence on the pleasure-unpleasure qualities of affects. *Bulletin of the American Psychiatric Association* 8: 235–236.

————(1953a). The affects and their pleasure-unpleasure qualities in relation to the psychic discharge processes. In: *Drives, Affects, Behavior,* ed. R. M. Loewenstein. New York: International Universities Press, vol. 1: 38–66.

————(1953b). Contribution to the metapsychology of cyclothymic depression. In: *Affective Disorders,* ed. P. Greenacre. New York: International Universities Press, pp. 49–83.

————(1954a). Contribution to the metapsychology of psychotic identification. *Journal of the American Psychoanalytic Association* 2: 239–262.

————(1954b). On psychotic identifications. *International Journal of Psycho-Analysis* 35: 102–108.

————(1954c). The self and the object world. *Psychoanalytic Study of the Child* 9: 75–127. New York: International Universities Press.

————(1954d). Transference problems in the psychoanalytic treatment of severely depressive patients. *Journal of the American Psychoanalytic Association* 2: 595–606.

————(1956). Interaction between psychotic partners: I. Manic-depressive partners. In: *Neurotic Interaction in Marriage,* ed. V. W. Eisenstein. New York: Basic Books, pp. 125–134.

————(1957a). Denial and repression. *Journal of the American Psychoanalytic Association* 5: 61–92.

————(1957b). Normal and pathological moods: Their nature and function. *Psychoanalytic Study of the Child* 12: 73–113. New York: International Universities Press.

————(1959). Depersonalization. *Journal of the American Psychoanalytic Association* 7: 581–610.

————(1961). Adolescent moods and the remodeling of psychic structures in adolescence. *Psychoanalytic Study of the Child* 16: 164–183. New York: International Universities Press.

————(1964). *The Self and the Object World.* New York: International Universities Press.

————(1966). Problems in the differentiation between schizophrenic and melancholic states of depression. In: *Psychoanalysis — A General Psychology: Essays in Honor of Heinz Hartmann,* ed. R. M. Loewenstein et al. New York: International Universities Press, pp. 499–518.

————(1967). *Psychotic Conflict and Reality.* New York: International Universities Press.

————(1971). *Depression.* New York: International Universities Press.

Jaques, E. (1970). *Work, Creativity and Social Justice.* New York: International Universities Press.

Jones, E. (1948). Early female sexuality. *International Journal of Psycho-Analysis* 16: 263–273.

Joseph, B. (1960). Some characteristics of the psychopathic personality. *International Journal of Psycho-Analysis* 41: 526–531.

Katz, D. and Kahn, R. L. (1966). *The Social Psychology of Organizations.* New York: John Wiley.

Katz, E. (1955). Skills of an effective administrator. *Harvard Business Review* vol. 33, 1: 33–42.

Kernberg, O. (1966). Structural derivatives of object relationships. *International Journal of Psycho-Analysis* 47: 236–253.

———(1969). A contribution to the ego-psychological critique of the Kleinian school. *International Journal of Psycho-Analysis* 50: 317–333.

———(1972). Early ego integration and object relations. *Annals of the New York Academy of Science* 193: 223–247.

———(1975). *Borderline Conditions and Pathological Narcissism.* New York: Jason Aronson.

———(1976a). *Object Relations Theory and Clinical Psychoanalysis.* New York: Jason Aronson.

———(1976b). Technical considerations in the treatment of borderline personality organization. *Journal of the American Psychoanalytic Association* 24: 795–829.

———(1977a). Clinical observations regarding the diagnosis, prognosis, and intensive treatment of chronic schizophrenic patients. In: *Traitements au Long Courses des États Psychotiques,* ed. C. Chiland and P. Bequart. New York: Human Science Press, pp. 332–360.

———(1977b). The structural diagnosis of borderline personality organization. In: *Borderline Personality Disorders,* ed. P. Hartocollis. New York: International Universities Press, pp. 87–121.

———(1978a). Contrasting approaches to the treatment of borderline conditions. In: *New Perspectives in Psychotherapy of the Borderline Adult,* ed. J. Masterson. New York: Brunner/Mazel, pp. 77–104.

———(1978b). The diagnosis of borderline conditions in adolescence. In: *Adolescent Psychiatry, vol. VI: Developmental and Clinical Studies.* Chicago: University of Chicago Press, 16: 298–319.

———(1979). Discussion of the paper, "The British Object Relations Theorists: Balint, Winnicott, Fairbairn and Guntrip" by J. L. Sutherland. Presented at a Scientific Meeting of the Association for Psychoanalytic Medicine, May, 1979. Unpublished.

———, Burstein, E., Coyne, L., Appelbaum, A., Horwitz, L., and Voth, H. (1972). Psychotherapy and psychoanalysis: Final report of the Menninger Foundations' psychotherapy research project. *Bulletin of the Menninger Clinic* 36: 1–275.

Kinsey, A., Pomeroy, W., Martin, C., Gebhard, P. (1953). *Sexual Behavior in the Human Female.* Philadelphia: W. B. Saunders.

Klein, M. (1927). The psychological principles of infant analysis. In: *The Psycho-Analysis of Children.* New York: Norton, pp. 29–39.

———(1932). *The Psycho-Analysis of Children.* New York: Norton.

Klein, M. (1935). A contribution to the psychogenesis of manic-depressive states. In: *Contributions to Psycho-Analysis,* 1921–1945. London: Hogarth Press, 1948, pp. 282–310.

——— (1940). Mourning and its relation to manic-depressive states. In: *Contributions to Psycho-Analysis,* 1921–1945. London: Hogarth Press, 1948, pp. 311–338.

——— (1945). The Oedipus complex in the light of early anxieties. In: *Contributions to Psycho-Analysis,* 1921–1945. London: Hogarth Press, 1948, pp. 339–390.

——— (1946). Notes on some schizoid mechanisms. In: *Development in Psycho-Analysis,* ed. J. Riviere. London: Hogarth Press, 1952, pp. 292–320.

——— (1948). On the theory of anxiety and guilt. In: *Developments in Psycho-Analysis,* ed. J. Riviere. London: Hogarth Press, 1952, pp. 271–291.

——— (1950). On the criteria for the termination of a psychoanalysis. *International Journal of Psycho-Analysis* 31: 78–80.

——— (1952a). Discussion of the mutual influences in the development of ego and id. *Psychoanalytic Study of the Child* 7: 51–68. New York: International Universities Press.

——— (1952b). Some theoretical conclusions regarding the emotional life of the infant. In: *Developments in Psycho-Analysis,* ed. J. Riviere. London: Hogarth Press, pp. 198–236.

——— (1957). *Envy and Gratitude.* New York: Basic Books.

——— (1961). *Narrative of a Child Analysis.* New York: Basic Books.

——— (1963). *Our Adult World.* New York: Basic Books.

Knight, R. P. (1954). Borderline states. In: *Psychoanalytic Psychiatry and Psychology,* ed. R. P. Knight and C. R. Friedman. New York: International Universities Press, pp. 97–109.

Kramer, S. (1979). The technical significance and application of Mahler's separation-individuation theory. *Journal of the American Psychoanalytic Association* 27 (suppl.): 241–262.

Lasswell, H. D. (1948). *Power and Personality.* New York: Viking Press.

Le Bon, G. (1895). *The Crowd.* New York: Penguin, 1977.

Levin, S. (1965). Narcissistic and object libido in the aged. *International Journal of Psycho-Analysis* 46: 200–207.

Levinson, D. J. (1978). *The Seasons of a Man's Life.* New York: Alfred A. Knopf.

——— and Klerman, G. L. (1967). The clinical-executive. *Psychiatry* 30: 3–15.

Levinson, H. (1968). *The Exceptional Executive: A Psychological Conception.* Cambridge: Harvard University Press.

Lewin, B. D. (1950). *The Psychoanalysis of Elation.* New York: Norton.

Lichtenstein, H. (1970). Changing implications of the concept of psychosexual development: An inquiry concerning the validity of classical psychoanalytic assumptions concerning sexuality. *Journal of the American Psychoanalytic Association* 18: 300–318.

————(1977). *The Dilemma of Human Identity.* New York: Jason Aronson.

Lidz, T. (1968). *The Person: His Development Throughout the Life Cycle.* New York: Basic Books.

Loewald, H. W. (1960). On the therapeutic action of psychoanalysis. *International Journal of Psycho-Analysis* 41: 16–33.

————(1978). Instinct theory, object relations, and psychic-structure formation. *Journal of the American Psychoanalytic Association* 26: 493–506.

Mahler, M. S. (1952). On child psychosis and schizophrenia: Autistic and symbiotic infantile psychoses. *Psychoanalytic Study of the Child* 7: 286–305. New York: International Universities Press.

————(1958). Autism and symbiosis. Two extreme disturbances of identity. *International Journal of Psycho-Analysis* 39: 77–83.

————(1971). A study of the separation-individuation process and its possible application to borderline phenomena in the psychoanalytic situation. *Psychoanalytic Study of the Child* 26:403–424. New York/Chicago: Quadrangle Books.

————(1972a). On the first three subphases of the separation-individuation process. *International Journal of Psycho-Analysis* 53: 333–338.

————(1972b). Rapprochement subphase of separation-individuation process. *Psychoanalytic Quarterly* 41: 487–506.

————(1975). On the current status of the infantile neurosis. *Journal of the American Psychoanalytic Association* 23: 327–333.

———— and Furer, M. (1968). *On Human Symbiosis and the Vicissitudes of Individuation.* New York: International Universities Press.

———— and Gosliner, B. J. (1955). On symbiotic child psychoses: Genetic, dynamic, and restitutive aspects. *Psychoanalytic Study of the Child* 10: 195–212. New York: International Universities Press.

———— and Kaplan, L. (1977). Developmental aspects in the assessment of narcissistic and so-called borderline personalities. In: *Borderline Personality Disorders,* ed. P. Hartocollis. New York: International Universities Press, pp. 71–85.

Mahler, M. S., Pine, F., and Bergman, A. (1975). *The Psychological Birth of the Human Infant.* New York: Basic Books.

Main, T. F. (1957). The Ailment. *British Journal of Medical Psychology* 30: 129-145.

Mann, T. (1924). *The Magic Mountain.* New York: Random House, 1969.

Masterson, J. (1967). *The Psychiatric Dilemma of Adolescence.* Boston: Little, Brown.

———(1972). *Treatment of the Borderline Adolescent: A Developmental Approach.* New York: Wiley-Interscience.

———(1976). *Psychotherapy of the Borderline Adult: A Developmental Approach.* New York: Brunner/Mazel.

———(1978). The borderline adult: Transference acting-out and working-through. In: *New Perspectives on Psychotherapy of the Borderline Adult.* New York: Brunner/Mazel, pp. 123-147.

May, R. (1969). *Love and Will.* New York: Norton.

Mellen, J. (1973). *Women and Their Sexuality in the New Film.* New York: Dell.

Meltzer, D. (1967). *The Psycho-Analytical Process.* London: Heinemann.

———(1973). *Sexual States of Mind.* Perthshire, Scotland: Clunie Press.

——— et al. (1975). *Explorations in Autism.* Aberdeen, Scotland: Aberdeen University Press.

Mendelson, M. (1974). Jacobson. In: *Psychoanalytic Concepts of Depression.* Second Edition. New York: Spectrum Publications, pp. 72-88.

Miller, E. J. and Rice, A. K. (1967). *Systems of Organization.* London: Tavistock Publications.

Montherlant, H. de (1936). Les Jeunes Filles. In: *Romans et oeuvres de fiction non theatrales de Montherlant.* Paris: Bibliotheque de la Pleiade, Editions Gallimard, 1959, pp. 1010-1012.

Offer, D. (1971). Rebellion and antisocial behavior. *American Journal of Psychoanalysis* 31: 13-19.

———(1973). *Psychological World of the Teen-ager: A Study of Normal Adolescent Boys.* New York: Harper & Row.

O'Neill, G. and O'Neill, N. (1973). *Open Marriage: A New Lifestyle for Couples.* New York: Avon Books.

Paz, O. (1974). *Teatro de Signos/Transparencias,* ed. Julian Rios. Madrid: Espiral/Fundamentos.

Person, E. (1974). Some new observations on the origins of femininity. In: *Women and Analysis,* ed. J. Strouse. New York: Viking, pp. 250-261.

Racker, H. (1968). *Transference and Countertransference.* New York: International Universities Press.

Rado, S. (1928). The problem of melancholia. In: *The Meaning of Despair,* ed. W. Gaylin. New York: Jason Aronson, 1968, pp. 70–95.

Rapaport, D. (1953). On the psychoanalytic theory of affects. In: *The Collected Papers of David Rapaport,* ed. M. M. Gill. New York: Basic Books, 1967, pp. 476–512.

Rascovsky, A. (1973). *El Filicidio.* Buenos Aires: Edicions Orion.

Reich, W. (1933–1934). *Character Analysis.* New York: Touchstone Books, 1974.

Rice, A. K. (1963). *The Enterprise and its Environment.* London: Tavistock Publications.

———(1965). *Learning for Leadership.* London: Tavistock Publications.

———(1969). Individual, Group and Intergroup Processes. *Human Relations,* 22: 565–584.

Richards, A. (1978). Discussion at a Panel on "The Technical Consequences of Object Relations Theory." Meeting of the American Psychoanalytic Association, New York, December, 1978. Unpublished.

Rinsley, D. (1977). An object-relations view of borderline personality. In: *Borderline Personality Disorders,* ed. P. Hartocollis. New York: International Universities Press, pp. 47–70.

Rioch, M. J. (1970a). The work of Wilfred Bion on groups. *Psychiatry 33:* 56–66.

———(1970b). Group relations: Rationale and techniques. *International Journal of Group Psychotherapy* 10: 340–355.

Riviere, J. (1936). A contribution to the analysis of the negative therapeutic reaction. *International Journal of Psycho-Analysis* 17: 304–320.

———, ed. (1952). *Developments in Psycho-Analysis.* London: Hogarth Press.

Rogers, K. (1973). Notes on organizational consulting to mental hospitals. *Bulletin of the Menninger Clinic* 37: 211–231.

Rohmer, E. (1969). *Ma Nuit Chez Maud. L'Avant-Scene,* No. 98, December, pp. 10–40.

Rosenfeld, H. (1959). An investigation into the psycho-analytic theory of depression. *International Journal of Psycho-Analysis* 40: 105–129.

———(1964a). Object relations of the acute schizophrenic patient in the transference situation. *Psychiatric Research Reports* 19: 59–68. Washington, D.C.: American Psychiatric Association.

———(1964b). On the psychopathology of narcissism: A clinical approach. *International Journal of Psycho-Analysis* 45: 332–337.

———(1965). *Psychotic States: A Psychoanalytic Approach.* New York: International Universities Press.

Rosenfeld, H. (1971). A clinical approach to the psychoanalytic theory of the life and death instincts: An investigation into the aggressive aspects of narcissism. *International Journal of Psycho-Analysis* 52: 169–178.

———(1975). Negative therapeutic reaction. In: *Tactics and Techniques in Psychoanalytic Therapy*, vol. II, Countertransference, ed. P. Giovacchini. New York: Jason Aronson, pp. 217–228.

———(1978). Notes on the psychopathology and psychoanalytic treatment of some borderline patients. *International Journal of Psycho-Analysis* 59: 215–221.

Ross, N. (1970). The primacy of genitality in the light of ego psychology: Introductory remarks. *Journal of the American Psychoanalytic Association* 18: 267–284.

Sanford, N. (1956). The approach of the authoritarian personality. In: *Psychology of Personality*, ed. J. L. McCary. New York: Logos Press.

Searles, H. F. (1963). Transference psychosis in the psychotherapy of chronic schizophrenia. In: *Collected Papers on Schizophrenia and Related Subjects*. New York: International Universities Press, pp. 654–716.

———(1965). *Collected Papers on Schizophrenia and Related Subjects*. New York: International Universities Press.

Segal, H. (1962). The curative factors in psycho-analysis. *International Journal of Psycho-Analysis* 43: 212–217.

———(1964). *Introduction to the Work of Melanie Klein*. New York: Basic Books.

———(1967). Melanie Klein's technique. In: *Psychoanalytic Technique: A Handbook for the Practicing Psychoanalyst*, ed. B. B. Wolman. New York: Basic Books, pp. 168–190.

———(1973). *Introduction to the Work of Melanie Klein*. Second edition. New York: Basic Books.

———(1977). Psychoanalytic dialogue: Kleinian theory today. *Journal of the American Psychoanalytic Association* 25: 363–370.

Shakespeare, W. (1977). *Romeo and Juliet*, ed. J. E. Hankins. New York: Penguin Books.

Singer, I. (1973). *The Goals of Human Sexuality*. New York: Schocken Books.

Smith, J. and Smith, L., ed. (1974). *Beyond Monogamy*. Baltimore: John Hopkins University Press.

Stanton, A. M. and Schwartz, M. (1954). *The Mental Hospital*. New York: Basic Books.

Stoller, R. J. (1973). Overview: The impact of new advances in sex research on psychoanalytic theory. *American Journal of Psychiatry* 130: 241–251.

Stoller, R. J. (1974). Facts and fancies: An examination of Freud's concept of bisexuality. In: *Women and Analysis,* ed. J. Strouse. New York: Viking, pp. 343-364.

————(1975). *Sex as Sin.* Unpublished.

Stone, L. (1951). Psychoanalysis and brief psychotherapy. *Psychoanalytic Quarterly* 20: 215-236.

————(1954). The widening scope of indications for psychoanalysis. *Journal of the American Psychoanalytic Association* 2: 567-594.

Sullivan, H. S. (1953). *The Interpersonal Theory of Psychiatry.* New York: Norton.

Sutherland, J. D. (1963). Object-relations theory and the conceptual model of psychoanalysis. *British Journal of Medical Psychology* 36: 109-124.

————(1965). Obituary: W. R. D. Fairbairn. *International Journal of Psycho-Analysis 46: 245*-247.

————(1979). The British object relation theorists: Balint, Winnicott, Fairbairn, and Guntrip. Presented at a scientific meeting of the Association for Psychoanalytic Medicine, May. Unpublished.

Ticho, E. A. (1972). Termination of psychoanalysis: Treatment goals, life goals. *Psychoanalytic Quarterly* 41: 315-333.

Turquet, P. (1975). Threats to identity in the large group. In: *The Large Group: Dynamics and Therapy,* ed. L. Kreeger. London: Constable, pp. 87-144.

Vaillant, G. E. (1977). *Adaptation to Life.* Boston: Little, Brown.

van den Haag, E. (1964). Love or marriage. In: *The Family Educated,* ed. R. L. Cosen. New York: St. Martins Press.

Van der Waals, H. G. (1965). Problems of narcissism. *Bulletin of the Menninger Clinic* 29: 293-311.

Wallerstein, R. D. (1965). The goals of psychoanalysis: A survey of analytic viewpoints. In: *Psychotherapy and Psychoanalysis: Theory-Practice-Research.* New York: International Universities Press, 1975, pp. 99-118.

———— and Robbins, L. L. (1956). The psychotherapy research project of The Menninger Foundation, Part IV: Concepts. *Bulletin of the Menninger Clinic* 20: 239-262.

Winnicott, D. W. (1953). Transitional objects and transitional phenomena. In: *Collected Papers: Through Paediatrics to Psycho-Analysis.* New York: Basic Books, 1958, pp. 229-242.

————(1958). *Collected Papers: Through Paediatrics to Psycho-Analysis.* New York: Basic Books.

Winnicott, D. W. (1960). Ego distortion in terms of true and false self. In: *The Maturational Process and the Facilitating Environment*. New York: International Universities Press, 1965, pp. 140–152.

———(1965). *The Maturational Process and the Faciliating Environment*. New York: International Universities Press.

———(1971). *Playing and Reality*. New York: Basic Books.

——— and Khan, M. M. R. (1953). Book review of *Psycho-Analytic Studies of the Personality* by W. R. D. Fairbairn. *International Journal of Psycho-Analysis* 34: 329–333.

Wisdom, J. O. (1962). Comparison and development of the psychoanalytical theories of melancholia. *International Journal of Psycho-Analysis* 43: 113–132.

———(1963). Fairbairn's contribution on object-relationship, splitting, and ego structure. *British Journal of Medical Psychology* 36: 145–159.

———(1971). Freud and Melanie Klein: Psychology, Ontology, and Weltanschauung. *Psychoanalysis and Philosophy,* ed. C. Hanley and M. Lazarowitz. New York: International Universities Press, pp. 327–362.

Zaleznik, A. (1974). Charismatic and consensus leaders: A psychoanalytic comparison. *Bulletin of the Menninger Clinic,* 38: 222–238.

Zetzel, E. (1955). Recent British approaches to problems of early mental development. *Journal of the American Psychoanalytic Association* 3: 534–543.

INDEX